Life Span Perspectives of Suicide

Time-Lines in the Suicide Process

Life Span Perspectives of Suicide

Time-Lines in the Suicide Process

Edited by
Antoon A. Leenaars, Ph.D.

Springer Science+Business Media, LLC

Library of Congress Cataloging-in-Publication Data

Life span perspectives of suicide : time-lines in the suicide process / edited by Antoon A. Leenaars.
p. cm.
Includes bibliographical references and index.
ISBN 978-1-4899-0726-4
1. Suicide--United States. 2. Life cycle, Human. I. Leenaars, Antoon A.
HV6548.U5L54 1990
362.2'82'0973--dc20 90-49557
CIP

ISBN 978-1-4899-0726-4 ISBN 978-1-4899-0724-0 (eBook)
DOI 10.1007/978-1-4899-0724-0

Originally published by Plenum Press, New York in 1991
Softcover reprint of the hardcover 1st edition 1991

To Edwin S. Shneidman,
who taught me about suicide's complexity

Contributors

W. D. G. Balance • 813 Pemberton, Grosse Pointe Park, Michigan 48230

John Benjafield • Department of Psychology, Brock University, St. Catharines, Ontario, Canada L2S 3A1

Alan L. Berman • Department of Psychology, American University, Washington, D.C. 20016

Allan Brooks • Department of Psychiatry, Albert Einstein Medical Center, Philadelphia, Pennsylvania 19141

Pamela Cantor • Department of Psychiatry, The Cambridge Hospital, Harvard Medical School, Cambridge, Massachusetts 02138

Bonnie Frank Carter • Department of Psychiatry, Albert Einstein Medical Center, Philadelphia, Pennsylvania 19141

Dorothy Counts • Department of Anthropology, University of Waterloo, Waterloo, Ontario, Canada N2L 3G1

Norman L. Farberow • The Suicide Prevention Center of the Family Services of Los Angeles, Los Angeles, California 90006

Antoon A. Leenaars • Private Practice, 880 Ouelette Avenue, Suite 702, Windsor, Ontario, Canada N9A 1C7

David Lester • Department of Psychology, Stockton State College, Pomona, New Jersey 08240

John T. Maltsberger • Boston Psychoanalytic Society and Institute, Boston, Massachusetts 02108

Ronald W. Maris • The Center for the Study of Suicide, University of South Carolina, Columbia, South Carolina 29208

John L. McIntosh • Department of Psychology, Indiana University of South Bend, South Bend, Indiana 46634

Jerome A. Motto • Department of Psychiatry and Langley Porter Psychiatric Institute, University of California, San Francisco, California 94143

David P. Phillips • Department of Sociology, University of California at San Diego, La Jolla, California 92093

Victor I. Reus • Department of Psychiatry and Langley Porter Psychiatric Institute, University of California, San Francisco, California 94143

Joseph Richman • Professor Emeritus, Albert Einstein College of Medicine, New York, New York 10461

Edwin S. Shneidman • Professor of Thanatology Emeritus, University of California, Los Angeles, California 90024

Daniel G. Smith • Department of Sociology, University of California at San Diego, La Jolla, California 92093

Steven Stack • Department of Sociology, Wayne State University, Detroit, Michigan 48202

Susanne Wenckstern • The Board of Education for the City of Windsor, Windsor, Ontario, Canada, N9A 6KI

Preface

In recent years, a great deal of interest has been focused on suicide in the elderly and in the young. However, in line with modern trends in psychology, sociology, psychiatry, anthropology, and other human health fields, interest has now shifted to suicide across the life span, from childhood through adulthood to old age. This book has been conceptualized within this developing tradition.

There are various ways in which life's timelines can be conceptualized. Developmental theory, we believe, should be open-ended. This has widened—and will continue to widen—our understanding of many complicated human acts including suicide. Though suicide is in many ways the same across the entire life span, understanding the time-lines in the suicidal process is imperative. To do so, however, is, we believe, challenging.

In this volume, we attempt to engage in the process of understanding suicide from a developmental perspective. To do this, we have been fortunate to obtain the cooperation of a highly competent group of contributors. One interesting footnote to our list of authorities is that they represent suicidologists from across the life span—a few who are at the beginning of their careers, a large number in their middle years, and a few who are in the Indian summer of their professional lives.

By way of background, the following introduces our contributors in order of their appearance in the text:

John Benjafield is professor of psychology, and director of the Institute for Applied Human Development at Brock University, St. Catharines, Ontario, Canada. Benjafield, a nonsuicidologist, has provided a larger metaperspective. He has published extensively on historical perspectives and developmental psychology.

David Lester is professor of psychology at Stockton State College, Pomona, New Jersey. Lester is current vice president of the International Association for Suicide Prevention (IASP). He has published a number of books and literally hundreds of papers.

Ronald W. Maris is professor of sociology and preventive medicine at the University of South Carolina, Columbia, South Carolina, where he directs the Center for the Study of Suicide. He is a past president of the American Association of Suicidology (AAS) and the current editor of *Suicide and Life-Threatening Behavior* (SLTB). Having published extensively, he has served as an expert witness on cases dealing with wrongful death and suicide.

Edwin S. Shneidman is professor of thanatology emeritus at the University of California at Los Angeles. He is one of the founding fathers of modern suicidology, having begun the AAS and its journal, SLTB. He has received numerous awards, most recently a Distinguished Professional Contributions Award from the American Psychological Association. Among his extensive list of publications is the recently published *Definition of Suicide*.

John L. McIntosh is associate professor of psychology at Indiana University at South Bend, Indiana, and a research associate at the Center for Gerentological Education, University of Notre Dame. He has published numerous papers and books, the latest being *Suicide and Its Aftermath*, coauthored by E. Dunne and K. Dunne-Maxim, and has received AAS's Edwin Shneidman Award for his research on the elderly.

David P. Phillips is professor of sociology at the University of California, San Diego in La Jolla, California. Having received the AAS's Edwin Shneidman Award for outstanding contribution in research in suicidology, his work on suicide and the contagion—Werther—effect has resulted in major reflections on the role of the media in suicide. Phillips has published extensively on the epidemiology of suicide and on the subject of motor vehicle fatalities.

Daniel G. Smith is a graduate student at the department of sociology, University of California, San Diego.

Antoon A. Leenaars is a psychologist in private practice in Windsor, Ontario, Canada. Leenaars has served as an expert witness in cases dealing with wrongful death and suicide. Currently he is president of the Canadian Association for Suicide Prevention (CASP) and a board member of AAS. Having received AAS's Shneidman Award, he has published extensively on suicide, including the recently released *Suicide Notes* (Human Sciences Press).

Susanne Wenckstern is a psychology consultant at the Windsor Board of Education, Windsor, Ontario, Canada. She is locally and nationally active addressing suicide in the schools, being a member of CASP's national school committee, and has published a number of papers and chapters on suicidology and co-edited a book, *Suicide Prevention in Schools*.

Alan L. Berman, a diplomate in clinical psychology, is a professor of psychology at American University, Washington, D.C. He is a past president of the AAS and the recipient of the Shneidman Award. Berman, recognized as an expert on youth suicide, has published over 50 professional articles and chapters and has served as an expert witness on cases dealing with wrongful death and suicide.

W. D. G. Balance, a psychology professor, has published extensively in a number of human health areas, most recently suicide and eating disorders. He is especially known in suicidology for his collaborative work with Leenaars on suicide notes.

Joseph Richman is professor emeritus at Albert Einstein College of Medicine, New York. He has been active, including as a board member, in AAS since its inception in 1969. Having received AAS's Dublin Award for a lifetime of contributions to suicidology, Richman has specialized in crisis intervention and family therapy. He is known for his focus on positive thinking, well-being, and humor throughout the life span, devoting special attention on the lifestyles of the elderly.

Jerome A. Motto, professor of psychiatry at the University of California, San Francisco, is also very active at the Medical Center as the associate director of its Psychiatric Consultation Service. Motto is a past president of AAS, past secretary-general of IASP, and the recipient of AAS's Dublin Award. His work in depressive and suicidal states has focused on risk assessment and clinical management.

Victor I. Rues, associate professor of psychiatry, University of California, San Francisco, also holds the position of medical director at the University's Langley Porter Neuropsychiatric Hospital. He is a Fellow of the American Psychiatric Association, has served as an editorial reviewer to 18 journals, and has published extensively in the area of biological aspects of depression, including the area of suicide.

Steven Stack is professor of sociology, Auburn University, Auburn, Alabama. Stack, a recipient of AAS's Shneidman Award for his outstanding contribution in research in suicidology, has recently focused on media impacts on suicide and the importance of the family in suicide.

Dorothy Counts is professor (and chairperson) of anthropology at the University of Waterloo, Waterloo, Ontario, Canada. She is known for her field research in West New Britain Province, Papua New Guinea, on its political and economic change, religious syncretism and cargo cult activities, aging and death, domestic violence, and suicide. Among many publications, she has produced a number of papers on suicide from an anthropological perspective.

Bonnie Frank Carter is director of research and program director for Youth Suicide Prevention Services and for the Violence Postvention Program, Albert Einstein Medical Center, Philadelphia. Her work and publications have dealt with the topics of human aggression, including repetitive interpersonal violence, war and other mass scale human violence, and suicide. Carter has been clinically active in addressing the problem of youth suicide including in the area of postvention.

Allan Brooks is director of child psychiatry and program medical director for Youth Suicide Prevention Services in the department of psychiatry, Albert Einstein Medical Center, Philadelphia. A practicing psychoanalyst, Brooks has collaborated with Carter to develop Youth Suicide Prevention Services with special emphasis on postvention in the aftermath of suicide (and other violence).

Norman L. Farberow, a past president of IASP and AAS, is co-director (and co-founder) of the Los Angeles Suicide Prevention Center, now a division of Family Services of Los Angeles. He is a clinical professor emeritus of the University of Southern California School of Medicine, Los Angeles, and is regarded as one of the fathers of modern suicidology, having received a large number of awards, including AAS's Dublin Award. Recently, he has been actively researching the survivors of suicide and the impact of disasters on children.

Pamela Cantor is a psychologist in private practice in Chestnut Hill, Massachusetts. A past president of AAS, she has received the Shneidman Award for her outstanding contributions. Having published extensively, Cantor is especially known for her work on youth suicide and the treatment of suicidal youngsters. Her film, *Young People in Crisis*, has received wide acclaim.

John T. Maltsberger, a psychoanalyst in private practice in Boston, is a lecturer of psychiatry at Harvard Medical School and staff psychiatrist at both Massachusetts General Hospital, Boston, and Cambridge Hospital, Cambridge. Well-recognized as a faculty member at the Boston Psychoanalytic Institute, he has also published extensively; his most recent book on suicide is titled *Suicide Risk: The Formulation of Clinical Judgment*.

It is my belief that these authors have an important contribution to make to suicidology and the developmental perspective in general. Understanding the time-lines in the suicidal process has a pivotal place in the study of the suicidal person. We hope that this book can assist us in preventing suicide, from childhood through adulthood to old age.

A.L.

Windsor, Ontario

Acknowledgments

First and foremost, I need to make explicit my debt to the contributors. They are the authorities in the field. I wish, with deepest gratitude, to thank them for their contribution. Obviously, without them, the book would not exist.

I am pleased to acknowledge the editorial contributions of David Lester, who worked with me from the conception of this volume.

Ed Shneidman has been a guiding light to me in my study of suicide in general. His support has been most helpful in my developing career.

I am extremely appreciative of the editorial guidance of Norma Fox, executive editor at Plenum Press, and her excellent staff.

Contents

I. INTRODUCTION

II. EPIDEMIOLOGY

III. SUICIDE BY TIME-LINES

IV. CORRELATES OF SUICIDE

V. SURVIVOR ISSUES

VI. PREVENTING SUICIDE

VII. CONCLUDING REMARKS

I

Introduction

There are various ways in which life's—including a suicidal person's—time-lines can be conceptualized. Though suicide is in many ways the same across the entire life span, understanding suicide from a developmental perspective is imperative. This volume introduces the reader to such a view of suicide across the life span. Part I consists of four chapters: a meta-outline of the process of development as open-ended, entitled, in line with the suicidal process as "The End of Development"; a brief review of the time-lines (or stages) of development; a developmental perspective of suicide; and an outline of the commonalities of suicide across the life span to make the point that "there is only human suicide."

1

The End of Development

John Benjafield

A recurrent theme in developmental theory has been that the process of development is intrinsically open-ended (e.g., Lerner, 1986, p.178f). The notion that development never ends has led to the kind of life-span psychology that is currently popular. Formerly, psychologists often felt differently. They sometimes talked as if one's character is crystallized early on in life, and has a fixed structure against which one may later have to struggle. Freud (1966) is often cited in this connection. Another example is James' (1890) famous discussion of habit.

> Habit . . . dooms us all to fight out the battle of life upon the lines of our nurture or our early choice . . . [Habit is something] from which a man can by-and-by no more escape than his coat sleeve can suddenly fall into a new set of folds . . . in most of us, by the age of thirty, the character has set like plaster, and will never soften again. (p.121)

There are numerous sources for the change in our beliefs about development. To some extent, it is the result of studies that have widened our perspective on the possibility of change later in the lifecycle. In part, it is also the result of a cultural metamorphosis. The 20th century has witnessed an explosion in the developmental alternatives open to people, contrasting sharply with the more rigid societal structure of earlier times. Perhaps more than ever before, development is the outcome of very complex interactions between historical, social, and personal variables (e.g., Benjafield, 1987; Benjafield & Muckenheim, 1989).

There is, however, another aspect to this issue that I want to consider in this

---

JOHN BENJAFIELD • Department of Psychology, Brock University, St. Catharines, Ontario, Canada L2S 3A1.

chapter. It may be an empirical fact that development in our culture and in our time is never-ending. However, is it a logical necessity that development must have no terminus? Why must we believe that development is something that can always go further? Might it not be possible to reach a point in development past which it is neither necessary nor desirable to go?

I will consider these questions in two ways. First, I will present two case histories of famous figures in 20th century thought who have considered these issues in a deep and serious way. Then I will contrast their thought with that of Piaget, and consider the virtues of alternative conceptions of the nature of development.

WITTGENSTEIN AND THE LIMITS OF INQUIRY

It is useful to begin a consideration of these issues by means of a paradigmatic "case history" of someone for whom they were very important—Ludwig Wittgenstein (1889–1951). It is customary to make a distinction between his early work, such as the *Tractatus Logico-Philosophicus* (1922/1974) and his later work, such as the *Philosophical Investigations* (1953). However, I am inclined to agree with those such as Drury (1973, p.189) who regard Wittgenstein's two periods as more similar than different. In discussing Wittgenstein, and subsequently others whose interests were similar to his, I am not at all interested in the philosophical merits of their work. Rather, I am interested in their work insofar as it illustrates certain states of mind. My approach to their work is psychological; I want to see what they tell us about the attitudes one has when one really asks "Where does life lead?" or "What does it all mean?"

In the question ending the last paragraph, the key word is the word *all*. Assume that you had attained an understanding of all the events in the world and their relations to one another. At that point, you might wish to understand what it was that you knew. The problem you would have is that there would be no place to look for further understanding, because everything in the world would have been understood. How would you understand what it is you understand if you understand everything? The question "makes the head swim," but it is an interesting question for us to ponder.

It has been the goal of modern science to understand everything. Certainly, many scientists have felt that their inquiries would eventually lead us to understand everything that could be known. Science gives us knowledge of the laws of nature, and 20th century man often "stops short of the laws of nature as something impregnable, as men of former times did at God and fate. . . The old ones are indeed clearer in the sense that they acknowledge a clear terminus, while in the new system it is supposed to look as if everything had a foundation" (Wittgenstein, 1969, p.72).

The ancients acknowledged a point past which mundane knowledge could not go; we tend to think that such knowledge could be exhaustive. It is true that some would say that contemporary science does not pretend that "everything has a foundation." Perhaps not, and we will discuss this point a little later on. In any case we can wonder what it would be like to grasp all possible events in the world; to "know it all." To imagine what this might be like we need first to consider what it is like when we do not know everything. That state is the state of our knowledge when we are children.

Piaget and the Development of a "Logical Space"

The study of the development of the ability to think logically owes more to Jean Piaget than to anyone else. When we are children, says Piaget (1957), we easily confuse class concepts. Suppose children of roughly 5 to 8 years of age are shown a box of wooden beads. The majority of the beads are brown and the rest white. They are asked if there are more brown beads or more wooden beads. We know that there are more wooden beads than brown ones, but the child is not at all sure of it. Rather, he is likely to say that there are more brown than wooden ones, because, after all, there are only a few white ones. This "logic" may strike us as puzzling until we realize that the child lacks the concept of a superordinate class that contains the other two classes. Thus, suppose we let A be the class of beads, and B1 be the class of brown beads and B2 be the class of white beads. As adults we immediately see that $A = B1 + B2$, and that $B2 < A$. The child does not yet appreciate that something can be the member of one class (B1) and of another (A) simultaneously. To him B1 is larger than A, because if you take B1 from A, then only B2 is left, and $B1 > B2$. The child lacks a stable concept of the superordinate class.

Eventually, however, the child will come to understand that an event may belong to both superordinate as well as subordinate classes. At that point he can go on to perform a "multiplication of classes." A multiplication of classes occurs when it is realized that an event can belong to (at least) two superordinate classes simultaneously. For example, people can be divided by height (A) into those who are tall (B1) and short (B2). Similarly, regarded from a different viewpoint, people can be classified by sex (A1) into men (B11) and women (B12). Multiplication of classes ($A \times A1$) yields the four classes given in Figure 1: short men; short women; tall men; tall women.

It is easy enough to imagine the result of multiplying only two dimensions, as in Figure 1. We may even imagine multiplying three dimensions, by adding Age (Old vs. Young) as a third distinction. Suppose we could go further, and imagine all possible distinctions, and combine these in all possible ways. If we could do this, then we would have a "logical space," which contained all conceivable events. The

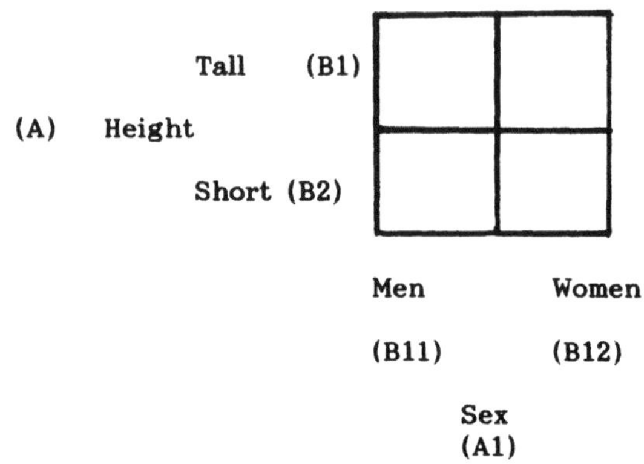

Figure 1. Multiplication of classes.

achievement of such a logical space would be the outcome of the process begun by multiplying two classes, and ending by multiplying all possible classes. Wittgenstein (1974) put it like this: "Logic deals with every possibility, and all possibilities are its facts. . . . If I know an object, I also know all its possible occurrences in states of affairs. . . . Each thing is, as it were, in a space of possible states of affairs. This space I can imagine empty, but I cannot imagine the thing without the space" (p.71). Without the logical space, which the multiplication of classes makes possible, I cannot imagine all possible states of affairs.

Logic thus describes "the scaffolding of the world." It delimits all the events we *could* observe. Once we know them, there is nothing left to know, even though we may feel that there is more that we WANT to know. Thus, any logical investigation appears to have a definite limit. The "sense of the world," the attainment of which is the reason for starting any investigation in the first place, is not given by any exhaustive description of the world. As Wittgenstein (1974) said, "In the world everything is as it is, and everything happens as it does happen. . . ."

If we think about things in this way, then we end up with a collection of possible facts, and there is no value inherent in these facts. Each one is of the same value as any other. Value is not in the world, "it must lie outside the world," said Wittgenstein (1974), outside the province of logic and observation.

Facts and Values

Values are nowhere in the logical space that we construct to represent the facts of the world. This is a hard thing to face since values are important to us, and we would like to be able to say something certain about them. Wittgenstein (1974) noted that "We feel that even when all possible scientific questions have been answered, the problems of life remain completely untouched." Since we can only describe what is in the world, and since values are not in the world, then about the problems of life there is nothing meaningful to be said.

In one form or another, the idea that ethics and aesthetics are "outside the world" is one that many psychologists share. These are often treated as "subjective" questions, not answerable in any "scientific" way. For Wittgenstein, however, this was not the end of the matter. When we contemplate the world as a whole, we can adopt an aesthetic attitude. Wittgenstein (1969), put it this way, "Aesthetically, the miracle is that the world exists. That what exists does exist. Is it the essence of the artistic way of looking at things, that it looks at the world with a happy eye? . . . And the beautiful IS what makes happy"(p.86).

There is no question that Wittgenstein is here expressing a mystical attitude to the world. While the deepest truths turn out to be inexpressible, "there is a feeling . . . to have had which is to have solved the meaning of life," as one of Wittgenstein's keenest students, McGuinness (1966) puts it. The "meaning of life" turns out not to be something that a delineation of the facts can give you. Rather, it is a "feeling" that does not reside in facts about the world.

Wittgenstein presents the distinction between Facts and Value, Truth and Beauty, as clearly as anyone. It is a feature of modern, as opposed to earlier, times that this distinction is worrisome, whether or not we formulate it as precisely as Wittgenstein did. How do we find happiness in the world? The answer may be that we do not. Rather, happiness comes from the attitude we take toward the world, rather than anything we may find in it. To have arrived at this attitude is to have reached the end of development.

SIMONE WEIL

A mystic like Wittgenstein, Weil (1909–1943) was one of the most brilliant and pure intellects of this century. We saw above how the nature of development and the nature of logic and mathematics are intertwined. Our concept of one will be in part determined by our concept of the other. Weil's view of mathematics is particularly sensitive to the contrast between ancient and modern conceptions of the purpose and value of mathematics.

Like Wittgenstein, Weil (1968) conveys a sense of the limits of what the world can give us.

> We are all aware that the good which we possess at present, in the form of wealth, power consideration, friends, the love of those we love, and so on is not sufficient; yet we believe that on the day when we get a little more we will be satisfied. We believe this because we lie to ourselves. If we really reflect for a moment, we know it is false. (p.148)

Neither our thought nor our desire can be fully satisfied in this world. Just as our understanding of this world, no matter how complete, is finally unsatisfying, so our attempts to gratify ourselves in this world, no matter how successful, are finally unsatisfying as well.

If we allow ourselves to reach this sort of conclusion, we can begin to adopt a different sort of attitude toward the world. This change is the one described by Plato in his famous image of the Cave, and is a transition from "darkness to the contemplation of the sun." What we seek is no less than a complete understanding of our situation. Such an understanding is contradicted in our experience by the disunity of the world of everyday life. Such a contradiction, felt by everyone at some level and at some time, is what begins the process of thought leading us to a higher level of understanding.

We are looking for a harmonious relationship between the contradictory tendencies, the opposing forces that rule our lives. Mathematics can express this relationship by means of the concept of proportion: the proper balance between opposites. Far from being an arcane pursuit, mathematics is the key to a practical understanding of the way the world actually works. Mathematics allows you to perceive the perfect forms we seek. Our everyday world is flawed and incapable of satisfying us, but through mathematical understanding we can find what we are actually looking for.

"Whenever the intelligence is brought up against a contradiction, it is obliged to conceive a relation that transforms the contradiction into a correlation, and as a result, the soul is drawn upwards . . . mathematics is the science of this kind of ratio."

The upward journey of the soul is a journey that requires what Weil (1977, p.363) calls *intermediaries*. Proportion, a statement of the relation between contraries is an intermediary. Weil's (1971, p.292) view is that the Ancients understood proportion in this way. "Proportions are found in the world. From the flash of genius of Thales until the time when they were crushed by the armed forces of Rome, they searched everywhere—in the regular recurrence of the stars, in sound, in equilibrium, in floating bodies—for proportions in order to love God." The observation of proportion in the world can give us the experience of contemplating necessity regulating the merely accidental. The function of this kind of observation was symbolic. "The mean proportional was in their eyes the image of the divine mediation between God and his creatures."

The Divine Proportion

To some readers this might all sound rather arcane. However, there are excellent examples of the sort of thing Weil has in mind. Consider the proportion in Figure 2. It was called the "Divine Proportion" by Kepler, and has been esteemed by a great many mathematicians and artists (Benjafield, 1985). The line is divided such that the smaller part is to the larger part as the larger part is to the whole, that

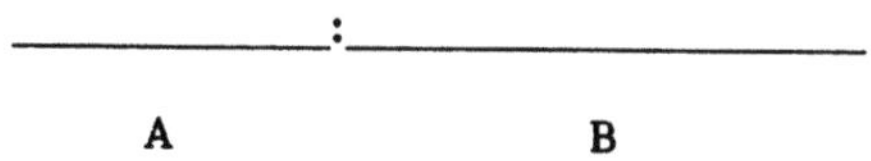

Figure 2. The divine proportion.

is, BC/AC = AC/AB. This proportion has a number of attractive mathematical properties, including a close relationship with the famous Fibonacci series of numbers, named after the 13th century mathematician. The sequence begins with 0 and 1, with each further term in the series being the sum of the previous two. Thus, the series goes:

$$0, 1, 1, 2, 3, 5, 8, 13, 21, 34, 55, \ldots$$

The ratio between any two consecutive terms of the sequence is an approximation to the Divine Proportion, an approximation that improves as the numbers increase. Thus: $1/2 = .5$; $2/3 = .67$; $3/5 = .6$; $5/8 = .63$; $8/13 = .62$; and so on.

The Divine Proportion appears in a number of natural forms (Stevens, 1974). One example will suffice. Consider Figure 3, which shows the head of a pine cone with 8 clockwise and 13 counterclockwise spirals. This is called Fibonacci phyllotaxis, and occurs in many plants. The Fibonacci sequence, and thus the Divine Proportion, describes the number of spirals displayed by the florets or leaves. Mitchison (1977), a Cambridge botanist, investigated several possible models of plant growth and concluded that: "Fibonacci phyllotaxis follows as a mathematical necessity . . . [and] . . . seems to be a robust and stable mathematical phenomenon, a finding which goes some way to explaining its widespread occurrence throughout the plant kingdom."

The importance of cases like the one illustrated in Figure 3 is that they constitute an example of development that has a final form. As the plant grows, it maintains the same proportion. In every instance, the organism reaches the same end. The Divine Proportion can stand as a *symbol* of the proper proportion, the "Golden Mean," which is the state of balance we seek (Thompson, 1929).

The Symbolic Function

Weil (1971, p.292) described in a particularly clear way how mathematics has a symbolic function. "Geometry thus becomes a double language, which at the same time provides information concerning the forces that are in action in matter, and talks about the supernatural relations between God and his creatures." She lamented the loss of the symbolic aspect of science and mathematics, but believed that we could recapture this way of doing them. "Concern for the symbol has completely disappeared from our science. And yet, if one were to give oneself the

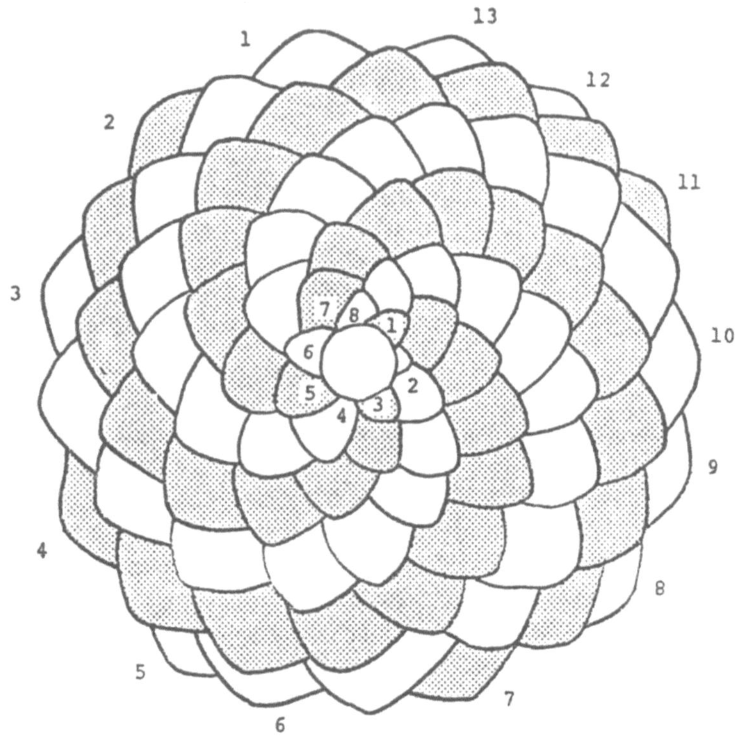

Figure 3. Fibonacci phyllotaxis.

trouble, we could easily find symbols as clear, as beautiful, and as full of spiritual meaning as that of the circle and mediation. . . . From modern thought to ancient wisdom the path would be short and direct if one cared to take it."

Weil commends us to adopt an older attitude; to recapture a world view that did not restrict science to the objective. One of the reasons for the appeal of the Divine Proportion, it seems to me, is that it can awaken us to this ancient attitude to the world. Simone Weil would have argued that the loss of this attitude is not a form of "progress" toward a great objectivity, but a turning away from Truth.

Weil's approach is strikingly different from that taken by most psychologists who specialize in the study of "moral development." However, Robert Coles (1981) has written a sensitive appreciation of her values. Perhaps the feminist theory of Gilligan (1982) raises the issues that are closest to the ones Weil thinks are important.

One difficulty lying in the way of those who would take the path Simone Weil demonstrates is that it presumes that there is an "eternal mathematics . . . that is the stuff of which the order of the world is woven." The idea that logic and mathematics are "eternal," that they describe immutable laws, has come into question in our time, and the sharp distinctions made by people like Weil and Wittgenstein in his early work are thus threatened with being blurred. This development has several sources, one of which we will now consider.

ETERNAL UNCERTAINTY

In his introduction to Wittgenstein's *Tractatus*, Russell (1974) suggested that the limitations Wittgenstein placed on scientific inquiry were not real. Wittgenstein's point was that the most important aspects of human existence can only be expressed, but not described in language. Russell agreed that ". . . every language has a . . . structure concerning which nothing can be said," but adds that "there may be another language dealing with the structure of the first language, and having itself a new structure and to this hierarchy of languages there may be no limit." Wittgenstein's theory applies to the "totality of such languages," and one could "deny that there is any such totality." Rather, once one level of understanding is achieved we recognize that it too needs to be understood, and move to a "higher" level of understanding that contains the former and explains it. Then this next level would itself require explanation, which can only be undertaken at a still higher level, and so on.

Brown (1969) puts the matter like this. A physicist who describes the world is himself made up of what he is describing. We are what we see, and this means that the world is constructed in such a way that it can see itself. However, in order to see itself, the world "must first cut itself up into at least one state which sees, and at least one other state which is seen. In this severed and mutilated condition, whatever it sees is only partially itself . . . In this condition it will always partially elude itself." What understands itself cannot itself be understood, unless there is something else that understands but cannot be understood, and so on, to infinity.

Piaget (1970) developed the theme we have been considering in the context of Godel's theorem, one of the most famous ideas in 20th century thought. Godel showed that

> all formal systems which are (1) consistent and (2) adequate for simple arithmetic—i.e., contain the natural numbers and the operations of addition and multiplication— . . . are incomplete, i.e., contain unprovable, though perfectly meaningful, formulae, some of which, moreover, we, standing outside the system, can see to be true. (p.112)

While an important and highly readable account of the implications of Godel's theorem can be found in a recent book by Hofstadter (1979), it is Piaget who has most clearly drawn out the implication of Godel's theorem for psychology.

The first important implication is that, as Russell intuited, any logical structure sufficiently powerful to generate arithmetic cannot be shown to be consistent without constructing a logical structure to contain the first one, and so on, ad infinitum. This applies to the stages of the development of human knowledge. At a particular stage of development, there will be things we know to be true which we cannot derive from within our existing logical structure. We must then move to the next higher stage in order to make what we know internally consistent. As Piaget (1970) describes it, this is a never-ending process.

> The idea of a formal system of abstract structures is thereby transformed into that of the construction of a never completed whole, the limits of formalization constituting the grounds for incompleteness, or . . . the incompleteness being a necessary consequence of the fact that there is no "terminal" or "absolute" form because any content is form relative to some inferior content, and any form the content for some higher form. . . . (p.140)

Thus, for Piaget, the idea that we can ever reach a complete state of knowledge is an illusion. "The idea of a structure of all structures is unrealizable. The subject cannot therefore be the a priori underpinning of a finished structure, rather it is a center of activity. And whether we substitute "society" or "mankind" or "life" or even "cosmos" for "subject," the argument remains the same." Wittgenstein's sharp contrast between what can be known and said and what cannot evaporates because the area subsumed by the former is continually expanding.

If Piaget is right, then the world is not to be regarded as complete and waiting to be understood in some final sense. Rather, we and the world are continually in the process of construction. There are no immutable Platonic forms hiding behind the veil of appearance. While, as Piaget says, it is "tempting to believe in Ideas . . . lying in God's lap from all eternity," such a hope must be put behind us.

Now we are to regard ourselves as continually growing toward a point ever receding from us. We can use the way that Fibonacci numbers tend toward the Golden Section as a symbol of such a process. Processes such as spiral phyllotaxis, which always give only an approximation of the Ideal of the Golden Section, can be compelling metaphors for our continual, yet perhaps vain, attempt at *complete* understanding. We are no longer to believe, however, in the existence of the Ideal. Before we could hope that the attempt to reach the Ideal just might succeed. Now we are to believe that it never can.

But do we really need to accept that our knowledge is necessarily only partial. Is it true that there is no "resting place" to be found? There is a point to such questions, because a sense of fulfillment, or completeness is something we desire. Its absence has been painfully noted in 20th century literature and philosophy, where attempts to attain certain knowledge are often seen as failures. Wisdom (1957) describes how metaphysical inquiry seems to let us down, and we may feel that his remarks about metaphysics may hold for all forms of inquiry.

> In the labyrinths of metaphysics are the same whispers as one hears when climbing Kafka's staircases to the tribunal which is always one floor further up. Is it because of this that when in metaphysics we seem to have arranged by a new technique a new dawn then we find ourselves again on Chirico's sad terraces where those whom we can never know still sit and it is neither night nor day? (p.282)

How depressing. Since Godel's theorem seems to be one of the ways in which uncertainty is justified as an eternal state of mind, let us have a closer look at it, and see if we are really condemned to such a fate.

In what follows, I will make extensive use of Lucas' (1961) account of Godel's proof. Suppose we want to know if a system that is logical is also complete. That is, we want to know if all true statements in the system are provable in the system. To do this we imagine a statement in the system such as "This statement is unprovable in the system." Call this statement G. On the one hand, suppose we prove that G is true. Then we have shown that a statement is true that itself asserts that it cannot be proven to be true in the system. On the other hand, suppose we show that G cannot be proven in the system. Then we have a true statement that cannot be proven in the system, and the system is therefore incomplete.

Godel's theorem has the same sort of effect on the mind as do paradoxes of the sort collected by Hughes and Brecht (1975). They make your head swim. Consider Figure 4, and see what happens to your thinking. Many people have taken such verbal devices very seriously, as revealing something central about the way the mind works. But do we really need to regard them as terribly important? Consider what Wittgenstein (1956) once said about the matter. He wondered if contradictions of the sort we have just been considering really do us any harm. Does it reflect on the rest of our thinking if in certain highly arcane contexts it generates something impossible? Since most of the time our thought works perfectly well, perhaps we should regard such contexts as Godel's theorem as merely games "with some similarity to the game of thumb-catching." Of course, I can hold the thumb of my right hand in my left hand, but I cannot then "catch" it in my right hand. However, I am not *upset* by this—I just see that it is impossible. Similarly, rather than being shocked into changing my world view because of Godel's theorem and its ilk, I can see instead how "tormenting problems grow out of language, and what kind of things can torment us." The remarkable thing is not Godel's theorem itself, but rather that we are the sort of creatures who can be *tormented* by problems like this.

We have covered a lot of ground. It is now time to recapitulate and connect these issues with suicide.

Suicide and the End of Development

Sometimes the concept of development may be understood as referring to a process that is open-ended, and sometimes it may best be understood as referring

Do not read this sentence

Figure 4. A paradoxical statement.

to a process that has a particular end. When people begin to think about an end to development, various problems and attempted solutions occur, among which are the following:

1. We live in an age of science, yet scientific inquiry appears to come up short of satisfying our most basic needs. This may be because science tells us nothing about human values. One can *know* a great deal, and still not be sure that one has attained anything of real importance.
2. Because our current preoccupation with science does not address the problems of life, people may despair of finding anything of value in the world. Perhaps they need to adopt what Wittgenstein described as an "aesthetic attitude" to the world.
3. Perhaps we need to acknowledge, as Weil did, that the world is incapable of satisfying us. This may begin a painful journey "upward," similar to the voyages of enlightenment described by Plato and other ancient sages.
4. However, there is nothing to guarantee that this journey will be successful. It might turn out to be endless, and endlessly disappointing. In this respect, development can be like the process described by Godel's theorem—a never-ending labor.

Each of the foregoing possibilities has suicidal potential. Spiritual journeys, of the sort described by Wittgenstein and Weil, are notoriously risky sources of salvation. Aesthetics and religion have their share of casualties. The concept of development is ambiguous, and that ambiguity allows for both positive and negative outcomes as people struggle to define the meaning of development in their own lives. The only thing we can be reasonably sure of is that the end of development will be a central issue in people's lives. Some of the ways in which people deal with this issue will be discussed in succeeding chapters.

In closing, it might be worth reminding ourselves of the difficulties in trying to say that a particular outcome is "good" or "bad." It is, I think, a deeply felt desire in human beings that there be an end to development, a point past which they neither should nor need to go. Simone Weil instantiated this desire as well as anyone, and it is instructive to consider the end of development for her. In 1943, in exile in England and dying of tuberculosis, she insisted on eating no more than what was then available to her French countrymen in her Nazi-occupied homeland. This amount of food was not enough to keep her from dying. She was 34.

> On September 3, 1943, the following headline appeared in a local English newspaper: "DEATH FROM STARVATION: FRENCH PROFESSOR'S CURIOUS SACRIFICE." The verdict of the coroner's court was "that the deceased did kill and slay herself by refusing to eat whilst the balance of her mind was disturbed" . . . Either this is madness or it is a vocation few are called to. Simone Weil's life and death compel us to face or to hide from such ultimate questions. (Cameron, 1981)

ACKNOWLEDGMENTS. The section dealing with Godel's theorem benefited from discussions with S. J. Segalowitz, and was composed while the author was supported by a grant from the National Sciences and Engineering Research Council of Canada.

REFERENCES

Benjafield, J. (1985). A review of recent research on the Golden Section. *Empirical Studies of the Arts, 3*, 117–134.

Benjafield, J. (1987). An historical, social analysis of imagery and concreteness. *British Journal of Social Psychology, 26*, 155–164.

Benjafield, J., & Muckenheim, R. (1989). A further historicodevelopmental study of the interpersonal circle. *Canadian Journal of Behavioural Science, 21*, 83–93.

Brown, G. S. (1969). *The Laws of Form*. London: Allen & Unwin.

Cameron, J. M. (1981). The life and death of Simone Weil. In G. A. White (Ed.), *Simone Weil: Interpretation of a life*. Amherst, MA: University of Massachusetts Press.

Coles, R. (1982). Simone Weil's Mind. In G. A. White (Ed.), *Simone Weil: Interpretation of a life*. Amherst, MA: University of Massachusetts Press.

Drury, M. (1973). *The Danger of Words*. London: Routledge & Kegan Paul.

Freud, S. (1966). Some thoughts on development and regression—aetiology. *New introductory lectures on psychoanalysis* (pp. 339–357). New York: W. W. Norton.

Gilligan, C. (1982). *In a different voice: Psychological theory and women's development*. Cambridge, MA: Harvard University Press.

Hofstadter, D. *Godel, Escher, Bach: An eternal golden braid*. New York: Basic Books.

Hughes, P., & Brecht, G. (1975). *Vicious circles and infinity*. New York: Penguin Books.

James, W. (1890). *The principles of psychology*. New York: Holt.

Lerner, R. M. (1986). *Concepts and theories of human development*. New York: Random House.

Lucas, (1961). Minds, machines and Godel. *Philosophy, 36*, 112.

McGuinness, B. (1966). The mysticism of the Tractatus. *Philosophical Review, 75*, 305–328.

Mitchison, G. J. (1977). Phyllotaxis and the Fibonacci series. *Science, 196*, 270–275.

Piaget, J. (1957). *Logic and psychology*. New York: Basic Books.

Piaget, J. (1970). *Structuralism*. New York: Harper & Row.

Russell, B. (1974). Introduction. In L. Wittgenstein (Ed.), *Tractatus logico-philosophicus*. New York: Routledge & Kegan Paul.

Stevens, P. S. (1974). *Patterns in nature*. Boston: Houghton-Mifflin.

Thompson, D. W. (1929). Excess and defect. *Mind, 38*, 43–55.

Weil, S. (1968). *On science necessity and the love of God*. New York: Oxford University Press.

Weil, S. (1971). *The need for roots*. New York: Harper & Row.

Weil, S. (1977). Metaxu. In G. Panichas (Ed.), *A Simone Weil reader*. New York: McKay.

Wisdom, J. (1957). *Philosophy and psychoanalysis*. Oxford: Blackwell.

Wittgenstein, L. (1953). *Philosophical investigations*. Oxford: Blackwell.

Wittgenstein, L. (1956). *Remarks on the foundations of mathematics*. Oxford: Blackwell.

Wittgenstein, L. (1969). *Notebooks 1914–1916*. New York: Harper & Row.

Wittgenstein, L. (1974). *Tractatus logico-philosophicus*. London: Routledge & Kegan Paul. (Original work published in 1922)

2

A Brief Introduction to the Stages of Development

David Lester

To bring some order into our discussion of suicidal behavior in people of different ages, we need some descriptive schema for how people change with age. Such schema are often called *stages of development*, and many developmental psychologists reject the notion of stages (Goodman & Feldman, 1975).

Such critics do not object to the notion that people change as they age. Rather, they object to specifying stages that imply an orderly sequence of periods of development with precise entrance and exit ages. So let us be clear at the beginning that the stages that I shall describe in this chapter are not meant to be precise.

For example, Erikson (1959) called the stage that we enter during middle adulthood "generativity versus stagnation" and saw the focus of this stage as caring for others. We must remember that some people enter this stage or deal with this issue at an earlier age, and perhaps some people never experience this stage. Furthermore, people do not neatly resolve the issues of earlier stages before passing onto this stage. Issues and concerns from earlier stages may continue to bedevil us during middle adulthood and, indeed, may continue to plague us for the rest of our lives.

The purpose of a stage theory is to describe briefly how the average person aged, say, 50 differs from the average person aged 20. So, with this caution in mind let us move on to a rough schema for development that will help us organize the information presented in this volume.

DAVID LESTER • Department of Psychology, Stockton State College, Pomona, New Jersey 08240.

STAGES OF DEVELOPMENT

In recent years, many schemata have been proposed for classifying time-lines or stages of life. The major psychologists proposing classifications have been Gould (1978), Levinson (1978), and Vaillant (1977), and a popular account of these stages has been written by Sheehy (1976). There is broad agreement on the stages, though disagreement on how to label them and exactly what ages they correspond to.

For example, Levinson tags early adulthood as ages 17 to 40 and includes the stages Early Adult Transition, Entering The Adult World, The Age 30 Transition and Settling Down. Gould proposes an age range of 16 to 34 for early adulthood and labels the stages Leaving Our Parents' World, I'm Nobody's Baby Now, and Opening Up To What's Inside. Sheehy labels the stages as Pulling Up Roots, the Trying Twenties, and Passage To The Thirties. Vaillant calls the whole period Intimacy And Career Consolidation.

Ignoring these fine distinctions, in this volume we will divide life into the following time-lines.

Infancy	0–2
Preschool years	2–6
Middle childhood	6–12
Adolescence	13–18
Young adulthood	18–25/30
Middle adulthood	25–55/60
Late adulthood	55/60 and older

We will see soon in chapter 6 that international suicide statistics take no account of this division. The World Health Organization publishes rates for 10-year age groups, proceeding from 5 to 14, 15 to 24, and onward. This illustrates the importance of a rough developmental schema for, if the one listed above makes psychological sense, perhaps national suicide rates should be given for the ages corresponding to those stages rather than for arbitrary 10-year groupings?

Individuals in these different stages differ in physical and physiological ways, have very different cognitive abilities and ways of interacting socially with others, and grapple with very different problems and issues. Some psychologists have explored some of these changes in detail. Erikson, for example, focused on the problems and issues at each stage while Kohlberg (1963) explored changes in moral development. In the following sections, I shall very briefly describe some of the characteristics of each stage.

Infancy

Infancy involves at first a profound physiological shock as the newborn must adjust to extra-uterine life. After birth, physical growth, perception, cognition (the acquisition of information about the world and the process of organizing it), and motor development all develop slowly.

More important, the infant also begins to interact socially with others, particularly parents and siblings. The first issue in Erikson's stages of development is that of *trust versus mistrust*. If the infant's caretakers are consistent and loving, the infant will acquire a basic trust in others. If the caretakers are cruel, abusive, inconsistent, and rejecting, the infant may never learn to trust others.

Preschool Years

From the age of 2 on, the child makes great progress in motor and cognitive skills, especially language. The child's sense of self begins to develop, and in Erikson's second stage the crisis involves the ability and desire to achieve self-control: *autonomy versus shame and doubt*. The child has to develop a sense of his or her own autonomy, yet parents and other caretakers have a lot of rules to impose. If the caretakers impose unrealistic and rigid demands on the child, the child may come to feel shame and doubt rather than developing a sense of autonomy. Parents know this stage as the "terrible twos" when the child's typical response to any request is "No!"

Preschoolers soon confront the next crisis: *initiative versus guilt*. They begin to be more assertive and to show initiative in pursuing their own interests and desires. They are much more willing to cooperate in endeavors with their caretakers. But their initiative often creates trouble. Their attempts to cook leave an incredible mess. Their tinkering with machines breaks them. As a result they often get punished for their activities rather than praised, which results in guilt.

Middle Childhood

The first 6 years of life described briefly above were the critical years for Sigmund Freud's psychoanalytic theory of development. Trauma in the first 6 years of life lays the groundwork for later psychological disturbance. After these early years, psychoanalysts saw the following period, which they called *latency*, as one for consolidation, during which little of interest happens.

Important changes take place during this period of middle childhood, however. The child begins to lose his or her egocentric perspective, and begins to understand other people's point of view a little.

In Kohlberg's (1963) description of moral development, the child shows Level I: *Preconventional Morality*. At this level, moral judgments are made on the basis of whether the actions will be rewarded or punished by those in authority. In Stage 1, the focus is on the punishment for not doing what you should. In Stage 2, the focus shifts more to the rewards for completing the task. Deeds are good if they are rewarded and bad if they are punished.

By the end of the middle childhood, the children may show elements of Level II: *Conventional Morality*. In this level, the moral guidelines set up by those in authority are adopted. If people in power accept and approve a behavior, then it is good. In Stage 3, the child focuses on the judgments of significant others. In Stage 4, the child begins to recognize the rules of the larger society.

For Erikson, the crisis here is *industry versus inferiority*. Children go off to school where they are required to work at academic tasks. In earlier years, they played and could abandon an activity whenever they chose to do so. Now they have to develop their skills and learn to persist at a task until it is completed. If they fail at these early tasks or are criticized for their performance, they may develop a sense of inferiority rather than coming to value achievements.

In recent years, as well shall see in later chapters, suicidal behavior has been recognized in children in this period of development. This raises the issue of the development of the child's concept of death. It had long been argued that, since children do not have a mature concept of death, they could not possibly attempt to kill themselves.

Goldstein (1940), for example, argued that suicide was possible only when a person understands what death is and consciously chooses to commit suicide. In contrast, Menninger (1938) allowed for unconscious suicidal desires and for behaviors only partially motivated by self-destructive impulses. For Menninger, then, children could show suicidal behavior.

The stages in the development of the child's concept of death have not been studied as intensively as, say, moral development. Nagy (1948) suggested that from ages 3 to 5, in early childhood, children deny death as a final process. Death is seen as a temporary departure, and the dead can come back in the same way that people go to sleep and wake up. From ages 5 to 9, in middle childhood, children personify death. Death is seen as someone or something coming to carry you off, and its permanence is recognized though the possibility remains of fighting off death. After age 9, the child begins to recognize that death involves the inevitable and permanent dissolution of the body, which will happen to all of us eventually.

As with other stage theories, this description is oversimplified, and children do not pass in an orderly fashion through the stages at the ages specified by Nagy. However, it is critical for understanding suicidal behavior in children to have some idea of what their concept of death is, for this knowledge will help us understand the intent of their self-destructive behavior.

Adolescence

Adolescence is marked, of course, by hormonal and morphological changes that result in an increasing concern with sexuality. The peer group becomes especially critical as an agent of socialization. Intimate friendships are formed now, and the adolescent's self-esteem is affected by his or her popularity. This stage also involves a gradual distancing from parents and, since gradual distancing is often difficult, this process is often marked by periods of great rebelliousness.

Erikson labeled the crisis during this stage as *identity versus confusion*. The adolescent's chief concern is to establish an identity and to make a career choice. The identity may be shaped by peers or by fashionable heros and ideals. Adolescents often experience anxiety, both at a general level as they search for decisions, but also cover more specific issues such as their academic abilities, their social skills, or their dating behavior.

As we shall see later, rates of both attempted suicide and completed suicide increase dramatically during adolescence in America. Most investigators note that the stresses for the suicidal adolescent are usually interpersonal. There appears to be a combination of chronic stress in the relationship with parents and acute stress in interpersonal relationships, often with a boyfriend or girlfriend.

Problems during adolescence will be especially marked in those who had difficulties making healthy resolutions during the earlier stages of development. If the adolescent has learned mistrust, shame and doubt and inferiority in these earlier times, then confusion may well be the resolution here.

It is probably true that education can play a large role in moving people out of adolescence. Not only does education develop intellectual skills that help the individual resolve some of the issues encountered during childhood and adolescent development, but also education helps disengage the individual from family and peer groups. Although modern society seems to have lengthened the period of immaturity and dependence beyond that found in nonliterate primitive societies, going away to college can stimulate the move to maturity.

Few adults remain fixated in the stages of childhood (unless they are mentally retarded or severely psychiatrically disturbed). However, many adults do not move much beyond the concerns and styles of adolescence. Thus, the behavior of some adults may resemble that of adolescents, while others regress to this phase of development when they experience stress.

Young Adulthood

As we move through the stages of life, we encounter greater variability. Infants have much in common. Adults, in contrast, are characterized by their diversity. In early adulthood, some individuals are still students while others have jobs. Some live at home with parents, others with roommates, while many are married and starting families.

Kohlberg reserved the final level of moral development for later adolescence and early adulthood. Level III: *Postconventional Morality* is based upon principles that people have thought about and accepted. In Stage 5, morality is based upon the social contract and basic human rights that do not need to be earned. Stage 6 rests upon individual conscience. Principled reasoning leads to the correct behavior, which in turn produces a feeling of being true to oneself.

For Erikson, the issue is *intimacy versus isolation*. Can the individual make a commitment to friends, lovers, and causes? Will he or she assume the responsibilities of adulthood, find an intimate lover or spouse, and work on building a healthy mutual relationship?

Erikson focused on interpersonal relationships, but career concerns also assume great importance during this stage. The young adult begins work and, in many cases, throws himself or herself into the pursuit for excellence. Often, the commitment is so great that the individual does not have time to consider whether the career goals are really desirable, foreshadowing the crises of middle adulthood.

Marcia (1980) has examined the crisis of early adulthood in a little more detail. He noted that not all people go through a crisis at this time. For some the path is smooth and without stress. In addition, some individuals show no commitment and remain indecisive about life decisions and values. This gives us a fourfold classification:

	Crisis	*No crisis*
Commitment	Identity achievers	Identity foreclosure
No commitment	Moratorium	Diffuse identity

Those who experience a crisis and make a personal decision based upon their own desires (rather than those of parents) are *identity achievers*. Those who follow along with parental desires, either because of dependence upon them or fear of striking out on their own, show *identity foreclosure*.

Other individuals remain indecisive about life decisions. If they remain in crisis, they continue to struggle with the issues, but postpone commitment to one solution. They are categorized as in *moratorium*. If they are not in crisis, then not only are they indecisive, but they seem to be unconcerned about their indecision, and they have a *diffuse identity*.

Middle Adulthood

By the time the individual has reached the mid 20s to 30s, he or she typically has married, started a family, and moved some way in their career. Erikson sees the person now beginning to confront *generativity versus stagnation*. The individual becomes concerned with future generations. He begins to be concerned with raising his children (now teenagers) and contributing to the culture through his work. If he remains concerned with himself, he stagnates.

In the latter stage of middle adulthood, the body beings to deteriorate, and concerns with physical health become more central. Cardiovascular disease and cancer become likely disorders now. Women face menopause, and men may experience a decrease in the level of sex hormones too. Even though research does not always show a decline in cognitive abilities, people begin to anticipate and fear the decline.

Other psychologists, such as Levinson (1978), see middle adulthood as a time for consolidation of the person's interests and goals. We begin to settle down, with an emphasis on stability and continuity. For Levinson, a successful middle age involves working through the discrepancies between what is and what might be.

Psychologists appear to reject completely the more popular descriptions of stressful life transitions proposed by Sheehy (1976) and others. However, the issues raised by such popular writers seem much more pertinent to the lives of real people than the more abstract writings of scholars.

Middle adulthood is often a time of great stress. Typically, many marriages break up around this time. One-third of all marriages end in divorce, and about a quarter take place after 15 years or more of marriage and so occur during middle adulthood.

People often question whether the career they have chosen is the one they really wanted. This is the time when the stockbroker quits and goes off to Vermont or Colorado and runs a farm or a ski resort. And even if few adults make such drastic changes, many make minor changes.

Erikson, writing in the 1950s, focused on the individual's connections with society versus unhealthy self-absorption. Since that time, America has become amazingly "psychologized." Psychotherapists turned from the treatment of the disturbed to helping people realize their potential. People began to visit psychotherapists because their lives felt empty and had no meaning. Psychological religions sprung up to focus people's searches, led, for example, by Zen, the Esalen Institute in California, and Erhard Seminars Training (Bry, 1976), and popularized by such famous personalities as John Denver and Shirley Maclaine.

Modern America has become increasingly self-contemplative, and it is common for the newly divorced 40-year-old to talk of being "selfish" and to embark on episodic searches for a new identity. It is interesting to talk to those in other cultures and realize how they view this as deviant. Most Europeans, for example, see the American penchant for psychotherapy as bizarre.

Modern America is also achievement oriented. There is only one gold medal awarded in each Olympic event. The other competitors are "failures." And so most people in middle adulthood have to come to terms with their failures. They weren't particularly good parents, they failed in their marriage, and they didn't advance quite as far in their career as they once had hoped.

Late Adulthood

In old age, physiological decline proceeds apace, with an increased risk of diseases, sensory decline, changes in physical appearance, and impaired mental functioning. Eventually, the older adult has to think about how to survive as he becomes increasingly impaired.

The older adult also has to face many external stresses. There is often abandonment by family members as they grow up and move away. Widowhood is frequent. Of women 75 years of age or older, 70% are widowed. The older adult retires from work, and the adjustment can be very stressful.

Erikson described the issue in this stage as *ego integrity versus despair*. Ego integrity means that you have found your life meaningful and that you are content with the way it has gone. The other extreme is characterized by despair, disgust, and bitterness.

CONCLUSIONS

Erikson's description of the stages has advantages for our goals in this book over other schemata because he discusses the *psychological* issues that we confront at each stage rather than focusing simply on the external stressors. We know that young adults are confronting issues of career and family while older adults confront issues of retirement, ill health, and impending death. Erikson explores the existential issues that we confront at each age, and so his scheme may have special relevance for the less superficial motives behind the suicides of people at different stages of life.

The goal in this chapter has been to introduce briefly the notion of stages and to describe some of the schemata that have been proposed. We will turn in later chapters to discussions of suicide by those in these various stages, and we will then be able to see whether this developmental framework helps us to understand the differences in the suicidal acts of those in these different stages of development.

REFERENCES

Bry, A. (1976). *EST*. New York: Avon.

Erikson, E. (1959). *Identity and the life cycle*. New York: International Universities Press.

Goldstein, K. (1940). *Human nature in the light of psychopathology*. Cambridge: Harvard University Press.

Goodman, N., & Feldman, K. A. (1975). Expectations, ideals, and reality. In S. E. Dragastin, & G. H. Elder (Eds.), *Adolescence in the life cycle* (pp. 147–150). Washington: Hemisphere.

Gould, R. L. (1978). *Transformations*. New York: Simon & Schuster.

Kohlberg, L. (1963). The development of children's orientations toward a moral order. *Vita Humana*, *6*, 11–23.

Levinson, D. (1978). *The season's of a man's life*. New York: Alfred A. Knopf.

Marcia, J. E. (1980). Identity in adolescence. In J. Adelson (Ed.) *Handbook of adolescent psychology* (pp. 159–187). New York: Wiley.

Menninger, K. (1938). *Man against himself*. New York: Harcourt Brace & World.

Nagy, M. (1948). The child's theories concerning death. *Journal of Genetic Psychology*, 73, 3–27.

Sheehy, G. (1976). *Passages*. New York: Dutton.

Vaillant, G. E. (1977). *Adaptation to life*. Boston: Little, Brown.

3

The Developmental Perspective of Suicide

Ronald W. Maris

> *Suicide is, in short, the one continuous every-day, ever-present problem of living*
>
> Daniel Stern

In 1981, I wrote:

> Virtually everyone engaged in suicide research agrees that it is time to move from static, structural, descriptive profiles of self-destructive behaviors to dynamic developmental models. Suicidal lethality (the probability of committing suicide) varies over time and among different types of individuals (and groups). It is argued here that the suicide's biography or "career" is always relevant to his or her self-destructive reaction to crises and that it is precisely this history, individual or group, which tends to be neglected. (Maris, 1981, p.9)

Regretably, almost 10 years later the study of suicide is still basically fragmented and nondynamic. For example, all of us are victims of our disciplinary training. Clinical psychologists and research psychiatrists routinely take careful case histories but often do not have scientific samples. Epidemiologists, on the other hand, tend to employ sound research methods but usually with a very narrow focus (as in the NIMH Epidemiological Catchment Area Program, Eaton, 1985). Physicians, interestingly, attend to the relationship of alcoholism, depressive

RONALD W. MARIS • The Center for the Study of Suicide, University of South Carolina, Columbia, South Carolina 29208.

illness, and suicide, but almost totally neglect other factors and often ignore the dynamic aspects of even alcoholism and depression. In short, no single discipline considers the full range of suicidal variables. We should remember that a disciplinary way of seeing is also a way of *not* seeing.

The developmental study of suicide is further fragmented by research costs. Most suicide research is cross-sectional with a focus on present conditions, with a few retrospective case-control designs (cf. Shneidman, 1971). Almost no suicide research is prospective, such as the cohort studies of Vaillant (1977) or Thomas (1969). One obvious reason for this relative lack of cohort studies of suicides is that suicide is a very rare behavior (1–3 in 10,000 in the general population each year). It would be extremely expensive to follow a large enough sample at high risk for suicide for 30 to 50 years to get meaningful data.

Suicidology is nondynamic when it examines discrete life stages in isolation from one another. Simply to investigate suicide among adolescents or the aged is clearly not the same thing as determining the interrelationships of suicidal stages in the entire life history of a single suicidal individual or group. It should be mentioned in passing that the middle stages of the suicidal life cycle typically have been understudied, even though the mean age for all suicide in 1980 was 40 years old. One should not forget that the proper developmental study of suicide includes systematic collection of family history data, especially on at least the parents and siblings of suicidal individuals (Andreasen et al., 1986, 1987). Many suicidologists have a crisis orientation or acute lethality bias. In the urgency of crisis intervention, we tend to forget that a patient's developmental history often determines who will and who will not respond suicidally to common stressors or negative life events.

When we think about suicidal behaviors, it is important to consider several different developmental connotations. For examples, individuals tend to go through life stages, each with different developmental tasks and meanings (Levinson, 1978). Relevant factors in individual suicidal development are parental or sibling suicides, prior suicide attempts of the individual, a history of depressive illness and alcoholism, and many more. A second connotation is social development. Societies themselves go through evolutionary stages, such as "hunting or gathering, industrial, or post-industrial," and so on (Lenski & Lenski, 1987). One might also note patterns of social support or of social isolation. The historical context is a third broad developmental connotation. Suicide and suicide rates are clearly affected by factors such as the Great Depression, the current world-wide AIDs crisis, or being in a World War II baby-boom cohort. Fourth, the economy is a developmental variable. For example, Brenner (1977) has argued that unemployment or inflation rate variations are related to suicide rates. A fifth developmental connotation is biological variation, such as the aging process or whether an individual has certain physical illnesses or not. Clearly, culture and basic values constitute a sixth developmental connotation. Some cultures are highly conducive to suicide in certain contexts (e.g., the Hindu cases of *suttee* or Japanese *hara-kiri*), while other cultures may discourage suicide under almost any circumstances (such as the Tiv of Nigeria). Some religions consider suicide a serious sin against God. Finally, there are legal connotations that vary with social development. For example, in about half of the United States, assisting suicide is a crime, while in the other half it is not or is uncertain (Battin & Mayo, 1980). In short, the developmental perspective of suicide has at least individual, social, historical, economic, biological, cultural, and legal connotations.

THE DEVELOPMENTAL LITERATURE

I saw the years of my life spaced along a road in the form of telephone poles, threaded together by wires. I counted one, two, three . . . nineteen poles, and then the wires dangled into space, and try as I would, I couldn't see a single pole beyond the nineteenth.

Sylvia Plath

The lives of human beings and social units are not just static structural phenomena, but can also be viewed as dynamic cycles of growth and development. Although we may debate whether stages in the human life cycle are more closely associated with biological or sociocultural factors, it is generally agreed that human beings progress through various developmental changes with relatively well-defined life stages (Dannefer, 1984; Birren, 1986; Erikson, 1950; Schlein, 1987). According to Erikson these life stages (note that Erikson's stages 7 and 8 are now too narrow in age range) may be said to include broadly:

1. Infancy (Ages 0–2)
2. Toddlerhood (2–4)
3. Early childhood (5–7)
4. Middle childhood (8–12)
5. Adolescence
    a. Early adolescence (13–17)
    b. Later adolescence (18–22)
6. Early adulthood (23–30)
7. Middle adulthood (31–50)
8. Later adulthood (51+)

Neugarten and Neugarten (1986) and Riley and Riley (1986) emphasize that role expectations ("developmental tasks") usually accompany these life stages and that rites of passage are often associated with moving from one role or stage to another (e.g., bar mitzvahs, graduations, marriages, or funeral ceremonies). Personal or social problems (including suicidal crises) can develop because individuals, groups, or societies age chronologically but not developmentally (i.e., they stagnate). Changing social roles is like dying and successfully grieving to be able to cathect new roles.

Most theories of human development can be collapsed into at least six broad types: (1) psychosexual and psychosocial stage theories (notably those of Freud, 1905; Jung, 1963; Erikson, 1950; Levinson et al., 1978); (2) life span theories (Baltes & Brim, 1979–1988); (3) cognitive theories (Piaget, 1952); (4) learning theories (Skinner, 1953; Bandura & Walters, 1963); (5) role theories (Kalleberg & Loscocco, 1983); and (6) cohort theories (Easterlin, 1980). Some of the basic issues in all theories of human development are whether the human life span can be divided into stages; what these stages are and when they occur; what crises, expectations, challenges, and so on are associated with these stages; and whether human life is teleological or ontogenetic (i.e., progresses to some natural end). Mussen, Conger, and Kagan (1984) comment as follows on the controversy concerning purposeful stages of human development:

> When the developmental psychologist addresses himself to the purpose, or the adaptive value of behavior, he becomes embroiled in one of the most controversial issues in human development, namely, does the theorist believe the child is growing toward some ideal goal? Put another way, should we conceive of psychological development as a sequence of stages that define progress toward a more "mature level" of functioning? (p.34)

The developmental theories of Freud, Erikson, Piaget, and, more recently, Levinson et al. (1978) and Dannefer (1984) assume various life stages and associate them with certain expectations or developmental tasks. In some theories, individual development depends on interaction with specific environmental conditions. Given a variance of about 4 to 5 years, these life stages can be dated only roughly. If one does not master the crises or challenges relevant to each life stage, then it is assumed that developmental debits will be acquired that could result in stagnation or the inability to mature normally (Coleman & Butcher, 1984):

> At each stage of development there are certain tasks or competencies to be mastered if the individual is to maintain a normal schedule of development. If developmental tasks are not mastered at the appropriate stage, the individual suffers from immaturities and incompetences and is placed at a serious disadvantage in adjusting at later developmental levels. (p.95)

In more formal sociological theories, focus is often not on individual development, but rather on the normal expected life courses of whole societies or cultures (Aldrich, 1979; Lenski & Lenski, 1987).

BASIC CONCEPTS IN SUICIDAL DEVELOPMENT

> *Life is impoverished, it loses in interest, when the highest stake in the game of living, life itself, may not be risked.*
>
> Sigmund Freud

It is argued here that we are particularly vulnerable to suicide when death, decay, and destruction, and the terror or anxiety that can accompany them, break through our defenses in systematic, patterned ways over a lifetime and dilute our will and ability to continue living, what I have designated elsewhere as *suicidal careers* (Maris, 1981). There are several separate but overlapping notions in the concept of a suicidal career. First, it is predicted that the profiles or models for completed suicides, nonfatal suicide attempters, natural deaths, living normals, and so on will differ on given sets of variables such as depressive illness, alcoholism, suicidal ideation, use of lethal methods, and social isolation. Second, the concept of suicidal careers implies that it is necessary to conceive of life-threatening behaviors as having relevant histories. Usually only a time-of-death profile is assumed, since the U.S. death registration system focuses on the situation at the time of death or the few weeks or months just before death. Third, suicidal deaths are never entirely reactive to present stressors. There is always a relevant set of biographies or "career contingencies" that mediates reaction to stress and helps to specify which individuals in so-called high-risk groups will be most likely to respond to life stress or negative life events with self-destructive behaviors. Fourth, it follows that suicide lethality can either be *acute* (the short-term probability of suicide) or *chronic* (the long-term probability of suicide) and that these types of lethality may be negatively associated (cf. Menninger, 1938; Farberow, 1980). For example, an individual or a group may have high acute lethality and low chronic lethality at the same time. Fifth, self-destructive behaviors need to be cast into causal models that span suicidal subjects' lives from birth to death (Mann & Stanley, 1988, p.425), adequate samples of cases and controls drawn, and analyzed with modern multivariate statistics (such as logistic regression or path analysis techniques). Finally, it is immensely helpful in the analysis of suicidal developmental models to specify both direct and indirect causal paths to suicide.

A second set of basic developmental concepts turn on suicide meaning different things at different ages, life stages, or for different types of suicide. In Chapter 4, Dr. Shneidman lists several "commonalities of suicide." These include seeking a solution to life problems, cessation of consciousness, intolerable psychological pain, ambivalence, constriction of perception, and so on. Suicidologists also have a short list of common predictors of suicide, such as depression, alcoholism, suicidal ideation, lethal methods, social isolation, hopelessness, anger, modeling, marital and work problems, prior suicide attempts, and so on (Brent, 1988). Developmental considerations can be thought of as in a sense the "noncommonalities" of suicide. For example, the weights of common factors or predictors change with age or life stage (Lyons, 1985; deCatanzaro, 1986). Ambivalence in general may lessen with age. The interpersonal factor in suicide, including hate and revenge, may be more salient at younger ages. Alcohol may actually protect one against suicide in the early phases of alcoholism. Depression and hopelessness without aggressive energy may also protect against a suicidal outcome. Finally, salient factors in suicide outcomes vary with the type of suicide (clearly not all suicides are alike). Escape suicides suggest that aggression is primary. Revenge suicides may feature interpersonal factors. Altruistic suicides

(Baechler's "oblative suicides," 1979) are usually not socially isolated. Risk-takers who suicide (Baechler's "ludic suicides") may actually be seeking to expand consciousness, not to die.

A third fairly obvious set of developmental concepts in suicide concerns variables or predictors of suicide with explicit temporal factors. Consider alcoholism. Clearly, alcoholism is a process, not a unitary state. If we assume Jellinek's disease model of development, then alcoholism evolves in three basic stages (1960). Some research has suggested that suicide is especially likely in Stage 3, namely, when alcoholic tolerance is lost. The developmental study of suicide requires us to specify the phase or stage of alcoholism. Another example might be the repeatability of depressive illness. The crucial suicidal consideration may be that the patient cannot tolerate the thought of yet another depressive episode. We might also need to know at what depressive episode does depression produce hopelessness, what phase of manic-depressive illness a person was in, or whether an individual's depression was lifting. Surely, just knowing if a subject is depressed or not, or even what kind of *DSM-III-R* depression they have, is not sufficient to predict a suicide outcome.

Many biological changes are also relevant to suicide. One immediately thinks of puberty or menopause, the onset of a terminal physical illness, or simply of aging. Predictors of suicide, such as social isolation or interpersonal relations, have temporal dimensions as well. I have argued elsewhere that social isolation is not as important as how one came to be alone (Maris, 1981). Aloneness by choice is very different from aloneness by necessity. Interpersonally, variation in the number of close friends is often critical. For example, having at least one significant other is quite different from having none at all. Suicidologists also need to be attentive to a potential suicide who exhausts social or community agency supports over time, so that at some point in time no viable helping resources are left for a particular individual—or at least he or she may perceive this to be the case.

A fourth set of developmental factors in suicide includes modeling, contagion, suggestion, and imitation. Modeling of prior suicides is a developmental factor, since the suicide always comes *after* the model or stimulus. The problem here is that often suicide does *not* come at all after a prior suicide. Thus, other factors interact with modeling to determine suicidal outcome and they need to be specified. Some candidates for relevant third variables include the similarity of the model and the would-be suicide, how often the model stimulus is presented, how close the potential suicide already was to suicide, and so on (Diekstra et al., 1989). Most of the work on imitation and suicide has been done by sociologists and most of that by Phillips (1974; Phillips & Carstensen, 1986). Oversimplifying many diverse pieces of research, Phillips argues that suicide rates tend to rise 1–7% over expected suicide rates 7 to 10 days after a publicized suicidal death. Teenagers seem to be especially suggestible. In one study Phillips noted a 6.9% rise in the teenage suicide rate after a televised suicide story. In my 1981 survey of Chicago suicides, I found that 11% of completed suicides had at least one suicide in their family of origin, while none of the natural death controls did. One needs to remember that modeling is only one developmental factor among many in the etiology of suicide and that it varies with suicidal type.

A fifth set of suicidal developmental considerations focuses on cohort studies or suicides among a group of people all born in some common time span, such as "baby-boom" births in the United States after World War II (Easterlin, 1980). One excellent, but costly and time-consuming developmental strategy is to follow a scientific sample of high-risk individuals over their lifetime and attempt to determine what factors distinguish those individuals who eventually suicide from those who do not (say, natural deaths). However, since suicides amount to only 1 to 3 people in 10,000 in the general population per year, this usually is not a very practical approach. Also, how can one even keep track of people for 30 to 50 years? The cohort approach has been done with some success by Thomas with 1,337 medical school graduates from the Johns Hopkins University between 1948 and 1964. Thomas (1969) found that the eventual suicides were distinguished by their difficulty sleeping, urge to be alone, irritability, not confiding in others, lack of appetite, and a few other factors. A modified cohort approach is to look backwards at suicides in a cohort and see how their earlier lives differed from other nonsuicides in the same cohort. Shneidman (1971) attempted such a "psychological autopsy" procedure with the Terman cohort data of high IQ Stanford students. Shneidman examined the files of 30 Terman subjects; 5 suicides, 10 natural deaths, and 15 living normals—after having removed all references to mode of death from their files. He then ranked all 30 cases from 1 (definite suicide) to 30 (definite nonsuicide). Shneidman got the first 4 cases right (all were suicides), case 5 was not a suicide, and case 6 was a suicide. Using clinical judgment he later speculated that the primary factors in distinguishing the suicides in the cohort were significant other problems (especially with nonsupportive spouses) and burnt-out affect. Other cohort suicide studies have focused on the competition for scarce resources of relatively large cohorts (Easterlin, 1980) and the fixed-number hypothesis (Lester, 1988). Lester argued that every cohort has a finite number of suicides, such that if they suicide early (as in Japan), they will have fewer suicides later in life (cf. Gouldney & Katsikitis, 1983).

A sixth set of suicidal developmental considerations concerns the various self-destructive acts leading up to the final act of completed suicide. Of particular interest are the dynamics of multiple suicide attempters and repeated self-harm patients. As I wrote in 1981:

> One commonly held belief about the development of suicides is that some lifelong precursors interact with acute stresses to "trigger" initial nonfatal suicide attempts. This initial attempt can be seen as having both benefits and costs to the attempter. On the positive side, nonfatal suicide attempters almost always get attention from family, friends, and professionals. The attempter is usually allowed to assume a "sick role," and

> ordinary responsibilities are often temporarily suspended. Suicide attempts may be cathartic, with even a short-term elevation of affect. Tension may be relieved and frustration reduced. On the negative side, the attention resulting from a suicide attempt is sometime stigmatizing and may make it more difficult for the individual to maintain a healthy identity. People may be sympathetic with suicide attempters, but they are also likely to be angry. Attempts inconvenience and manipulate people. After a period of recuperation the attempter is expected to give up the sick role and reassume a more normal, preattempt social role. In short, suicide attempters incur costs. Nevertheless the problems that were associated with the first attempt tend to recur, in part because of the suicide attempt itself. Attempting suicide may then become a conditioned reaction. When old problems return, the attempter may recall the positive response to his or her first attempt. The attempter may learn to adapt to stress through repeated self-destructive behaviors. However, second suicide attempts may be made with more lethal methods. In part this could be because the attempter is older and more hopeless. Furthermore, to get a positive response from significant others, the attempter may have to appear more serious the second time. Of course, more lethal attempts may provoke elevated anger and frustration from those individuals being manipulated or otherwise affected. Potentially stigmatizing hospitalization may be unavoidable. Resources may begin to dry up and supportive individuals may become increasingly impatient with the suicide attempter. Finally, perhaps after a few more nonfatal attempts, there may appear to be no way out of this increasingly intolerable situation except to actually complete suicide. (pp. 266–67)

Noting the important caveat that as many as 85% to 90% of older males make only one fatal suicide attempt and that even young females seldom attempt suicide more than four times before completing, it is obviously important for the developmental study of suicide to determine if the above profile of the multiple suicide attempter is correct. Why do some individuals make repeated suicide attempts? An important theme of this chapter is that one is usually not simply suicidal or nonsuicidal. Suicidal outcomes are contingent upon many interacting factors. Oversimplifying, we know that multiple suicide attempters tend to be younger and female. Probably multiple nonfatal suicide attempters are often making desperate efforts to resolve interpersonal problems. Barnes (1986) found that about 66% of the suicide attempters she studied were repeaters. Female repeaters had more sexual maladjustment and problems of loneliness while male suicide attempt repeaters reported more alcohol problems, family stress, and dropping out of school problems. Clearly, the method one chooses for attempting suicide is critical as is the subjective meaning of the method. Suicide repeaters almost by definition are less likely to use firearms. Numerous research studies have found that suicide attempt repeaters are more likely to be among attempters with personality disorders (especially antisocial and borderline patients), multiple personalities, and sexual masochists (Pattison & Kahan, 1983; Favazza, 1989). Kessel further argued that impulsive suicide attempts were more likely to be repeated. In a recent study, Steer et al. (1988) reported a curious result that nonfatal suicide attempters who were interrupted were about three times more likely to eventually suicide than attempters who were not interrupted. Whatever the particular contingencies, the developmental study of suicide needs to include concepts and measurements of factors related to repeated self-harm or multiple life-threatening attempts in suicidal careers.

THREE SUICIDE STUDIES IN THE DEVELOPMENTAL PERSPECTIVE

It will generally be found that as soon as the terrors of life reach the point where they outweigh the terrors of death, a man will put an end to his life
Arthur Schopenhauer

It remains to review a few major developmental studies of suicide and to determine what results can be gleaned. If we require book-length research on the development of completed suicides, it is surprising how little exists. Most of the work has been done by social-psychiatrists with a research orientation and even that focuses on the suicidal process just a few months before suiciding. A good example of this genre is Robins's *The Final Months: A Study of the Lives of 134 Persons Who Committed Suicide* (1981).

Robins and associates at the Washington University School of Medicine studied the lives of 134 suicides from St. Louis in 1956 and 1957. They used coroners' informants and records. The primary predictors of suicide were alcoholism (25% of the cases) and depressive illness (47%). Thus, 72% of the suicides were either alcoholic or depressed; 92% of the suicides had psychiatric disorders at the time of death. The most frequent symptoms in the suicidal subjects were weight loss, nervousness, insomnia, weekly to daily drinking of alcohol, and loss of interest in usual activities.

Although 18% of the sample had made a prior suicide attempt, attempted suicide was not a very strong predictor. Perhaps more interesting was that 73% of the suicides had sought professional clinical help in the last year of their life. Sixty-nine percent of the suicides communicated their suicidal intent to others, 25% had suffered a loss of an important relationship in the year before suicide, and 46% of the suicides had a medical illness.

Despite some important descriptive statistics Robins's research has some serious flaws as well. To begin with, the sample is relatively small and nonsystematic. There is no control group, so the reader often does not know how to evaluate the percentages cited for the cases. Robins limits the developmental perspective to the final months of the completed suicide—especially to the last year of life. The Robins research is not good at detecting interactions among suicide predictors and incorporates no analytical statistics. Finally, Robins's types of suicide are not all that general or imaginative. In fact they are extremely literal (e.g., depressives or alcoholics).

A second developmental study that improves upon Robins's methodology is that of British psychiatrist Barraclough, *Suicide: Clinical and Epidemiological Studies* (1987, with Jennifer Hughes). Barraclough investigated 100 suicides committed from 1966 to 1968 in West Sussex and Portsmouth, England. Unlike Robins, Barraclough also obtained a control group of 150 age-matched depressed patients. The research design was a retrospective case-control study involving interviews with relatives and friends of the suicides—what has come to be called a "psychological autopsy." As in the Robins's research, mental illness was of overwhelming importance as a precursor to suicide. Ninety-three of Barraclough's 100 suicides were mentally ill. A second comparison with Robins's data revealed that 70% of the suicides were depressed and 15% were alcoholic. A history of prior suicide attempts was about ten times more common among the suicides as among depressed controls (i.e., 41% vs. 4%).

We also know that seven times more suicides than controls lived alone (42% vs. 6%). Of the 15 suicides who were alcoholic, the mean duration of their alcoholism was 25 years. We know from a large series of studies by Roy (in Maris, 1986) that about 18% of all alcoholics eventually die by suicide. Thirty-four percent of the suicides (55%, if ambiguous statements are included) made unequivocal threats of suicide before the actual suicide. Fifty-nine percent of the suicides saw a family physician the month before they died. However, by itself the influence of physical disease on suicide was modest. Life events occurred five times more frequently among the suicide cases than among the nonsuicidal controls.

Despite improvements in Barraclough's research over that of Robins, problems still exist. For example, the analysis remains descriptive, not analytic. A multivariate analysis is clearly required to determine the joint effect of predictors on suicide. Barraclough, too, examines primarily the developmental period just before the suicide. There is no data on all stages of the suicides' life history. Finally, one could argue with the appropriateness of Barraclough's control group. Perhaps what we are most interested in is the contrast of suicides with living normals.

A final developmental study of suicide is *Pathways to Suicide: A Survey of Self-Destructive Behaviors* (Maris, 1981). This research investigated 266 cases of completed suicide in Cook County (i.e., mainly Chicago), Illinois and compared them with 64 nonfatal suicide attempter controls and 71 natural death controls (mainly cancer, heart disease, and respiratory deaths). The dependent variable was (in effect) low (i.e., natural deaths), moderate (i.e., nonfatal suicide attempters), and high (completed suicides) suicidality. Multiple Nominal Scale Analysis was made of 15 to 34 basic predictors of the suicidality outcome. Survivors (viz., coroner's informants) were interviewed and records were collected. The predictors were examined over the entire life span of both cases and controls. Usually predictors were broken up into background, early life, midlife, and late-life sets of independent variables. Major predictors included age, sex, race, early trauma, multiproblem family of origin, social isolation, negative interaction, socioeconomic status, occupational mobility, alcohol and drug use, physical illness, depression and hopelessness, religion, concepts of death, and prior suicide attempts. The fact that the mean age for completed suicides was 51 years old (it dropped to 40 years old in the United States in 1980) suggested that suicide was related to gradual developmental stagnation. It was hypothesized that the inability of suicides to react or adapt to life stresses was associated with the accumulated burden and magnitude of stress and the relative absence of the usual supports of meaningful work and loving people.

Among the major research results of the Maris study were the following. Early trauma (including the psychoanalyst's concept of "object loss") tended not to differentiate cases from controls, but suicide in one's family of origin did. Suicides were also more socially isolated than controls. For example, suicides were significantly more likely to score zero on the Chapin Social Participation scale than controls were. Fifty percent of the completed suicides had no close friends versus 20% of the attempted suicides. There was significant downward intragenerational work mobility just before death among the suicides. Additionally, there was more developmental stagnation in work for completed suicides. Rates of alcoholism among cases were about two times the alcoholism rate in the U.S. general population. Alcohol use often defended against suicide in the short run, but not in the long run. Seventy-five percent of the natural death controls had no major mental disorder but only 27% of the suicides did not. Forty percent of the completed suicides were hospitalized for mental disorder at least one time in their lives. The Beck Depression Inventory items that differentiated the completed and attempted suicides from the natural deaths were hopelessness, dissatisfaction, wanting to die, loss of interest in other people, sleep disturbance, and preoccupation with physical health. As in prior studies, suicide rates were highest for white, Protestant males. Suicide completers were more likely than controls to conceive of death as escape. Finally, among males aged 45 and older 88% of the first suicide attempts were fatal.

Of course, the Maris research could be improved too. A better case-control design could have been used. Such an improved design would involve consistent use of third-party informants, larger numbers of controls from more similar geographical regions, perhaps adding a control group of living normal subjects, use of power equations to assist in the calculation of sample size, and employing logistic regression techniques to estimate models. It would also help to have more explicit temporal models for all basic suicidal types, more data on mid-life suicides, and more interdisciplinary, biopsychosocial models.

NEEDS AND PROSPECTS

Ivan Ilyach locked the door and then began to examine himself in the glass, first full face, then in profile. He took up a portrait of himself taken with his wife, and compared it with what he saw in the glass. The change in him was

immense. Then he bared his arms to the elbow, looked at them, drew the sleeves down again, sat down on an ottoman and grew blacker than night.
Tolstoy

Typically we do the doable, rather than what needs to be done. The study of suicide is no exception. For the most part we have focused in our research on the moment of death, not on suicide across the life span. It is past time in suicidology to establish chronological patterns for various suicidal types. For example, what are the predictor variables of suicide and their relationships to different life stages—such as childhood, youth, adolescence, young adulthood, middle age, the young-old, the old-old, etc.? We especially need much more understanding of midlife suicide, its types and dynamics. What are the developmental aspects of escape, altruistic, male versus female, multiple versus single suicide attempters, organic versus nonorganic suicidal types, etc.? On the continuum of ideators, gesturers, nonfatal suicide attempters, and suicide completers, we need to know much more about suicide completers. There are both social and individual developmental types. For example, in the study of heart disease there are type A societies as well as type A individuals. Relatively little is understood about social development and suicide.

Of course, a major conclusion of this chapter is that we should have more prospective and cohort research designs in the study of suicide. Interaction effects of developmental variables need to be specified (e.g., more attention should be given to co-morbidity or multi-morbidity). For example, what are the combined effects of alcoholism and other variables on suicide under different circumstances or of depression and other predictors? The individual case history paradigm should be extended to include basic types of suicide—a kind of typological history. To be sure, adequate methods, sampling, research designs, control groups, and analysis all help guarantee good basic suicidological science. Finally, a greater melding of professional research perspectives is needed. The developmental study of suicide requires interdisciplinary teams of clinical psychiatrists, epidemiologists, biostatisticians, pharmacologists, sociologists, psychologists, and others. The suicidal act is a process, a convergence of many factors over time. It is a process that varies by suicidal type. Suicide is not one thing and is not the simple product of an acute crisis. Our research needs to reflect that.

REFERENCES

Aldrich, E. (1979). *Organization and environments*. Englewood Cliffs, NJ: Prentice-Hall.
Andreasen, N. C., Rice, J., Endicott, J., Reich, T., & Coryell, W. (1986). The family history approach to diagnosis. *Archives of General Psychiatry*, *43*, 421–429.

Andreasen, N. C., Rice, J., Endicott, J., Coryell, W., Grove, W. M., & Reich, T. (1987). Familial rates of affective disorder. *Archives of General Psychiatry, 44* (May), 461–469.

Baechler, J. (1979). *Suicides*. New York: Basic Books.

Baltes, P. B., & Brim, O. G., Jr. (Eds.). (1979–1987). *Life-span development and behavior* (Vols. 1–7). New York: Academic Press.

Baltes, P. B., Featherman, D. F., & Lerner, R. M. (1988). *Life-span development and behavior* (Vol. 8). Hillsdale, NJ: Lawrence Erlbaum.

Bandura, A., & Walters, R. H. (1963). *Social learning and personality development*. New York: Holt, Rinehart & Winston.

Barnes, R. (1986). The recurrent self-harm patient. *Suicide and Life-Threatening Behavior, 16-4*, 399–408.

Barraclough, B. (1987). *Suicide: Clinical and epidemiological studies* (with Jennifer Hughes). London: Croom Helm.

Battin, M. P., & Mayo, D. J. (1980). *Suicide: The philosophical issues*. New York: St. Martin's Press.

Birren, J. E. (1986). The process of aging: Growing up and growing old. In A. Pifer & L. Bronte (Eds.), *Our aging society* (pp. 263–282). New York: W.W. Norton.

Brenner, M. H. (1977). Health costs and benefits of economic policy. *International Journal of Health Services, 7*, 611.

Brent, D. A., Perper, J. A., Goldstein, C. E., Kolko, D. J., Allan, M. J., Allman, C. J., & Zalenak, J. P. (1988). Risk factors for adolescent suicide. *Archives of General Psychiatry, 45* (June), 581–588.

Coleman, J. C., & Butcher, J. N. (1984). *Abnormal psychology and modern life*. Chicago: Scott, Foresman.

Dannefer, D. (1984). Adult development and social theory. *American Sociological Review, 49*, 100–116.

DeCatanzaro, D. (1986). A mathematical model of evolutionary pressures regulating self-preservation and self-destruction. In R. W. Maris (Ed.), *Biology of suicide* (pp. 84–100). New York: Guilford Press.

Diekstra, R. F. W. (1989). *Suicide and its prevention: The role of attitude and imitation*. Leiden: E. J. Brill.

Easterlin, R. A. (1980). *Birth and fortune: The impact of numbers on personal welfare*. London: Grant McIntyre.

Eaton, W. W., & Kessler, L. G. (1985). *Epidemiologic field methods in Psychiatry: The NIMH epidemiologic catchment area program*. New York: Academic Press.

Erikson, E. H. (1950). *Children and society*. New York: W.W. Norton.

Farberow, N. L. (1980). *The many faces of suicide: Indirect self-destructive behavior*. New York: McGraw-Hill.

Favazza, A. R. (1989). Why patients mutilate themselves. *Hospital and Community Psychiatry, 40-2*, 137–145.

Freud, S. (1905). In J. Strachy (Ed.), *The standard edition of the complete psychological works of Sigmund Freud*. London: Hogarth Press.

Gouldney, R. D., & Katsikitis, M. (1983). Cohort analysis of suicide rates in Australia. *Archives of General Psychiatry, 40*, 71–74.

Jellinek, E. M. (1960). *The disease of alcoholism*. Highland Park, NJ: Hillhouse Press.

Jung, C. G. (1963). *Memories, dreams, and reflections*. New York: Pantheon Books.

Kalleberg, A., & Loscocco, K. A. (1983). Age, values, and rewards: Explaining age differences in job satisfaction. *American Sociological Review, 48*, 78–90.

Lenski, G. E., & Lenski, J. (1987). *Human societies: An introduction to macro-sociology*. New York: McGraw-Hill.

Lester, D. (1988). Birth cohort suicide rates in Canada. *Suicide and Life-Threatening Behavior, 18-4*, 372–378.

Levinson, D. J., Darrow, C. N., Klein, E. B., Levinson, M. H., & McKee, B. (1978). *The seasons of a man's life*. New York: Alfred A. Knopf.

Lyons, M. J. (1985). Observable and subjective factors associated with attempted suicide in later life. *Suicide and Life-Threatening Behavior, 15-3*, 168–183.

Mann, J. J., & Stanley, M. (Eds.). (1988). Suicide. In A. J. Frances, & R. E. Hales (Eds.), *Review of Psychiatry* (Vol. 7, pp. 278–430). Washington, DC: American Psychiatric Press.

Maris, R. W. (1981). *Pathways to suicide: A survey of self-destructive behaviors*. Baltimore: Johns Hopkins University Press.

Maris, R. W. (1986). *The biology of suicide*. New York: Guilford Press.

Menninger, K. (1938). *Man against himself*. New York: Harcourt, Brace & World.

Mussen, P. H., Conger, J. J., & Kagan, J. (1984). *Child development and personality*. New York: Harper & Row.

Neugarten, B. L., & Neugarten, D. A. (1986). Changing meanings of age in aging society. In A. Pifer & L. Bronte (Eds.), *Our aging society* (pp. 33–52). New York: W.W. Norton.

Pattison, E. M., & Kahan, J. (1983). The deliberate self-harm syndrome. *American Journal of Psychiatry, 140*, 867–872.

Phillips, D. P. (1974). The influence of suggestion on suicide. *American Sociological Review, 39*, 340–354.

Phillips, D. P., & Carstensen, L. L. (1986). Clustering of teenage suicides after television stories about suicide. *New England Journal of Medicine, 315-11*, 685–689.

Piaget, J. (1952). *The origins of intelligence in children*. New York: International Universities Press.

Robins, E. (1981). *The final months: A study of the lives of 134 persons who committed suicide*. New York: Oxford University Press.

Riley, M. W., & Riley, J. W. (1986). Longevity and social structure: The potential of added years. In A. Pifer & L. Bronte (Eds.), *Our aging society* (pp. 53–78). New York: W.W. Norton.

Schlein, S. P. (Ed.). (1987). *A way of looking at things: Selected papers of Erik H. Erikson from 1930-1980*. New York: W.W. Norton.

Shneidman, E. S. (1971). Pertubation and lethality as precursors of suicide in a gifted group. *Suicide and Life-Threatening Behavior, 1*, 23–45.

Skinner, B. F. (1953). *Science and human behavior*. New York: MacMillan.

Steer, R. A., Beck, A. T., Garrison, B., & Lester, D. (1988). Eventual suicide in interrupted and uninterrupted attemptors. *Suicide and Life-Threatening Behavior, 18*(2), 119–128.

Thomas, C. B. (1969). Suicide among us: Can we learn to prevent it? *Johns Hopkins Medical Journal, 125*, 276–285.

Vaillant, G. E. (1977). *Adaptation to life*. Boston: Little, Brown.

4

The Commonalities of Suicide across the Life Span

Edwin S. Shneidman

To be a pristine suicidologist, one may have to be a radical mentalist. In other words—given the obvious (and perhaps banal) fact that there are biological structures and physiological concomitants—suicide is an act of volition and frustrated psychological needs, and that the very core of suicide always relates to overwhelming psychological pain.

Of course, conation and affect are not all there is to suicide, but they are the most there is. Psychological pain and the urge (and will) to stop that pain are the core of suicide. I do not believe that I can be charged with disregarding the wide panoply of relevant etiology, having written explicitly about the various legitimate approaches to suicide. These approaches include literary, philosophical, theological, demographic, sociocultural, sociological, dyadic, familial, psychodynamic, psychological, psychiatric, constitutional, genetical, political, and supernational, as well as personal documents (Shneidman, 1984, 1985, 1986, 1987).

 Portions of this chapter have appeared previously in: *Definition of suicide* (New York: John Wiley, 1985); "Suicide," in R. Corsini (Ed.), *Encyclopaedia of psychology* (New York: John Wiley, 1984); "Some essentials of suicide and some implications for response," in A. Roy (Ed.), *Suicide* (Baltimore: Williams & Wilkins, 1986); and "A psychological approach to suicide," in G. R. VandenBos and B. K. Bryant (Eds.), *Cataclysms, crises, and catastrophes: Psychology in action* (Washington, DC: American Psychological Association, 1987).

EDWIN S. SHNEIDMAN • Professor of Thanatology Emeritus, University of California, Los Angeles, California 90024.

I am one of those who early and constantly have advocated the multidisciplinary nature of suicide. But I certainly do not believe that the mind's decision to stop its unbearable flow of painful consciousness is to be understood in terms of chemical formulae, and I believe that it borders on being quaint to assert so.

Another point: *Of course*, blacks, females, unemployed, AIDS patients—and, apropos, the human life course—children, youth, adults, and oldsters commit suicide, and it is often useful to group suicides under these rubrics. But it is meaningful only if one goes further and looks at underlying patterns. In my analyses of suicide, there are no separate youth suicides, adult suicides, gerontologic suicides; there is only human suicide and all of it is to be understood in terms of the same principles.

In this sense I may fail to qualify as a wholehearted participant in a volume largely dedicated to the proposition that each decade of life is created unequal. The psychological pains of being adolescent or adult, or middle aged or old—or being black, or female, or widowed—are, of course, phenotypically different, but, paradoxically (and this is the key), just as each suicidal event is exquisitely idiosyncratic, so also all suicidal events, by virtue of their human quality, have a number of important psychological characteristics in common.

With this view in mind, "suicidology" can be divided into the following subfields: (1) the mentalistic stuff of suicide—the heart of the matter; (2) the biological concomitants of suicide; (3) the sociological concomitants of suicide; (4) the nomothetical aspects (statistics and demography) of suicide; and (5) the issues—theoretical, philosophical, moral, ethical—surrounding suicide.

THE TEN COMMONALITIES OF SUICIDE

My purpose is to speak about the introspective act of suicide, i.e., of suicide considered on its own. I now turn to those psychological characteristics of suicide, 10 in number (Table 1).

I. The common *purpose* of suicide is to seek a *solution*.

First of all, suicide is not a random act. It is never done pointlessly or purposelessly. It is a way out of a problem, a dilemma, a bind, a challenge, difficulty, crisis, an unbearable situation. It has an inexorable logic and impetus of its own. It is the answer—the only available answer—to a real puzzler: How to get out of this? Its purpose is to solve a problem.

The English novelist and essayist, John Fowles, early in his career, wrote a brilliant set of aphorisms called *The Aristos* (1964/1975). The Greek word *aristos* means the best possible solution in a given situation. The half dozen individuals whom I have talked to, who, in one way or another, committed suicide and fortuitously survived—immolating, jumping, shooting—have all, to paraphrase them, said something like this: It was the only thing I could do. It was the best way

Table 1. The Ten Commonalities of Suicide[a]

I.	The common purpose of suicide is to seek a solution.
II.	The common goal of suicide is cessation of consciousness.
III.	The common stimulus in suicide is intolerable psychological pain.
IV.	The common stressor in suicide is frustrated psychological needs.
V.	The common emotion in suicide is hopelessness-helplessness.
VI.	The common cognitive state in suicide is ambivalence.
VII.	The common perceptual state in suicde is constriction.
VIII.	The common action in suicide is egression.
IX.	The common interpersonal act in suicide is communication of intention.
X.	The common consistency in suicide is lifelong coping patterns.

[a]From Shneidman, E. S. (1985). *Definition of Suicide*. New York: Wiley.

out of that terrible situation. It was the answer to the problem I had to solve. I couldn't see any other way.

In this sense every suicide is an *aristos*; every suicide has as its purpose the seeking of a solution to the perceived problem. To understand what a suicide was about, one has to know the problem it was intended to solve.

II. The common *goal* of suicide is *cessation* of consciousness.

In a curious and paradoxical way, suicide is both a moving toward and a moving away from something; the something that it is moving toward, the common practical goal of suicide is the stopping of the flow of consciousness. Suicide is best understood not so much in relation as a moving toward the idea of a reified Death, as it is in terms of the idea (in the mind of the chief protagonist) of "cessation," specifically when cessation—the complete stopping of one's consciousness of unendurable pain—is seen by the suffering individual as a solution, indeed the perfect solution, of life's painful and pressing problems. The moment that the idea of the possibility of stopping consciousness—death, in ordinary terms—occurs to the anguished mind as the answer or the way out in the presence of unusual constriction and elevated perturbation and high lethality—the three essential ingredients of suicide—then the igniting spark has been added and the active suicidal scenario has begun.

III. The common *stimulus* (or information input) in suicide is intolerable psychological *pain*.

If cessation is what the suicidal person is moving toward, pain is what that person is seeking to escape. In any close analysis, suicide is best understood as a combined movement toward cessation and as a movement away from intolerable emotion, unendurable pain, unacceptable anguish. No one commits suicide out of joy; no suicide is born out of exaltation. The enemy to life is pain and, when pain does not come from one's own soma, then the threateners of life are those who cause the pain. But here, it is psychological pain of which we are speaking; metapain; the pain of feeling pain. The clinical rule is: Reduce the level of suffering, often just a little bit, and the individual will choose to live. *Psychological pain is the key to suicide*. All suicide is reflected psychological pain.

IV. The common *stressor* in suicide is frustrated psychological *needs*.

Suicide is best understood not so much as an unreasonable act—every suicide seems logical to the person who commits it given that person's major premises, style of syllogizing, and constricted focus—as it is a reaction to frustrated psychological needs. A suicide is committed because of thwarted or unfulfilled *needs*. Psychological needs are the very color and texture of our inner life.

To understand suicide in this kind of context, we have to ask a much more broad question, which, I believe, is the key: What purposes do most human acts in general intend to accomplish? The best nondetailed answer to that question is that, in general, human acts are intended to satisfy a variety of human *needs*. There is no compelling a priori reason why a typology (or classification or taxonomy) of suicidal acts might not *parallel* a classification of *general* human needs. Indeed, such a classification of needs exist. It can be found in Murray's *Explorations in Personality* (1938). These needs—some 20 in number—include the need for abasement, achievement, affiliation, aggression, autonomy, counteraction, defendence, deference, dominance, exhibition, harmavoidance (including painavoidance), avoidance of shame, inviolacy, nurturance, order, play, rejection, sentience, succor, and understanding. There, in Murray's list of human needs, is a ready-made, viable, useful taxonomy of suicidal behaviors.

Each need can be related to a specific (psychological) kind of suicidal act. In Murray's discussion of needs, he further refines their place in human psychology by distinctions between covert and overt needs, between focal and diffuse needs, proactive and reactive needs, random and focused activities.

Most suicides represent combinations of various needs, so that a particular case of suicide might be subsumed under at least two or three different need categories. The point is: We shall understand suicide only when we have mastered an understanding of psychological needs. There are many pointless deaths, but there is never a needless suicide. Address the thwarted psychological needs, the pain will shrink, and the suicide will not occur.

V. The common *emotion* in suicide is *hopelessness–helplessness*.

At the beginning of life the common emotion is probably randomized general excitement. In the suicidal state it is a pervasive feeling of hopelessness-helplessness. The suicidal person says: There is nothing that I can do (except to commit suicide) and there is no one who can help (with the pain that I am suffering). I believe that this formulation permits us somewhat gracefully to withdraw from the (sibling) rivalry among the various emotions, each with the proponents to assert that *it* is the central of them all. Historically—in the 20th century, that is—hostility was the eldest brother. Stekel said so in the 1910 meeting of the Psychoanalytic

Society in Vienna; no one kills himself except as he has fantasized the death of another. And then, in a somewhat more ornate phrase: Suicide is essentially hostility directed toward the (ambivalently viewed) introjected love object (Friedman, 1967). One would plunge a knife into one's chest in order to expunge or kill the internalized homunculus of the loved-hated father within—what I once called murder in the 180th degree.

But today we suicidologists know that there are other deep basic emotions: shame, guilt, frustrated dependency. The early psychoanalytic formulations are seen as a brilliant hypothesis, more pyrotechnical than universal. But underlying all of these—and others that might be mentioned—is that emotion of active, impotent ennui, the feeling of hopelessness-helplessness.

VI. The common *cognitive state* in suicide is *ambivalence*.

One does not ordinarily think of Freud as a giant in the history of logic but, in a way, he made as enormous an impact in extending our understanding of our cognitive maneuvers as perhaps Bacon, Mill, and Russell. In a word, Western logic is Aristotelian. (The topic of Eastern logic—see Nakamura's [1960] *The Ways of Thinking of Eastern Peoples*—does not occupy us here; that is one reason why I have never said anything about Japanese and other Eastern suicides.) Aristotle's logic is dichotomous; more accurately, it is binary. A term is either A or non-A. An inference either true or false; a mood of the syllogism is either valid or invalid. Except when one is arguing with one's spouse, as Aristotle did with Xantippe, the life of the mind is supposed to be rather straightforward; black or white, you might say. And that is what most people believe.

Freud brought to our unforgettable attention a psychological truth that transcends the Aristotelian appearance of the neatness of logic. Something can be *both* A and non-A. We can both like and dislike the same person; we can both love and hate a parent, a spouse, a child. It is an Aristotelian question to say, "Make up your mind!" The answer is that we are of two minds, at least. We can now assert that the prototypical suicidal state is one in which an individual cuts his throat and cries for help at the same time, and is genuine in both of these acts. This non-Aristotelian accommodation to the psychological realities of mental life is called ambivalence. It is the common internal attitude toward suicide: To feel that one has to stop the pain (and die) and, simultaneously, to yearn (and even plan) for rescue and intervention.

VII. The common *perceptual state* in suicide is *constriction*.

I am not one who believes that suicide is best understood as a psychosis, a neurosis, or a character disorder—borderline or otherwise. I believe that a suicide is much more accurately seen as a more-or-less transient psychological constriction of affect and intellect. Synonyms for "constriction" are a tunnelling or narrowing or focusing of the range of options usually available to *that* individual's consciousness when the mind is not panicked into dichotomous thinking. In constriction, the range of choices has been narrowed to two—not very much of a range. The usual life-sustaining images of loved ones are not disregarded; worse, they are not even within the range of what is in the mind. One of the most dangerous aspects of a suicidal state (high lethality/high perturbation) is the active presence of crippling constriction. Any attempt at rescue or remediation has to deal almost from the first with the pathologic constriction.

People are often critical, prejudiced, and unforgiving about suicide; they forget that, for the victim it is (also) a narrow-minded decision. This fact, that suicide is committed by individuals who are in a special constricted condition, leads us to suggest that no one should ever commit suicide while disturbed. (The psychological oxygen of life is self-acceptance, as opposed to self-loathing or self-abnegation, and when there is a critical deprivation of this life-necessary psychological element then there is dizziness, shortness of breath, and tunnel vision—exactly as occurs with the deprivation of oxygen itself.) Suicide is not a thing to do while one is not in one's best mind. Never kill yourself when you are suicidal. It takes a mind capable of scanning a range of options greater than two to make a decision as important as taking one's life. Dichotomous slogans like "Death before dishonor" or "Give me liberty or give me death" all have some emotional appeal, but they are not sensible or wide-ranged enough to be prescriptions for making it through life.

It is vital to counter the suicidal person's constriction-of-thought by attempting to widen the mental blinders and to increase the number of options, certainly beyond the two options of either having some magical resolution or being dead.

VIII. The common *action* in suicide is *escape* (egression).

Egression is a person's intended departure from a region of distress. Suicide is the ultimate egression, besides which running away from home, quitting a job, deserting an army, or leaving a spouse are relatively pale actions. Then there are "unpluggings": having a good read, darting into a movie, or going for a weekend to Las Vegas or Atlantic City, which are benign egressions. It is important to distinguish between one's wish to get away and the need to end the distress forever. The point of suicide is a radical and permanent change of scene; the action to effect it is to leave.

In 1921, Violet Keppel Trefusis wrote to her lover Vita Sackville-West, who was then in the 8th year of her bisexual marriage to Harold Nicholson. "I am dead with grief. I am utterly alone. You cannot want me to suffer so. You had to choose between me and your family, and you have chosen them. I do not blame you. But you must not blame me if one day I seek for what escape I can find" (Nicholson, 1972, pp. 149–150).

That passage is an operational definition of what suicide is from the suicidal person's point of view: "what escape I can find." In that brief quotation from the letter, one can see intimations of several common characteristics of suicide: the wish for cessation, the need to stop pain, the sense of hopelessness, the presence of constriction, and the search for escape, as well as the communication of the intent.

IX. The common *interpersonal act* in suicide is *communication of intention*.

One of the most interesting findings from large numbers of "psychological autopsies" of unequivocal suicidal deaths was that there were clues to the impending lethal event in approximately 80% of the cases studied (Shneidman, Farberow, & Leonard, 1961). Individuals intent on committing suicide consciously or unconsciously emit signals of distress and pleas for response, in the usually dyadic interplay that is an integral part of the suicidal drama. It is sad and paradoxical to note that the common interpersonal act of suicide is not hostility, destruction, withdrawal, or depression, but communication of intention.

Suicidologists now know the usual verbal and behavioral clues of suicide. The verbal statements are tantamount to saying, "I am going away" (i.e., egression), "You won't be seeing me," "I cannot endure the pain any longer." The behavioral signs are such unusual acts as putting affairs in order, giving away prized possessions, and, more generally, behaving in ways that are different from one's usual patterns.

The communication of suicidal intention is not always a cry for help. First, it is not always a cry; it can be a shout, a murmur, or silence. Second, it not always for help; it can be for autonomy, inviolacy, or any of a number of needs. Nevertheless, in most cases of suicide, the common penultimate act is some interpersonal communicative exchange related to that intended final act.

X. The common *consistency* in suicide is with *lifelong patterns*.

People who are dying over weeks and months of a disease, i.e., cancer, are very much themselves, even exaggerations of themselves. Contrary to some currently popular notions, there do not appear to be any standard group or set stages of the dying process through which we are marched by Nature, lock-step, to our deaths. In terms of emotions displayed (rage, acceptance, etc.) or mechanisms of psychological defense manifested (projection, denial, etc.) one sees a full panoply of both of these arranged in almost every conceivable number and order. What one does sees in almost every case, I believe, are certain constellations of display of emotion and uses of defense that are consistent with *that* individual's microtemporal, mesotemporal, and macrotemporal reactions to pain, threat, failure, powerlessness, and duress in previous earlier episodes of that life. People dying are enormously consistent with themselves. So are suicidal people. So are people who are neither dying nor suicidal.

In suicide, we are initially thrown off the scent because suicide is an act, which by definition, that individual has never done before so there is no precedent. And yet there are some consistencies with lifelong coping patterns. We must look to previous episodes of disturbance, to capacity to endure psychological pain, to the penchant for constriction and dichotomous thinking, for earlier paradigms of egression.

I speak with a tiny bit of experimental authority on this issue, at least with a sense of conviction that flows from the data I examined. Very briefly, in a study of a group of men who were about 55 years old, each of whom had been studied rather intensively on a continual basis since he was about 6 years old—I am referring here to the well-known Terman longitudinal study of the gifted, begun in 1921 and continuing to this date at Stanford University. In my bite-sized study, other than the demonstration that it was possible (way beyond chance expectation) to select the five subjects who had committed suicide from a group of 30 cases, the main finding was that—working as I did, from a detailed life chart that I constructed for each individual—the determination that the person would (or would not) commit suicide at around age 55 often could be made before the 30th birthday in each man's life. There were already certain psychological consistencies within the life, certain characteristics or habitual patterns of reaction for that person to threat, pain, pressure, and failure that made dire predictions of a tragic suicidal outcome at age 55 an almost straightforward, logical (and perhaps psychological) extrapolation (Shneidman, 1971).

Who, reading the adolescent entries in the diary of the great 20th century Italian writer, Cesare Pavese, and his detailed notations in his 20s, is then truly surprised at his last entry—"Not words. An act. I'll write no more"—and his suicide at age 42? In the sight of the enormous unpredictability of life, what impresses and excites me as a psychologist is how much of a person's life, in some of its more important aspects, is reasonably predictable. In general, I feel this way about suicide. It is enormously complicated, but it is not totally random and it is amenable to some prediction. That is our main handle on individual prevention.

A CUBIC MODEL OF SUICIDE

What are some of the implications of this approach for a possible overarching theoretical model of suicide into which data on a large range of variables might be placed to build an empirical science of suicidology? Briefly, I shall attempt to outline a proposal.

Imagine a cube made up of 125 cubelets, with 25 cubelets on each plane, and 5 cubelets in each row and each column. As we look at the cube, we see three planes, each with 25 small squares. I call these three factors or components of this model (A) press, (B) pain, and (C) perturbation (Figure 1).

A. *Press*. Murray (1938) might have had the word pressure in mind when he decided to use the word press to represent those aspects of the inner and outer world, or environment, that move, touch, impinge on, or affect an individual and make a difference. Press refers to the events done to the individual to which he or she reacts. There is positive press (e.g., good genes and happy fortune) and negative press (e.g., conditions and events that perturb, stress, threaten, or harm the individual). It is the latter—even success is negative if it is threatening—that are relevant to suicide. Press includes both actual and imagined events. There are

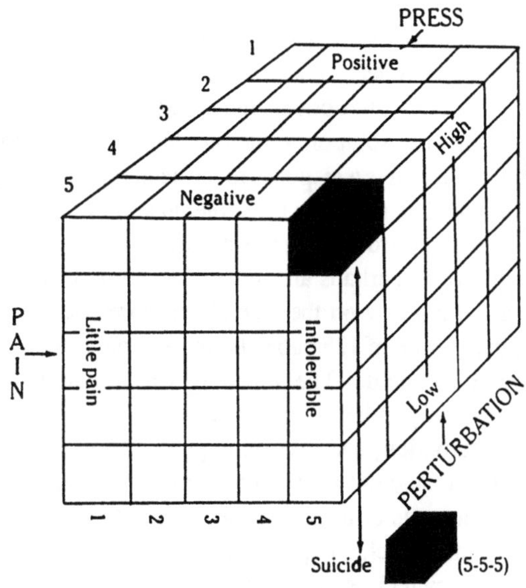

Figure 1. A theoretical cubic model of suicide.

all sorts of negative press: belittlement by an insult, being rejected or humiliated, a real or imagined slight, a loss of a loved one, real or magnified failure, a diagnosed cancer, powerlessness, humiliation, loss of control, poverty, bigotry, oppression, or persecution. But I am referring to the press—the self-abnegation—that comes as the mind mediates, exaggerates, or even imagines the negative press that it perceives or misperceives. In this cubic model, press ranges from positive (in the back row at the top plane) to negative, in the front row of the top plane.

B. *Pain* refers to psychological pain resulting from thwarted psychological needs. Pain is the front plane of the cube. The left column of cubelets represents little or no pain; the next column over, some bearable pain, and so on up, until the right column represents intolerable psychological pain. Pain comes from thwarted or frustrated needs.

Murray's (1938) list of psychological needs (given above) are especially relevant in suicide. The rule is: Redress the thwarted needs of a suicidal person and the willingness to live resurges.

C. *Perturbation* (arbitrarily assigned to the side plane of the large cube) is a general term meaning the state of being perturbed or upset. Perturbation, ranked on a 9-point scale, includes everything that is in *DSM-III*. In relation to suicide, perturbation includes, especially, (a) constriction and (b) the self-harming *penchant for precipitous* or ill-advised *action*. Constriction is the reduction of the individual's perceptual and cognitive range. At its worst, the individual cuts the viable options down to two, then to one. On this plane the bottom row reflects open-mindedness, wide mentational scope, and clear syllogistic (and nonsyllogistic) reasoning. The top row reflects constriction of thought, tunnel vision, and a narrowing of focus to one or two options, including cessation, death, and egression and, ultimately, as the only solution to the problem of pain and frustrated needs.

The penchant for action is a response to the needs for inviolacy and autonomy. The bottom row of cubelets reflects a high tolerance for ambiguity, a capacity for patience. As we move forward (up) on this plane, we come closer to this penchant for consummatory action, perhaps an irreversible action that is inimical to one's self. That is what the top row on the side plane represents.

In this imaginary cube of 125 cubelets, there is only *one* shaded cubelet that represents a committed suicide. The upper right-hand corner—cubelet 5-5-5 in this example—is the only cubelet that contains the concatenation of maximum pain, maximum perturbation, and maximum press. When egression is added as a lethal complement, the suicidal setting has come into being.

Although most aspects of press represent the outer world, the 5-5-5 cubelet represents a totally intrapsychic experience. Suicidal individuals are in special, almost autistic state; they feel totally alone. They may know or vaguely remember that there are others somewhere in their lives, but they are, at that moment, simply not connected with them. For the connections to be re-established, there must first be some diminution of the crippling pain, or press, or perturbation, or push for action.

As for possible research: Studies related to pain might include studies of pain thresholds or studies of levels of psychological disturbance, including anxiety. Research related to perturbation might include studies of perceptual sharpeners and levelers, intense concentration, tunnel vision, styles of scanning, dichotomous thinking, impulsiveness, and acting out. Studies related to press might include studies of traumatic life events, studies of disaster, defeat, and death. It would be useful to examine the literature of psychiatry and psychology (e.g., sensation, perception, emotion, learning, and personality) to find nonsuicide studies that have related one of these aspects with another and then ponder the possible implications of those *general* psychological findings for this suicide model.

These three aspects of suicide—press, pain, and perturbation—are closely interconnected. One can address either the topic of suicide or an individual case of suicide by beginning with any of the three planes of cubic model. Conceptually, the three separate aspects are, in some ways, synonymous with each other. For instance, pain grows out of perturbation, perturbation makes the pain, there is neither pain nor perturbation without negative press, and some negative press grows out of perturbation. One can come in on the concatenating suicidal drama during any one of its three linked acts. Even so, I believe the central feature of suicide is pain, and the key to suicide prevention lies in the reduction of that individual's psychological pain. All else—age, demographic variables, family history, previous suicidal history—is peripheral except as those factors bear on the commonly felt pain. Ultimately, suicide occurs when there is the coexistence of intolerable pain, intense negative press, and extreme perturbation with perceptual constriction and an irresistible penchant for life-ending action. It is the future task of a scientific suicidology to explicate—with empirical studies on intrapsychic variables (thoughts, feelings, bodily sensations), on interpersonal aspects, and on situational stressors—the several cubelets of this larger model. The goal is to stitch suicide into the body of academic psychology—perception, memory, cognition, conation, emotion, motivation, and consciousness.

IMPLICATIONS FOR PREVENTION AND RESPONSE

One can hardly fail to infer the implications for treatment in the real life-and-death situation of a suicidal crisis. They follow logically from the explication of the suicidal state of mind. Thus, psychologically speaking, the simply stated prescriptions are (a) reduce the hurt, (b) widen the blinders, (c) pull back from action, and (d) lighten the pressure, even just a little bit. (Get the person out of the 5-5-5 cubelet.) Any of these actions can save a life. In terms of this model, this is how suicide is prevented. The underlying rule is: Lower the pain, perturbation, and press, and the lethality will decrease with it.

Following this model, some key questions for a potentially suicidal person would include: Where do you hurt? What is going on? What do you feel that you have to solve or get out of? Do you have any plans to do anything harmful to yourself and what might you do? What would it take (to keep you alive)? Have you ever been in a similar situation before, what did you do, what happened, and how was it resolved? The next step is to state (not in a question, because the suicidally constricted mind usually cannot formulate an answer): Let me help you generate more possibilities, to rethink and restate the problem and then look at possible courses of action other than the only one that you have in mind; although these new ideas might not totally solve the problem the way you had thought of it, they can provide some solution that you can live with.

An example will be useful: A university senior who made straight A's for 3½ years received a B and was determined to kill himself. Friends around him pointed out to him that he still had a 3.98 grade point average. That had no effect. They were attempting to dissuade him by talking about grades. That was on the phenotypic level and missed the genotypic point. He could have been better addressed by saying, "I understand your anguish, your need for a perfect performance, this blemish on your academic record, and your problem." His problem, like a man who committed suicide after having lost the tip of a finger in an industrial accident, was how to live with an imperfection. His pain, perturbation, and negative press were, as he perceived and conceptualized them, more than he could live with. His problems did not relate to age; they related to psychological hurt, and his distortion of how he would then be viewed and what he would see in the eyes of others looking at him. What he thought—about himself, about his options, about others' reactions—was unsafe to believe at any age.

The mental pain of the suicidal person relates to the frustration or blocking of important psychological needs, that is, needs deemed to be important by that person. It should be the therapist's function to help the patient in relation to those thwarted needs. Even a little bit of improvement can save a life. Oftentimes just the possibility of a small amount of reduction of pain gives the perturbed individual enough hope and comfort to divert the suicidal course. In general, the goal of psychotherapy is to increase the patient's psychological *comfort*. One way to operationalize this task is to focus on the thwarted needs. To repeat: Questions such as "What is going on?" "Where do you hurt?" and "What would you like to have happen?" can usefully be asked by a therapist helping a suicidal person.

The psychotherapist can focus on feelings, especially such distressing feelings as guilt, shame, fear, anger, thwarted ambition, unrequited love, hopelessness, helplessness, loneliness. The key is to improve the external and internal situations a J.N.D. (Just Noticeable Difference). This can be accomplished through a variety of methods: ventilation, interpretation, instruction, behavior modification, and realistic manipulation in the world outside the consultation room. That last means to do things, involve significant others and agencies. All this implies—when working with a highly lethal person—a heightened level of interaction and intervention during the period of elevated lethality. The therapist needs to work diligently, always giving the suicidal person realistic transfusions of hope until the perturbation intensity subsides enough to reduce the lethality to a tolerable, life-permitting level.

Another example may be useful. A teenage college student, demure, rather elegant (and somewhat wealthy), was encouraged to come to see me. She was single, pregnant, and suicidal, with a formed suicidal plan. Her challenge to me was that I somehow, magically, had to arrange for her to be the way she was before she was pregnant (virginal in fact), or she would have to commit suicide. Her being pregnant was such a mortal shame to her that she simply could not "bear to live." At that moment suicide seemed the *only* possibility to her.

I did several things. For one, I took out a sheet and—to begin to "widen her blinders"— said something like, "Now, let's see: You could have an abortion here locally." ("I couldn't do that.") (It is precisely the "can'ts" and the "won'ts" and "have to's" and "nevers" and "always" and "onlys" that are negotiated in psychotherapy.) "You could go away and have an abortion." ("I couldn't do that.") "You could bring the baby to term and keep the baby." ("I couldn't do that.") "You could have the baby and adopt it out." ("I couldn't do that.") "We could get in touch with the young man involved." ("I couldn't do that.") "We could involve the help of your parents." ("I couldn't do that.") "You can always commit suicide, but there is obviously no need to do that today." (No response.) "Now, let's look at this list and rank them in order of your preference, keeping in mind that none of them is perfect."

The very making of this list, my nonhortatory and nonjudgmental approach, already had a calming influence on her. Within a few minutes her lethality had begun to de-escalate. She actually rank-ordered the list, commenting negatively on each item. What was of critical importance was that suicide was no longer ranked first or second. We were then simply "haggling" about life—a perfectly viable solution.

The point is not how the issue was eventually resolved or what interpretations were made as to why she permitted herself to become pregnant, other aspects of her relationships with men, etc. What is important is that it was possible to achieve the assignment of that day: To lower her lethality by reducing her perturbation by widening her range of visible and realistic options from the choice between suicide and only one other choice.

I am suggesting no less than the idea that there is *a* way to prevent suicide. That way is to understand the model of suicide that is being proposed in this chapter and then to work with individual suicidal patients to seek to mollify—to reduce a little bit—the psychological pain as that person perceives it; to widen the person's perceptual blunders and remove the method of death as decided upon by that person; to reduce the risk of impulsiveness by doing the opposite of isolating that person; by reducing the negative push within the mind; by removing "death" as the philosophic solution and postponing thoughts of reunion with dead loved ones; and by realistically and effectively changing the negative press of unemployment, poverty, homelessness—and the frustrated needs of selfness, pride-in-self, achievement, autonomy, self-reliance, self-worth that make livable for most of us.

That is the formula for prevention of suicide. It will work because it is tailor-made—without regard to race, sex, or age—to the contours of a viable suicide model.

REFERENCES

Fowles, J. (1975). *The Aristos*. New York: New American Library. (Original work published 1964)

Friedman, P. (Ed.) (1967). *On suicide*. (Discussion of the Vienna Psychoanalytic Society, 1910). New York: International Universities Press.

Murray, H. A. (1938). *Explorations in personality*. New York: Oxford University Press.

Nakamura, H. (1960). *The ways of thinking of Eastern peoples*. New York: UNESCO.

Nicholson, A. (1972). *Portrait of a marriage*. New York: Atheneum.

Shneidman, E. S. (1971). Perturbation and lethality as precursors of suicide in a gifted group. *Life-Threatening Behavior, 1*, 23–45.

Shneidman, E. S. (1973). Suicide. In *Encyclopaedia Britannica*. Chicago: William Benton.

Shneidman, E. S. (1984). Suicide. In R. Corsini (Ed.), *Encyclopaedia of psychology*. New York: Wiley.

Shneidman, E. S. (1985). *Definition of suicide*. New York: Wiley.
Shneidman, E. S. (1986). Some essentials of suicide and some implications for response. In A. Roy (Ed.), *Suicide*. Baltimore: Williams & Wilkins.
Shneidman, E. S. (1987). A psychological approach to suicide. In G.R. VandenBos & B.K. Bryant (Eds.), *Cataclysms, crises and catastrophes: Psychology in action*. Washington, DC: American Psychological Association.
Shneidman, E. S., Farberow, N. L., & Leonard C. V. (1961). Some facts about suicide: Cause and prevention (PHS Publication #852). Washington, DC: U.S. Government Printing Office.

II
Epidemiology

An American dies by his or her own hand on the average of every 17 minutes. However, this differs depending on the time-line/age (as well as major demographic factors, sex, gender, race/ethnicity, and so on). Age, in line with this volume, is a noteworthy factor: Why should the rate of suicide be higher at one developmental age than that at other ages? Part II presents three chapters: the epidemiology of suicide in the United States; a look at international trends; and suicide at symbolic ages (subtitled "Death on Stocktaking Occasions").

5

Epidemiology of Suicide in the United States

John L. McIntosh

An American dies by his or her own hand on the average of every 17 minutes (1986, data calculated from figures in National Center for Health Statistics [NCHS]; 1988a) or approximately 85 self-inflicted deaths per day. The more than 30,000 suicides in 1986 (30,904) represent a rate of 12.8 per 100,000 population. In other words, if a representative sample of 100,000 Americans had been chosen on January 1 of 1986 and followed through the year, by the end of the day on December 31 about 12 or 13 would have died by suicide. This number of deaths places suicide currently as the eighth leading cause of death in the United States. The present chapter will focus on the epidemiological factors associated with these 30,000 annual suicide deaths.

Trends in suicide rates for the United States indicate increases over the last several decades (see Figure 1). These increases have been slight, however. As observed for most cultures, suicide rates tend to remain somewhat stable over time. As Lester shows elsewhere in this book, the United States ranks among those cultures with moderate levels of suicide, and this has not changed over time. Although the number of suicides has steadily increased (see bottom of Figure 1), the change in number has only slightly outpaced increases in the number of individuals in the country.

JOHN L. McINTOSH • **Department of Psychology, Indiana University at South Bend, South Bend, Indiana 46634.**

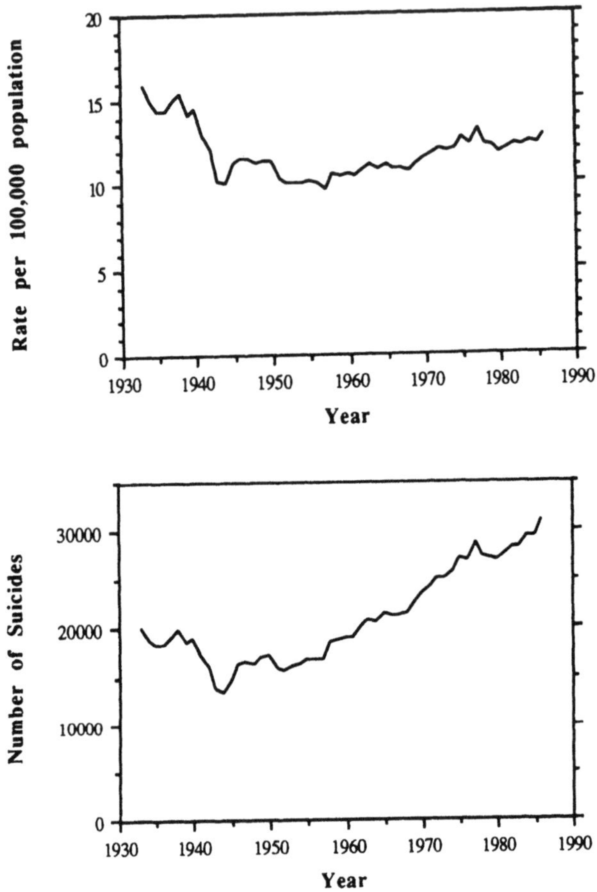

Figure 1. U.S. suicide rates and number of suicides, 1933 to 1986.

Suicide, the fatal self-inflicted act, is only one dimension of the entire spectrum of self-destructive behaviors. It is conservatively estimated that in addition to the deaths occurring each year there are at least 600,000 nonfatal suicide attempts or "parasuicides" ("suicide-like") in the United States. Furthermore, the loved ones of those who die by their own hand, individuals called "suicide survivors," also pay a heavy emotional toll in altered grief and bereavement processes. Although these two groups (attempters and survivors) are also immensely important in the total picture of suicidal behavior and in their own right (e.g., Dunne, McIntosh & Dunne-Maxim, 1987; Kreitman, 1977), this chapter will focus on the epidemiology (i.e., characteristics, levels, and trends) of those whose deaths are by suicide.

Before proceeding to the major demographic factors associated with elevated suicide risk, it is important to realize that the figures discussed thus far and in the information to follow are derived from official statistics for suicide mortality. This means that the numbers and rates presented result from the compilation (by the NCHS) of individual deaths for which the official cause of death was designated as suicide. Only in the case of this definitive classification would the death be included in the official statistics reported by NCHS in its many reports and annual volumes of *Vital Statistics of the United States*.

Official statistics have a longstanding history in the study of suicide, including most famously the classic work of sociologist Émile Durkheim (1897/1951). This long history notwithstanding, these official data have frequently been criticized and questioned as indices of the actual levels and number of suicides that occur (Atkinson, 1978, Chapter 3; Douglas, 1967, Chapter 12; Lester, 1972). Among the criticisms that have been leveled against the accuracy of official suicide data are bias and stigma resulting in underreporting and even blatant and intentional misclassification; variability in classification depending on several factors such as the training of the medical examiner or coroner, the use of different definitions, or the lack of a clear, generally accepted definition of suicide.

These and other criticisms and shortcomings of official figures should be taken seriously such that the consumer of suicide data realizes that numbers and rates are imperfect. At the same time, although the imperfect nature of suicide data has been generally accepted, others (e.g., Sainsbury & Barraclough, 1968; Sainsbury & Jenkins, 1982) have argued that the bias so often attributed to suicide classifications may not be as great as claimed. In any event, official suicide statistics are the most reliably and consistently maintained indices of suicide levels, trends, and high-risk factors that exist. If properly recognized as an indication of the most conservative estimates of actual suicide occurrence (Allen, 1984), they provide a useful index of the extent to which suicide is a mental health problem within a particular culture and its subgroups.

MAJOR DEMOGRAPHIC FACTORS IN SUICIDE

Within its large literature (e.g., Farberow, 1972; McIntosh, 1985a), suicide has been studied in association with a large number of factors. Many of these factors have proven unreliable or the data or methodologies associated with them have been poor (e.g., weather conditions, time of day, occupations, socioeconomic levels, etc.). This chapter will focus on the major factors for which U.S. data are both consistent and more reliable. Such factors are most often derived from the official mortality data (and the death certificates from which they are taken) mentioned above and include: sex/gender, race/ethnicity, age, marital status, temporal factors (day of week, monthly variations), geographic differences (states, regions), and the method employed in the suicide. Official statistics, on which this presentation will rely, are published after data collection and reliability checks have been made that necessitate a time-lag. Generally, official suicide figures are available for the United States from NCHS that are approximately 2 to 3 years old. Thus, until approximately September of 1989, the most current suicide data available are for the year 1986 (NCHS, 1988a,b).

Sex/Gender

One of the single most important factors with respect to suicide is the sex or gender of the individual. Males as a group kill themselves more than three times more often than do females both in numbers as well as for rates. For example, in 1986 there were on the average 66 male and 18 female suicides each day. In that same year the male rate of suicide was 20.6 per 100,000 population compared to 5.4 for females (a ratio of 3.8). The number of male suicides was 24,226 whereas for females the figure was 6,678 (a ratio of 3.6). Predictions in recent years (e.g., Neuringer, 1982) have suggested that because of the women's movement, increased numbers of women in the work force, and increased stress for women, female suicide rates would increase and become closer to those for males. In reality, however, differences between the sexes have actually *increased* rather than decreased since the early 1970s (e.g., McIntosh & Jewell, 1986; Steffensmeier, 1984). There was a slight tendency toward decreased differences during the 1960s, but the rates were at their closest ratio in 1971 at 2.46. Since that time female rates have been either stable or displayed a slight tendency toward decline whereas male rates have increased (see Figure 2).

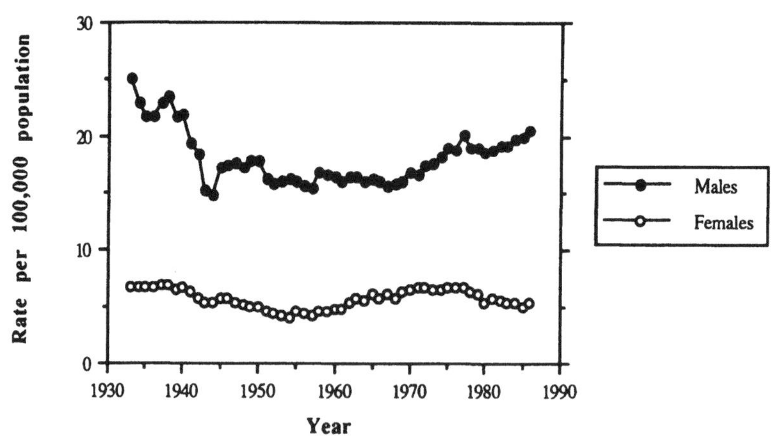

Figure 2. U.S. male and female suicide rates, 1933 to 1986.

Race/Ethnicity

Race Suicide, as measured by either rates or numbers, is a white phenomenon when compared to nonwhites as a whole. For example, whites committed 28,347 of the 1986 suicides for a rate of 13.9 per 100,000 population. By contrast, nonwhites accounted for 2,467 suicides for a rate of 6.7 (a ratio of 2.1 for rates). On an average day in 1986, 78 whites and 7 nonwhites died by their own hand. Although some suggestions of increases in nonwhite rates of suicide and a lessening of racial differences in suicide have been made, the data show no real change in this white predominance (e.g., McIntosh, 1989) (see Figure 3).

When considering race and sex, males are at highest risk within each racial grouping. In 1986 white males had a suicide rate of 22.3 while white females' rate was 5.9. Among nonwhites the rates were 11.1 and 2.7 for males and females, respectively. As can be seen, overall racial differences of 2:1 (white:nonwhite) are consistent for both males and females. Clearly the group at highest risk therefore is white males and the lowest risk is among nonwhite females.

Ethnicity Little attention has been given to ethnic differences in suicide other than among blacks and Native Americans (American Indians). There is evidence, however, that there is tremendous diversity among the various ethnic groups that comprise the nonwhite as a whole population. It is likely that some differences would also exist among white ethnic groups if data were available, but presently only partial data (only 18 states report such data) for Hispanics (who may be of any race but are most often white) are available. Rates of suicide are not available annually for the specific ethnic groups in the United States, but in 1986 blacks

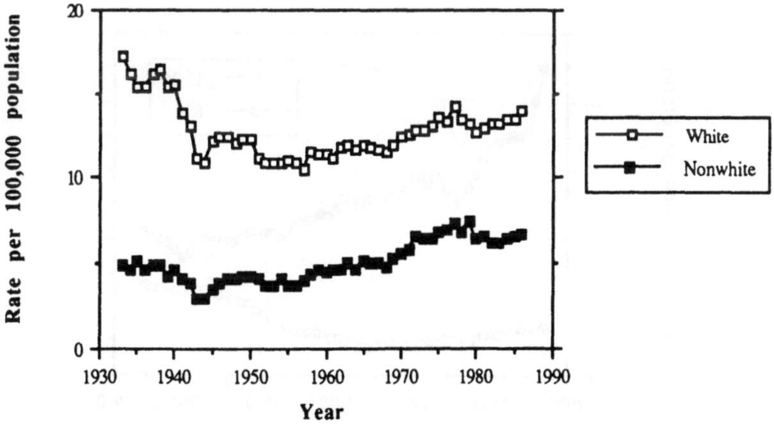

Figure 3. U.S. white versus nonwhite suicide rates, 1933 to 1986.

accounted for 1,892 of the 2,467 nonwhite suicides while Native Americans, Chinese-Americans, Japanese-Americans, Filipino-Americans, and other Asian or Pacific Islanders committed 218, 65, 81, 36, and 173 suicides, respectively. McIntosh (1985b, 1986, 1987a) reported age-adjusted suicide rates for these groups for the years 1979 to 1981. Age-adjusted suicide rates control for the differences in the distributions of the populations of the groups by age. McIntosh found that the highest rates were among Native Americans (18.1), followed by whites (16.7), Hispanics from 10 southwestern, midwestern, and eastern states (10.8), Japanese-Americans (10.7), Chinese-Americans (10.6), blacks (9.0), and Filipino-Americans (4.9).

Age

Suicide rates have shown increases with increasing age for as long as U.S. figures have been kept (and indeed in many other cultures as well). There have been two major trends in suicide rates by age that have slightly altered that characterization, however (see Figure 4). First, as highly publicized, there has been an increase in suicide rates among the young. Although the media and research literature have focused on the 15 to 24 age group, these increases have been seen for all age groups younger than 45 years of age. Among 15- to 24-year-olds there has been an increase of approximately 200% from the mid-1950s to the early 1980s. For example, in 1953 the suicide rate for those 15 to 24 was 4.4 compared to 13.1 in 1986 (an increase of 198%).

The second major trend with respect to age and suicide has been the decline in suicide among all age groups older than 45 and especially those older than age 65. This trend has received far less attention but for the elderly has occurred over a

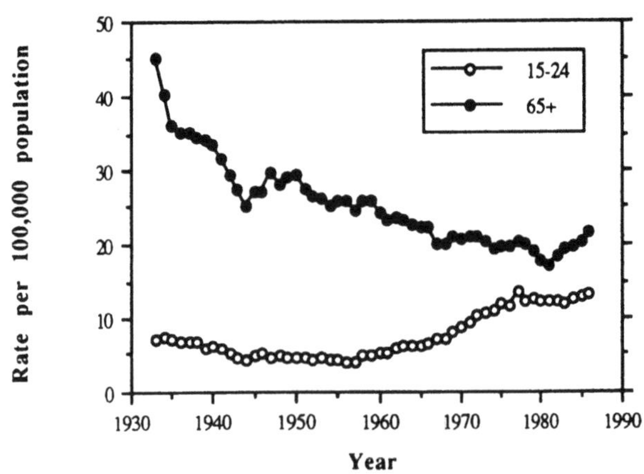

Figure 4. Suicide among U.S. young (15–24) and old (65+), 1933 to 1986.

longer time period and has been as dramatic as the youth increases, simply in the opposite direction. For instance, suicide rates for those 65 and older were 45.3 per 100,000 population in 1933, declined to 26.2 for 1953, and to 21.5 in 1986. The decline from 1933 to 1986 has therefore been 52%. Despite these large declines, however, the suicide rate for older adults remains at a level more than 50% above those for the 15 to 24 age group (21.5 vs. 13.1 in 1986).

There are reasons then to target both the young and old as high risks for suicide. Among the young we see (1) a pattern of increased suicide risk over the last several decades (even though a slowing in this trend may have already occurred and declines are predicted to continue until the mid-1990s, e.g., [Holinger, Offer, & Zola, 1988]) to levels greatly elevated over earlier times and currently at levels similar to those for the nation as a whole, (2) suicide is a higher ranking cause of death than for any other age group or the nation as a whole (3rd in 1986 behind accidents and homicide compared to 13th for those 65 and older), (3) suicide accounts for a much higher proportion of deaths than in the nation as a whole and other age groups (suicides were 12.8% of deaths for those 15-24 in 1986 compared to 1.5% in the nation as a whole and 0.4% for those 65 years of age and older), and (4) there annually have been more than 5,000 young people 15 to 24 years of age who officially committed suicide (5,120 in 1986 and an additional 255 younger than the age of 15).

Among the elderly, on the other hand, although suicide ranks relatively low among the many causes from which older adults die and represents a much smaller proportion of deaths compared to young people, there are several reasons that demand attention to the phenomenon of elderly suicide. Despite long-term declines in elderly suicide (1) suicide rates for older adults have increased each year through 1986 from their lowest point ever recorded in 1981 (from 17.1 to 21.5, respectively; an increase of 25.7%), (2) several writers have predicted long-term increases in elderly suicide (e.g., Manton, Blazer, & Woodbury, 1987; Pollinger-Haas & Hendin, 1983), (3) the elderly remain the highest risk group for suicide by age, and (4) the elderly commit greater proportions of the suicides than their proportion in the population (20.3% of suicides and 12.1% of the U.S. population, U.S. Bureau of the Census, 1988, compared to 16.2% and 16.6%, respectively, for those 15–24 years of age).

The net result of these two trends in suicide rates is a slight tendency toward characterizing the U.S. rates by age as bimodal. That is, suicide rates increase with age reaching an early life peak followed by slight decreases in successive age groups and an increase again to a second, highest peak after age 65 (see Figure 5). Although still not pronounced, this bimodal pattern in U.S. suicide is perhaps closer to characterizing current U.S. rates by age than is the earlier unimodal pattern with rates strictly increasing with age to a peak in older adulthood.

The factor of sex is also important when looking at suicide risk and age. Male suicide rates follow the increases with age (or more recent bimodal pattern) described above at even higher rates than for the nation as a whole (see Figure 6).

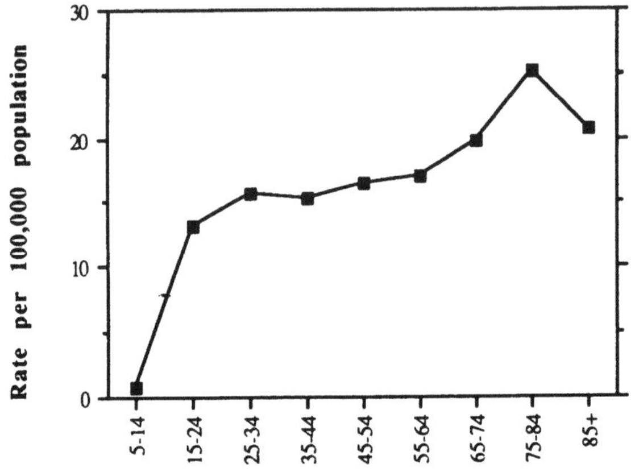

Figure 5. U.S. suicide rates by age groups, 1986.

Female rates, on the other hand, increase with advancing age until "middle age" (the mid-40s to mid-50s) and then decline thereafter in older age groups. Therefore, after age 65 male and female suicide rates are most divergent because male rates continue to increase in old age whereas female rates decline throughout older adulthood. The smallest differences between the sexes across the life span are in middle age when female rates reach their peak.

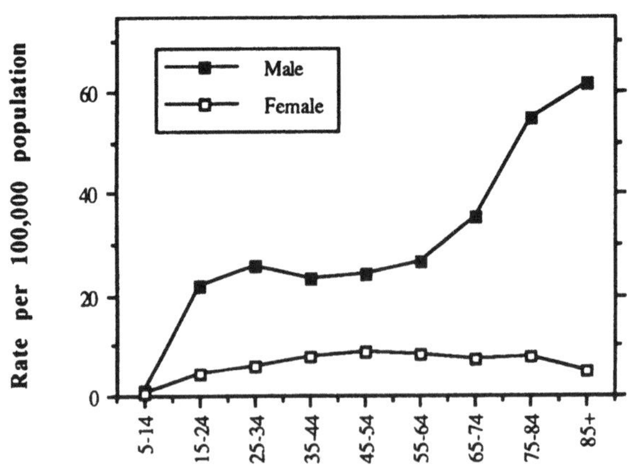

Figure 6. U.S. suicide rates by age and gender, 1986.

The age characterization of suicide as increasing with age and peaking in old age is particularly true when white suicide is studied (as well as among Chinese-, Japanese-, and Filipino-Americans) (see Figure 7). Among nonwhites as a whole, however, and particularly blacks, Native Americans, and Hispanics, suicide rates are highest in young adulthood and decline to low levels in old age (e.g., McIntosh, 1985b, 1986, 1987a; McIntosh & Santos, 1981).

Marital Status

The majority of suicides occur among the married population. However, when taking into account the number of individuals in this group within the total

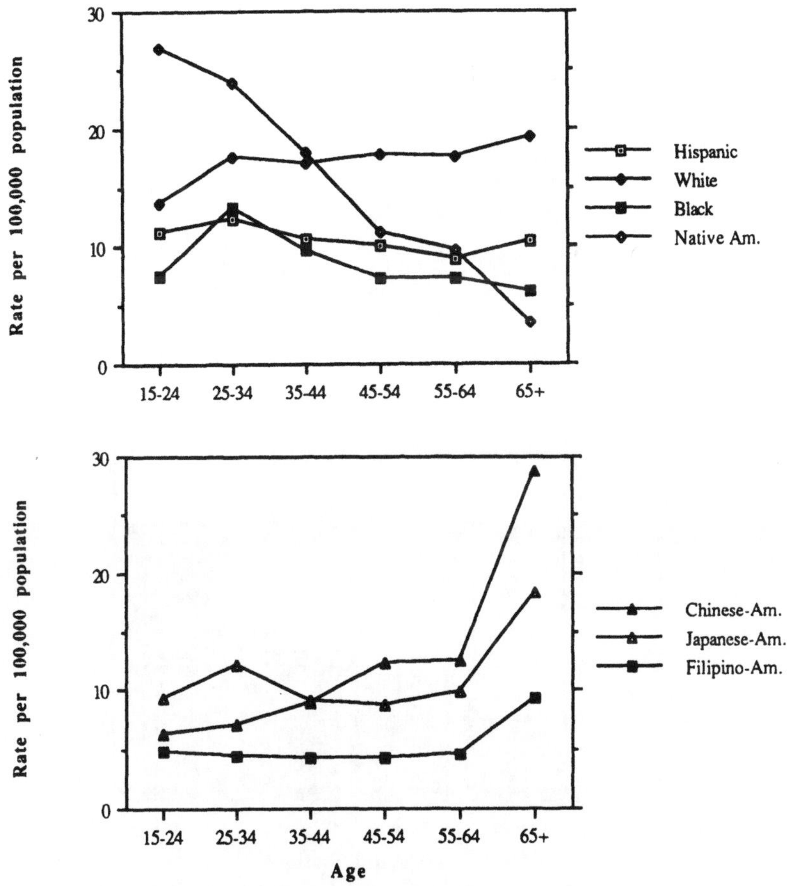

Figure 7. U.S. suicide rates by ethnic groups and age, 1979 to 1981 average.

population (i.e., by calculating suicide rates), the married are actually the lowest risk group for suicide. For example, in 1986 the married committed 13,526 of the 30,637 suicides above the age of 15. Those who were single and never married represented 8,921 suicides followed by 5,049 for the divorced, and 2,925 among the widowed. When rates are calculated, highest risk is among the divorced with lower rates among the widowed and single and lowest rates for the married (see Figure 8). With few exceptions these levels of risk are seen among those of both sexes (e.g., McIntosh, 1987b). It might also be kept in mind that the married category includes those who are married but separated. It is likely that this

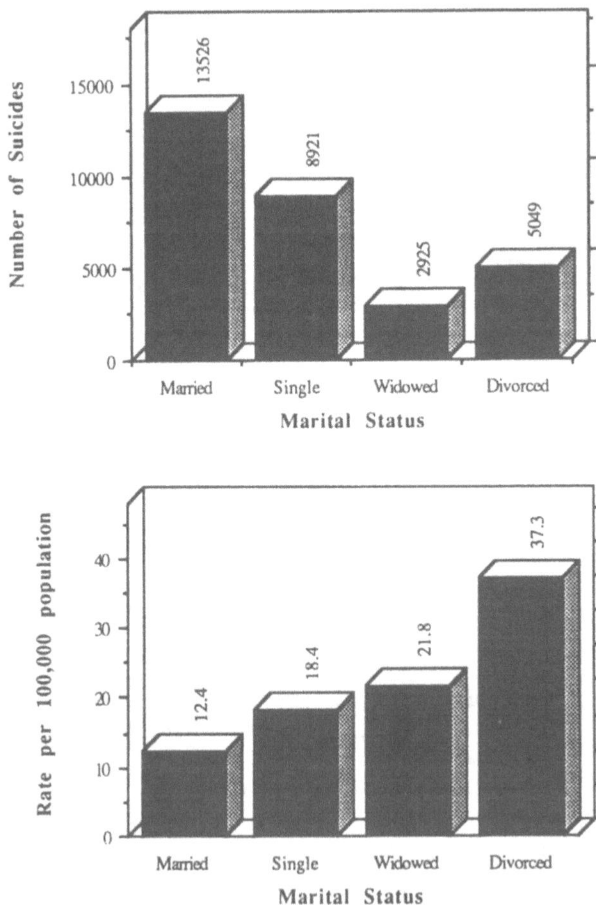

Figure 8. U.S. suicide rates and number of suicides by marital status (15+ years of age), 1986.

subgroup has higher risk than the married, spouse-present category, and inclusion of the separated in the calculation of rates probably increases the overall rate of the married population.

Methods

Suicide in the United States is most often committed with firearms. In 1986 firearms were utilized in 18,153 of the 30,904 suicides (58.7%) compared with 4,606 by hanging (14.9%), 3,070 by solid and liquid poisons (9.9%), and 2,966 by gas poisoning (9.6%). Indeed, the use of firearms is now ranked first among both males (64.1%) and females (39.5% vs. 25.3% by solid and liquid poisons) and have increased among all age, sex, and race groups over time (e.g., McIntosh & Santos, 1982, 1985–1986).

Temporal Factors

Although winter is often thought to be associated with high suicide risk (e.g., McIntosh, Hubbard, & Santos, 1985), the highest time of year for suicide is consistently observed in spring (see Figure 9). In general, fall has most often been second in suicide risk followed by summer and winter. Although these differences are relatively consistent they are usually small from one season or month to another. The same could be said for the small but consistent differences by day of the week. Monday and Tuesday are nearly always the highest days for suicides, with Wednesday, Thursday, Friday, and Sunday lower (but similar) and lowest risk of all for Saturdays (see Figure 10).

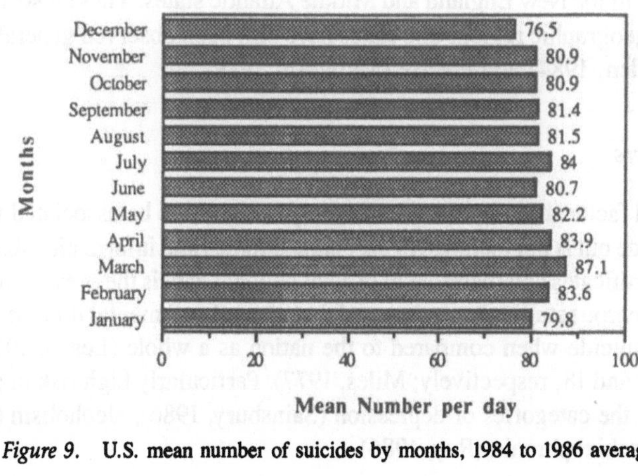

Figure 9. U.S. mean number of suicides by months, 1984 to 1986 average.

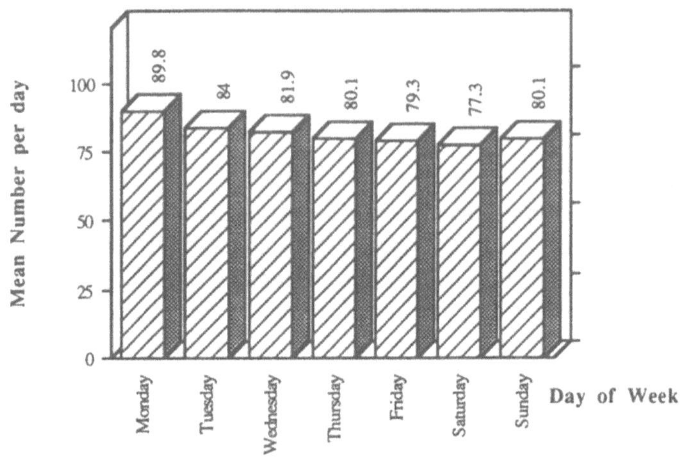

Figure 10. U.S. mean number of suicides by day of week, 1984 to 1986 average.

Geographic Differences: States and Regions

Suicide rates are highest in the western divisions of the United States (see Table 1 and Figure 11). The Mountain Region has the highest rates and among the 8 states that comprise this region were the top 7 in the United States in 1986 with the 8th tied for 12th. The Pacific states had the next highest rates, and all but 1 of its 5 states were in the top 13 in 1986. Central and southern states had lower rates, with lowest rates in the New England and Middle Atlantic states. These distributions of suicide by geographic regions and states have also been observed generally for the young (Seiden, 1984) and elderly (McIntosh, 1988).

Other Factors

A final factor that has been consistently observed to be associated with high risk of suicide but is not included in the characteristics and information that appears on death certificates and therefore in official national data is the presence of mental illness. Numerous studies have observed that virtually all mental illnesses increase the risk of suicide when compared to the nation as a whole (Lester, 1972, 1983, Chapters 17 and 18, respectively; Miles, 1977). Particularly high risk of suicide is observed in the categories of depression (Sainsbury, 1986), alcoholism (Murphy, 1986), and schizophrenia (Roy, 1986).

Table 1. Rates and Rankings of Suicide for Each State, 1986[a]

Rank	State	Rate	Rank	State	Rate
1	Nevada	24.1 [M][b]	—	U.S. Total	12.8
2	Montana	21.7 [M]	31	Minnesota	12.8 [WNC]
3	New Mexico	19.4 [M]	32	Wisconsin	12.5 [ENC]
4	Arizona	19.3 [M]	33	Alabama	12.4 [ESC]
5	Wyoming	19.1 [M]	34	Michigan	12.3 [ENC]
6	Idaho	17.7 [M]	35	North Carolina	12.2 [SA]
7	Colorado	17.6 [M]	35	Pennsylvania	12.2 [MA]
8	Oregon	16.7 [P]	35	Maryland	12.2 [SA]
9	Florida	16.0 [SA]	38	Washington, D.C.	12.0 [SA]
10	Washington	15.3 [P]	39	Indiana	11.7 [ENC]
11	Alaska	14.8 [P]	40	Ohio	11.6 [ENC]
12	California	14.7 [P]	41	South Carolina	11.4 [SA]
12	Utah	14.7 [M]	42	Maine	11.1 [NE]
14	Oklahoma	14.6 [WSC]	42	Mississippi	11.1 [ESC]
15	South Dakota	14.3 [WNC]	44	Illinois	11.0 [ENC]
15	Nebraska	14.3 [WNC]	45	North Dakota	10.8 [WNC]
17	Missouri	14.2 [WNC]	45	Hawaii	10.8 [P]
17	Louisiana	14.2 [WSC]	47	Rhode Island	10.2 [NE]
17	West Virginia	14.2 [SA]	48	Connecticut	9.6 [NE]
17	Kentucky	14.2 [ESC]	49	Massachusetts	9.2 [NE]
21	Virginia	14.1 [SA]	50	New Jersey	7.6 [MA]
22	Vermont	14.0 [NE]	50	New York	7.6 [MA]
23	Texas	13.6 [WSC]			
23	Kansas	13.6 [WNC]			
25	Arkansas	13.5 [WSC]			
26	Delaware	13.3 [SA]			
27	Georgia	13.0 [SA]			
27	New Hampshire	13.0 [NE]			
29	Tennessee	12.9 [ESC]			
29	Iowa	12.9 [WNC]			

[a]From the National Center for Health Statistics (1988b, pp. 45–46, Table 18) (data are by place of residence).
[b]Region: Mountain [M]; Pacific [P]; West South Central [WSC]; South Atlantic [SA]; West North Central [WNC]; East South Central [ESC]; East North Central [ENC]; New England [NE]; Middle Atlantic [MA].

CONCLUSIONS

Based on the most consistent data, therefore, the modal suicide victim is an elderly white male who commits suicide with a firearm. Although those with the opposite demographic characteristics may also consider and commit suicide, individuals with these modal and other psychological (e.g., hopelessness, helplessness), physical (e.g., illness, pain), and social circumstances (e.g., social isolation, loneliness) should be targeted for special suicide prevention efforts.

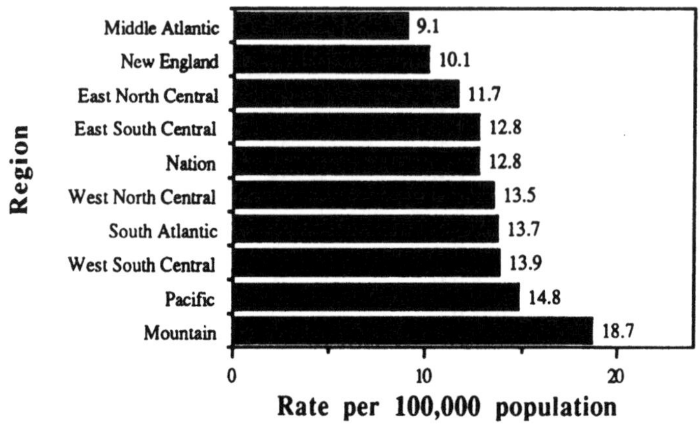

Figure 11. U.S. suicide rates by geographic regions, 1986.

REFERENCES

Allen, N. H. (1984). Suicide statistics. In C. L. Hatton & S. M. Valente (Eds.), *Suicide: Assessment and intervention* (2nd ed., pp. 17–31). Norwalk, CT: Appleton-Century-Crofts.

Atkinson, J. M. (1978). *Discovering suicide: Studies in the social organization of sudden death.* Pittsburgh: University of Pittsburgh Press.

Douglas, J. D. (1967). *The social meanings of suicide.* Princeton, NJ: Princeton University Press.

Dunne, E. J., McIntosh, J. L., & Dunne-Maxim, K. (Eds.). (1987). *Suicide and its aftermath: Understanding and counseling the survivors.* New York: W. W. Norton.

Durkheim, É. (1951). *Suicide.* New York: Free Press. (Original work published 1897)

Farberow, N. L. (1972). *Bibliography on suicide and suicide prevention, 1897–1957, 1958–1970* (DHEW Publication No. (HSM) 72-9080). Washington, DC: United States Government Printing Office.

Holinger, P. C., Offer, D., & Zola, M. A. (1988). A prediction model of suicide among youth. *Journal of Nervous and Mental Disease, 176,* 275–279.

Kreitman, N. (1977). *Parasuicide.* New York: Wiley.

Lester, D. (1972). *Why people kill themselves: A summary of research findings on suicidal behavior.* Springfield, IL: Charles C Thomas.

Lester, D. (1983). *Why people kill themselves: A 1980s summary of research findings on suicidal behavior* (2nd ed.). Springfield, IL: Charles C Thomas.

Manton, K. G., Blazer, D. G., & Woodbury, M. A. (1987). Suicide in middle age and later life: Sex and race specific life tables and cohort analysis. *Journal of Gerontology, 42,* 219–227.

McIntosh, J. L. (1985a). *Research on suicide: A bibliography.* Westport, CT: Greenwood Press.

McIntosh, J. L. (1985b, November). *Suicide among minority elderly.* Paper presented at annual meeting of the Gerontological Society of America, New Orleans, LA.

McIntosh, J. L. (1986, April). *Cross-ethnic suicide: U.S. trends and levels.* Paper presented at the annual meeting of the American Association of Suicidology, Atlanta, GA.

McIntosh, J. L. (1987a, May). *Hispanic suicide in ten U.S. states.* Paper presented at the joint meeting of the American Association of Suicidology and the International Association for Suicide Prevention, San Francisco, CA.

McIntosh, J. L. (1987b, May). *Marital status and suicide: Recent U.S. data*. Paper presented at the joint meeting of the American Association of Suicidology and the International Association for Suicide Prevention, San Francisco, CA.

McIntosh, J. L. (1988, April). *Geographic changes in U.S. elderly suicide*. Paper presented at the annual meeting of the American Association of Suicidology, Washington, DC.

McIntosh, J. L. (1989). Trends in racial differences in United States suicide statistics. *Death Studies*, *13*, 275–286.

McIntosh, J. L., Hubbard, R. W., & Santos, J. F. (1985). Suicide facts and myths: A study of prevalence. *Death Studies*, *9*, 267–281.

McIntosh, J. L., & Jewell, B. L. (1986). Sex difference trends in completed suicide. *Suicide and Life-Threatening Behavior*, *16*, 16–27.

McIntosh, J. L., & Santos, J. F. (1981). Suicide among minority elderly: A preliminary investigation. *Suicide and Life-Threatening Behavior*, *11*, 151–166.

McIntosh, J. L., & Santos, J. F. (1982). Changing patterns in methods of suicide by race and sex. *Suicide and Life-Threatening Behavior*, *12*, 221–233.

McIntosh, J. L., & Santos, J. F. (1985–1986). Methods of suicide by age: Sex and race differences among the young and old. *International Journal of Aging and Human Development*, *22*, 123–139.

Miles, C. P. (1977). Conditions predisposing to suicide: A review. *Journal of Nervous and Mental Disease*, *164*, 231–246.

Murphy, G. E. (1986). Suicide in alcoholism. In A. Roy (Ed.), *Suicide* (pp. 89–96). Baltimore: Williams & Wilkins.

National Center for Health Statistics. (1988a; and annual volumes, 1937–1985). *Vital Statistics of the United States, 1986* (and other annual volumes). *Volume II—Mortality*. Washington, DC: U.S. Government Printing Office.

National Center for Health Statistics. (1988b). Advance report of final mortality statistics, 1986. *NCHS Monthly Vital Statistics Report*, *37*(6, Suppl.).

Neuringer, C. (1982). Suicidal behavior in women. *Crisis*, *3*, 41–49.

Pollinger-Haas, A., & Hendin, H. (1983). Suicide among older people: Projections for the future. *Suicide and Life-Threatening Behavior*, *13*, 147–154.

Roy, A. (1986). Suicide in schizophrenia. In A. Roy (Ed.), *Suicide* (pp. 97–112). Baltimore: Williams & Wilkins.

Sainsbury, P. (1986). Depression, suicide, and suicide prevention. In A. Roy (Ed.), *Suicide* (pp. 73–88). Baltimore: Williams & Wilkins.

Sainsbury, P., & Barraclough, B. (1968). Differences in suicide rates. *Nature*, *220*, 1252.

Sainsbury, P., & Jenkins, J. S. (1982). The accuracy of officially reported suicide statistics for purposes of epidemiological research. *Journal of Epidemiology and Community Health*, *36*, 43–48.

Seiden, R. H. (1984). Death in the West—A regional analysis of the youthful suicide rate. *Western Journal of Medicine*, *140*, 969–973.

Steffensmeier, R. H. (1984). Suicide and the contemporary woman: Are male and female suicide rates converging? *Sex Roles*, *10*, 613–631.

U.S. Bureau of the Census. (1987). Marital status and living arrangements: March 1986. *Current Population Reports*, Series P-20, No. 418.

U.S. Bureau of the Census. (1988). United States population estimates, by age, sex, and race: 1980 to 1987. *Current Population Reports*, Series P-25, No. 1022.

6

Suicide across the Life Span
A Look at International Trends

David Lester

Scholars in one nation sometimes write as if they believed that the data from their own nation are typical of all nations at all times, and this belief is not always valid. A cross-cultural perspective helps us to identify which aspects of a phenomenon are unique to the nation in which the phenomenon was first identified and which have generality beyond that limited region.

The two most striking epidemiological features of suicide in America are the increasing suicide rates with age and the rising adolescent suicide rate in recent years. This chapter will explore the extent to which each of these features is found in other nations of the world.

PREVIOUS RESEARCH

The Variation of Suicide Rates with Age

Fuse (1980) described three patterns for the variation of suicide rates with age. The Hungarian pattern is one in which the suicide rate increases regularly with age. The Japanese pattern is one with two peaks, a lesser peak in young adulthood and a major peak in old age. The Scandinavian pattern is one that peaks in middle age and is an inverted U-shaped curve.

DAVID LESTER • Department of Psychology, Stockton State College, Pomona, New Jersey 08240.

Lester (1982) examined the validity of Fuse's hypothesis for suicide rates of nations of the world in 1975. The patterns Lester identified are shown in Table 1.

Lester concluded that Fuse's patterns were useful for describing the variation of suicide rates with age, but that his labels for them were not the best since, for example, Japanese males had the Hungarian pattern rather than the Japanese pattern. Furthermore, not all patterns could be fitted to one of the three proposed by Fuse. (For example, Danish and Swedish males fell into none of the three patterns.)

Lester also divided the nations into four groups on the basis of their gross national product per capita. In general, male suicide rates increased with age for all four groups of nations. For females, the peak age for suicide rose (from the age group 55–64 to 75+) with decreasing gross national product per capita from the first to the third quartile and then dropped dramatically to the 15-to 24-year-old group for the poorest nations (those in the fourth quartile).

Table 1. Patterns of Suicide in Males and Females

Pattern	Males	Females
Hungarian	Austria	Austria
	Bulgaria	Czechoslovakia
	Chile	Germany
	Cuba	Hungary
	Czechoslovakia	Italy
	England & Wales	Singapore
	France	West Germany
	Hong Kong	
	Italy	
	Japan	
	Portugal	
	Spain	
	West Germany	
Scandinavian (peak for age 45–54 or 55–64)	Canada	Australia
	Norway	Canada
	Poland	Denmark
		Netherlands
		Poland
		Sweden
		USA
Japanese (minor peak for age 15–24, 25–34, or 35–44)	Belgium	Bulgaria
	Greece	Hong Kong
	Puerto Rico	Japan
	Singapore	Portugal
	Uruguay	Spain
	Venezuela	
	USA	

[a]From Lester, D. (1982). The distribution of sex and age among completed suicides. *International Journal of Social Psychiatry*, *28*, 256–260.

Youth Suicide Rates

Lester (1988) examined changes in the suicide rates of youths in nations of the world. The nations with the greatest increases from 1970 to 1980 for the group aged 15 to 24 were Norway, Spain, and Switzerland. In contrast, several nations experienced a drop in the youth suicide rate: Guatemala, Chile, and Venezuela, for example.

Closer examination revealed that sometimes the changing youth suicide rate paralleled the changing total suicide rate, but sometimes did not. Differences were also found for male and female youths.

Lester examined the association between some social indicators and youth suicide rates and found that the associations for youth suicide rates were sometimes different than for overall suicide rates. For example, whereas Lester found that the overall suicide rate was greater in nations with a higher quality of life, youth suicide rates were not related to the quality of life. In addition, whereas the overall suicide rate rose more from 1970 to 1980 in nations with the higher suicide rates in 1970, this was not true for youth suicide rates.

Looking at the suicide rates of those aged 5 to 14, Barraclough (1987) found that the female rates were as high or higher than the male rates in 14 nations, mainly in South America and Asia. This is surprising since the overall male suicide rates are higher than female suicide rates in almost all nations of the world.

To explore these phenomena further, suicide rates by age were extracted for 1970 and 1980 from the annual volumes of *Statistics Annual*, published each year by the World Health Organization in Geneva. To obtain reasonable stable estimates of the suicide rates by age, only nations with data available for both 1970 and 1980, with a population of more than 1 million, and with more than 250 suicides a year were selected. The data are shown in Table 2.

THE PEAK SUICIDE RATE

Previous research had identified three patterns for the variation of suicide rates with age: monotically increasing, a peak in middle age, and bimodal. Let us examine the nations whose data are shown in Table 2.

Monotically Increasing

Several nations have suicide rates that rise with age for both sexes: Austria, Bulgaria, France, Greece, Hong Kong, Hungary, Italy, Japan, Portugal, Singapore, and Spain. It is obvious that this is a diverse group of nations, European and Asian, relatively rich and relatively poor.

In some of these nations, the peak in old age is striking. For example, in Hungary the suicide rate for men aged 75 and older in 1980 was 202.2 per 100,000

Table 2. Suicide Rates by Age in Countries of the World in 1970 and 1980

	Age (yr)							
	5–14	15–24	25–34	35–44	45–54	55–64	65–74	75+
Australia								
1970 male	0.3	12.4	20.1	26.1	33.6	30.9	31.9	38.5
1980 male	0.3	17.6	22.9	23.4	22.3	24.0	22.4	31.9
1970 female	0.3	4.7	7.8	11.8	14.6	17.0	14.4	9.5
1980 female	0.2	4.5	6.9	9.8	9.2	7.9	7.1	9.1
Austria								
1970 male	0.7	27.0	31.7	46.6	58.5	64.6	72.7	77.7
1980 male	3.9	28.8	36.3	43.9	59.3	56.3	72.6	85.7
1970 female	0.0	5.7	8.2	16.4	22.3	25.7	27.6	29.4
1980 female	0.7	6.7	11.1	14.3	20.7	23.0	29.1	33.9
Bulgaria								
1970 male	1.1	9.0	11.6	11.3	19.3	27.1	53.2	108.3
1980 male	1.1	11.1	12.9	16.3	21.9	26.8	52.2	108.7
1970 female	0.8	4.8	4.9	5.3	9.8	15.9	18.4	34.5
1980 female	0.6	7.4	5.8	5.7	8.2	14.4	17.0	31.9
Canada								
1970 male	0.6	15.6	20.1	26.6	27.9	31.9	28.0	24.6
1980 male	0.8	24.8	29.5	25.1	30.7	28.5	26.9	38.1
1970 female	0.1	4.8	8.6	10.6	14.5	11.4	9.5	4.6
1980 female	0.3	5.4	8.1	8.8	13.7	12.1	9.5	5.9
Chile								
1970 male	1.1	14.3	17.7	14.9	16.6	13.9	22.1	19.9
1980 male	0.3	10.8	12.1	13.9	12.5	15.3	10.6	21.2
1970 female	0.5	6.1	3.4	1.6	3.2	2.9	3.0	3.5
1980 female	0.1	2.9	1.9	0.9	1.7	2.9	1.3	2.4
Denmark								
1970 male	0.5	11.1	25.4	39.5	55.9	48.8	45.7	55.0
1980 male	0.3	16.3	42.7	61.8	70.7	71.8	60.4	81.3
1970 female	0.0	5.7	10.6	22.6	30.2	34.1	26.7	19.1
1980 female	0.3	7.7	16.7	35.8	42.8	39.3	32.9	31.6
Finland								
1970 male	1.3	22.5	41.5	55.8	60.9	62.6	66.5	50.5
1980 male	0.6	37.5	55.7	55.0	60.3	54.9	62.1	60.1
1970 female	0.3	6.7	9.4	11.2	20.6	15.9	12.2	7.4
1980 female	0.3	9.1	9.5	11.4	16.8	16.2	22.8	9.7
France								
1970 male	0.7	9.4	17.1	25.5	36.2	51.1	55.3	74.4
1980 male	0.7	15.7	27.4	32.7	39.7	41.2	57.1	99.6

(continued)

Table 2. (Continued)

	Age (yr)							
	5–14	15–24	25–34	35–44	45–54	55–64	65–74	75+
France (*Cont.*)								
1970 female	0.0	4.4	7.4	8.0	11.3	16.3	17.9	18.6
1980 female	0.2	5.4	9.6	13.2	14.9	17.2	22.6	24.4
Greece								
1970 male	0.0	1.7	3.9	6.1	6.7	10.6	10.7	11.6
1980 male	0.7	3.0	5.4	5.6	5.2	5.4	10.1	16.6
1970 female	0.1	1.4	1.7	1.0	3.2	4.3	1.7	5.6
1980 female	0.1	0.6	1.1	1.9	2.8	2.9	4.5	6.1
Hong Kong								
1970 male	0.6	7.2	27.3	23.8	33.8	41.5	50.5	88.7
1980 male	0.0	7.9	18.7	17.2	27.6	31.4	53.8	63.0
1970 female	0.4	8.2	11.1	18.9	13.2	26.8	46.4	89.1
1980 female	0.5	7.6	12.4	11.8	14.3	21.4	44.4	64.6
Hungary								
1970 male	1.9	27.8	48.6	63.6	78.4	85.1	104.9	146.4
1980 male	3.6	31.5	58.3	86.8	106.4	96.7	116.3	202.2
1970 female	0.4	9.6	11.0	17.5	23.8	33.8	46.2	76.4
1980 female	0.8	8.0	16.4	26.7	36.2	42.2	52.9	90.6
Italy								
1970 male	0.3	3.5	5.9	7.4	11.4	18.3	24.3	33.3
1980 male	0.3	5.3	8.3	9.1	14.0	17.3	26.5	37.4
1970 female	0.2	2.3	2.7	3.5	5.2	7.0	7.5	7.8
1980 female	0.1	2.4	3.3	4.2	6.8	8.2	10.2	10.2
Japan								
1970 male	0.5	14.0	20.1	17.8	20.1	32.3	50.4	82.1
1980 male	0.4	16.6	24.9	28.9	33.3	32.2	40.9	73.3
1970 female	0.2	11.9	13.8	10.0	13.5	20.6	40.5	66.3
1980 female	0.2	8.2	11.4	12.5	15.1	17.8	35.5	60.2
Netherlands								
1970 male	0.7	5.8	6.4	11.1	15.7	24.0	25.4	42.5
1980 male	0.2	8.3	14.9	15.1	17.1	22.3	26.1	41.1
1970 female	0.1	2.1	5.5	7.5	11.0	12.6	14.9	17.5
1980 female	0.0	3.7	8.0	8.9	12.4	14.1	14.3	12.0
New Zealand								
1970 male	1.0	12.1	10.4	23.1	24.5	16.8	34.6	31.2
1980 male	0.7	19.5	17.8	17.4	17.3	22.2	24.4	35.6
1970 female	0.0	3.8	2.9	8.5	12.1	21.1	19.2	11.1
1980 female	0.0	8.1	9.3	6.8	15.6	4.4	13.1	17.8

(continued)

Table 2. *(Continued)*

	Age (yr)							
	5–14	15–24	25–34	35–44	45–54	55–64	65–74	75+
Norway								
1970 male	0.3	5.4	15.0	17.4	19.2	24.7	19.6	13.3
1980 male	1.2	20.4	18.2	20.6	28.6	31.8	25.5	24.0
1970 female	0.0	2.0	4.5	10.1	10.4	8.9	6.9	1.9
1980 female	0.3	3.3	9.0	6.7	14.2	12.1	9.6	4.7
Portugal								
1970 male	0.1	5.6	6.2	17.5	14.5	27.6	43.4	72.2
1980 male	0.2	5.2	7.9	14.7	18.6	24.1	31.0	53.7
1970 female	0.1	3.6	2.1	3.0	3.8	6.7	9.2	11.7
1980 female	0.8	4.1	5.4	3.8	4.2	5.4	5.6	11.0
Singapore								
1970 male	0.3	9.1	8.1	13.3	23.2	39.0	56.5	137.9
1980 male	1.3	9.0	17.7	8.1	17.5	32.9	40.9	107.4
1970 female	0.7	6.3	15.7	0.0	14.1	14.5	39.9	53.6
1980 female	0.4	11.7	10.1	8.3	12.3	17.1	34.5	57.3
Spain								
1970 male	0.1	2.0	4.1	7.0	9.6	15.7	21.9	29.0
1980 male	0.2	4.3	6.2	6.6	9.7	12.4	18.6	28.5
1970 female	0.1	0.9	1.4	1.6	3.8	5.4	5.7	6.9
1980 female	0.0	1.1	1.3	2.1	3.3	4.9	4.7	6.4
Sweden								
1970 male	0.5	18.5	27.9	44.9	52.5	54.6	46.3	48.8
1980 male	0.5	16.9	33.3	37.6	43.9	35.3	39.3	48.9
1970 female	0.6	7.9	15.3	19.3	26.0	17.8	15.6	13.0
1980 female	0.0	5.8	11.3	16.2	17.8	21.2	14.5	11.4
Switzerland								
1970 male	0.8	21.3	27.6	31.2	46.2	49.9	49.5	74.1
1980 male	1.5	34.2	36.5	42.2	46.1	63.4	58.9	80.7
1970 female	0.0	4.7	10.2	8.8	19.5	19.1	21.7	16.0
1980 female	0.7	12.3	14.8	17.6	21.7	20.8	26.8	23.2
Thailand								
1970 male	0.3	7.2	5.7	9.0	8.5	11.7	9.5	10.7
1980 male	0.7	12.8	11.1	11.6	13.8	12.9	12.6	
1970 female	0.3	9.9	3.4	3.8	3.0	2.8	2.2	1.1
1980 female	1.2	19.6	8.6	7.4	7.1	4.8	3.3	
United Kingdom: England & Wales								
1970 male	0.0	6.0	9.1	11.3	14.1	17.5	20.7	23.9
1980 male	0.1	6.4	13.0	15.5	15.4	17.9	18.2	21.6

(continued)

Table 2. (Continued)

	Age (yr)							
	5–14	15–24	25–34	35–44	45–54	55–64	65–74	75+
United Kingdom: England and Wales (*Cont.*)								
1970 female	0.1	2.6	4.4	7.4	10.3	12.9	15.3	9.7
1980 female	0.0	3.0	4.2	8.1	10.9	11.8	13.3	11.0
United Kingdom: Scotland								
1970 male	0.0	5.8	8.6	15.6	13.1	24.0	12.9	21.7
1980 male	0.0	9.6	15.2	19.1	23.4	17.8	18.8	23.2
1970 female	0.0	1.8	5.8	8.2	15.1	12.7	5.7	5.6
1980 female	0.0	3.1	7.0	9.6	14.3	14.3	10.9	8.1
United States								
1970 male	0.5	13.5	19.6	22.2	27.8	32.8	36.5	41.8
1980 male	0.7	20.2	24.8	22.3	23.0	24.4	30.2	43.5
1970 female	0.1	4.2	8.6	12.1	12.5	11.4	9.3	6.7
1980 female	0.2	4.3	7.0	8.4	9.4	8.4	6.5	5.4
Venezuela								
1970 male	0.3	14.5	12.6	17.8	19.0	28.8	42.5	47.5
1980 male	0.3	10.4	13.9	13.1	18.5	20.6	24.9	46.8
1970 female	1.1	11.3	5.6	4.1	4.1	3.0	7.6	5.3
1980 female	0.4	3.5	3.2	3.3	2.8	2.4	1.8	2.8
West Germany								
1970 male	1.4	19.6	27.0	35.1	43.2	51.6	53.9	75.2
1980 male	1.6	19.0	26.9	33.0	42.0	38.9	54.0	72.8
1970 female	0.5	6.9	11.5	15.9	25.4	27.2	26.1	27.0
1980 female	0.3	5.6	9.9	14.0	20.4	23.6	27.1	25.9

per year compared to 31.5 for men aged 15 to 24. The rate for the elderly men was double that in Bulgaria and Singapore, the nations with the next highest suicides for elderly men.

Peak in Youth

Three nations have the peak suicide rate for women in the age range 15 to 24: Chile, Thailand, and Venezuela. In Chile and Venezuela, the male suicide rate peaks in the oldest group (75 and older), while in Thailand the male suicide rate peaks in those aged 45 to 64. These three nations are all relatively poor, and this suggests that the phenomenon of peak rates of suicide in young women is a feature of less developed nations.

Peak in Middle Age

The rest of the nations have peak suicide rates in age groups that vary from decade to decade and for men and women. For example, the peak suicide rate for Australian women was in those aged 55 to 64 in 1970 and in those aged 35 to 44 in 1980. In New Zealand, the peak age for men rose from 65 to 74 in 1970 to 75 and older in 1980, while in Scotland the peak age for men dropped from 55 to 64 in 1970 to 45 to 54 in 1980.

The United States

The U.S. pattern is unimodal, with the peak at 75 and older for men and 45 to 54 for women. No other nation in the sample has exactly this pattern.

CHANGES IN THE YOUTH SUICIDE RATE DURING THE 1970S

The suicide rates in 1970 and 1980 for the total population and for those aged 15 to 24 years of age are shown in Table 3. It can be seen that there is great variation among the nations of the world in the change in youth suicide rates.

Nations with the highest increases in youth suicide rates are Norway (+224%), Spain (+93%), Switzerland (+80%), and Thailand (+78%). In addition, New Zealand, Finland, Canada, and the Netherlands have experienced large increases in the youth suicide rate from 1970 to 1980.

In contrast, several nations have witnessed decreases in the youth suicide rate, including Chile (−32%), Venezuela (−28%), and Sweden (−13%). West Germany and Japan also experienced decreases during this period.

More detailed examination shows that many nations have witnessed increasing suicide rates in general from 1970 to 1980. Thus, it perhaps makes more sense to compare the increase in youth suicide rates with those of the total population. Furthermore, the rise varies with sex.

Using a criterion that the percentage increase in the youth suicide rate must be 10% or greater than the percentage increase in the overall suicide rates, the following nations had a rising youth suicide rate in both males and females: Finland, the Netherlands, New Zealand, Norway, Scotland, Spain, and Switzerland. Nations with a rising youth suicide rate in only males were Australia, Canada, France, Greece, Italy, Thailand, and the United States. Nations with a rising youth suicide rate in only females were Austria, Bulgaria, England and Wales, and Singapore.

It is clear that there is no universal pattern. Different nations are experiencing very different changes in the rates of male and female youth suicide as compared with the suicide rate of the total population.

Table 3. Suicide Rates (per 100,000 per year) in 1970 and Changes by 1980 for the Total Population and for Those Aged 15–24

	Total population		Youth	
	1970	% change by 1980	1970	% change by 1980
Australia	12.4	−11.2	8.6	+30.2
Austria	24.2	+6.2	16.5	+9.1
Bulgaria	11.9	+14.3	6.9	+34.8
Canada	11.3	+23.9	10.2	+50.0
Chile	6.0	−18.3	10.1	−31.7
Denmark	21.5	+47.0	8.5	+42.4
Finland	21.3	+20.7	14.7	+60.5
France	15.4	+26.0	7.0	+52.9
Greece	3.2	+3.1	1.5	+20.0
Hong Kong	13.6	−0.7	7.7	+1.3
Hungary	34.8	+29.0	18.9	+5.8
Italy	5.8	+25.9	2.9	+34.5
Japan	15.2	+15.8	13.0	−3.8
Netherlands	8.1	+24.7	4.0	+50.0
New Zealand	9.6	+12.5	8.0	+73.7
Norway	8.4	+47.6	3.7	+224.3
Portugal	7.5	−1.3	4.5	+2.2
Singapore	8.9	+25.8	7.8	+32.1
Spain	4.2	+4.8	1.4	+92.9
Sweden	22.3	−13.0	13.3	−13.5
Switzerland	18.6	+38.2	13.0	+80.9
Thailand	4.2	+76.2	7.2	+77.8
United Kingdom: England and Wales	8.0	+10.0	6.0	+6.7
United Kingdom: Scotland	7.6	+31.6	5.8	+65.5
United States	11.5	+2.6	8.8	+39.8
Venezuela	6.8	−23.5	14.5	−28.3
West Germany	21.3	−1.9	13.4	−6.7

DISCUSSION

The data presented in this chapter have indicated that the rising youth suicide rate is not found in every nation of the world. Some nations are experiencing a decrease in the youth suicide rate while others are witnessing a rise in the youth suicide rate in only one sex.

In addition, the data have indicated that the variation in suicide rates with age varies greatly from nation to nation and from decade to decade. In general, though, the most common pattern is for suicide rates to peak in old age in men and in late age in women.

REFERENCES

Barraclough, B. M. (1987). Sex ratio of juvenile suicide. *Journal of the American Academy of Child & Adolescent Psychiatry, 26*, 434–435.

Fuse, T. (1980). To be or not to be. *Stress, 1*, 18–25.

Lester, D. (1982). The distribution of sex and age among completed suicides. *International Journal of Social Psychiatry, 28*, 256–260.

Lester, D. (1988). Youth suicide: A cross-cultural perspective. *Adolescence, 23*, 955–958.

7

Suicide at Symbolic Ages
Death on Stocktaking Occasions

David P. Phillips and Daniel G. Smith

More than 50 years ago, when Freud was about to turn 80, he asked Ernest Jones, "What is the secret meaning of celebrating the big round numbers of one's life?" (Sampson & Sampson, 1985, p.152). Freud's question has not been answered, or even addressed, since he first posed it, despite the widespread recognition that some ages have more symbolic significance than others. Professional works on the life cycle (Erikson, 1959; Birren, 1964; Riley, Abeles, & Teitelbaum, 1982; Kakar, 1979; Levinson, 1978; Colarusso & Nemiroff, 1981; Falicov, 1988; Karp, 1988) have not systematically discussed the psychological consequences of reaching symbolic ages like 40, 50, 60, 70, or 80 (aside from attention to the psychological impact of retirement at age 65). The topic of symbolic ages also seems to have been largely overlooked in literary works and entirely overlooked in research on suicide and in popular psychological discussions of aging (Sheehy, 1976). Failure to address this subject is puzzling in view of the very general tendency to regard certain ages as symbolic milestones, sometimes approached with celebration, but often regarded with dread and foreboding.

For many people, the birthday seems to be an occasion of "stocktaking," when one evaluates past achievements and future prospects; this seems to be particularly true of symbolic birthdays, like 40, 65, or 70. For many people, "boundary ages" of this sort may serve as a signal that one promising period of life

---

DAVID P. PHILLIPS and DANIEL G. SMITH • Department of Sociology, University of California at San Diego, La Jolla, California 92093.

is over and another less promising one is about to begin. Many persons reaching boundary ages reflect on whether they have achieved the goals they set for themselves earlier in life. Some persons taking stock on these occasions are likely to consider that they have failed themselves and their families. The recognition that one has failed to achieve longstanding goals (and is unlikely to achieve them in the future) often elicits feelings of depression and hopelessness. These psychological states have frequently been associated with suicide (Beck, Steer, Kovacs, & Garrison, 1985; Dyer & Kreitman, 1984; Black, Winokur, & Nasrallah, 1987; Tsuang, 1978) and thus one would expect suicides to be abnormally frequent at "symbolic" or "boundary" ages.

In this chapter we will show that suicides (but not passenger deaths) display noticeable peaks at almost all symbolic ages. This type of analysis, which examines short-term fluctuations in mortality before and after important social events, has shed light on other aspects of suicide (Phillips & Carstensen, 1986; Phillips & Paight, 1987; Phillips, 1974; Phillips & Wills, 1987; Schmidtke & Hafner, 1988; Ganzeboom & de Haan, 1982), motor vehicle fatalities (Phillips, 1977, 1979), and general mortality (Phillips & King, 1988). But this approach does not seem to have been used to analyze suicides and motor vehicle fatalities around symbolic ages; perhaps this is because of the near-universal tendency for researchers to group ages into 5-year intervals (e.g., 40–44, 45–49, 50–54) rather than to study mortality at each age separately.

METHODS

We analyzed computerized records of all California suicides and motor vehicle fatalities for a 17-year period, 1969 to 1985. The study period ends in 1985, because this was the latest year for which mortality was available at the beginning of the investigation. As the starting point of the study, 1969 was chosen because it is the first year for which the Eighth Revision of the International Classification of Diseases took effect in California (the Seventh Revision employed somewhat different criteria for classifying suicides).

There is a widespread popular supposition that ages ending in 0 and 5 are considered more "symbolic" than others. But it is not evident a priori which of these symbolic ages are particularly critical. In the absence of theory to identify these ages, we chose to examine all decadal and mid-decadal ages from 20 to 80, i.e., 20, 25, . . . , 80. Age at death was calculated by subtracting the decedent's birthdate from his deathdate. Individuals lacking a recorded birth date or death date were excluded from the analysis (suicides excluded on these grounds constitute less than .6% of all cases). It should be emphasized that we are here analyzing the *calculated* rather than the reported age at death; this allows us to rule out the possibility that age-heaping in mortality is merely an artifact of misreporting of age on the death certificate.

To assess the possibility that our findings were due to other types of artifact or bias, we examined a control group of motor vehicle passenger deaths. This comparison group was chosen for the following reasons. The potential suicide can control the timing of his death more than any other decedent. At the opposite extreme is the passenger about to die in an automobile accident. He can control the timing of his death less than almost any other decedent (we know of no study providing systematic evidence of a suicidal component in passenger deaths). If deaths peak at symbolic ages because the decedent adjusts the timing of his death to achieve this, suicides should show such peaks and passenger deaths should not. On the other hand, if deaths peak at symbolic ages because of misreporting of the birth date or death date, then suicides *and* passenger deaths should show such peaks, since both types of death are subject to misreporting of birth dates and death dates. The influence of misreporting and other potential biases is further analyzed at the end of this paper.

To determine whether deaths peaked at symbolic ages, we compared the observed number of deaths at the symbolic age with an estimate of the number expected under the null hypothesis. This estimate was calculated as

$$(n(a - 2) + n(a - 1) + n(a + 1) + n(a + 2))/4$$

where n(a) is the number of deaths at age a. Thus, for a = 50, the expected number of deaths was estimated by averaging the number of deaths at ages 48, 49, 51, and 52. This is algebraically equivalent to fitting a linear regression line to deaths at ages 48, 49, 51, 52 and interpolating the expected number of deaths at age 50. (One might be tempted to fit a curvilinear regression line to these four data points, but such a procedure is inappropriate: With such a small number of data points, the use of a curved regression line results in "overfitting." Furthermore a graph of mortality for the four ages—a − 2, a − 1, a + 1, a + 2—generally approximated a straight line.) It is worth noting that the data used to estimate the expected number of deaths for one symbolic age do not overlap with the data used for any other symbolic age. Thus, for example, the ages 48, 49, 51, 52 are used to estimate the expected number of deaths at age 50, while the ages 53, 54, 56, 57 are used for the next symbolic age, 55. This procedure helps to ensure that the estimated expected number of deaths for one symbolic age is not statistically dependent on the estimated expected number of deaths for any other symbolic age. We tested for dependence of this sort (Durbin, 1970) and for heteroscedasticity (Glejser, 1969) of the residuals (observed number of deaths-estimated expected number of deaths).

The *t*-test for paired comparisons was used to test the significance of the difference between the observed number of deaths at each symbolic age and the expected number. Some of the assumptions required by the *t*-test are not met by our data; to increase confidence in the statistical significance of our findings, we also used the randomization test for paired comparison (Conover, 1971), a nonparametric procedure that requires very few assumptions about the data under study. As will be evident in Tables 1 and 2, the t-test and the randomization test both indicate the statistical significance of our findings.

RESULTS

Table 1 displays the overall results of the analysis. Column 1 lists the symbolic ages, column 2 the observed number of suicides at that age, and column 3 the expected number of suicides using the estimation techniques described above. The differences between the observed and expected number of suicides is expressed numerically in column 4 and as a percent in column 5. For example, at age 60 there are 884 reported suicides and 827.75 expected (calculated from the observed suicides at ages 58, 59, 61, and 62). Thus, at age 60, there is an excess of 56.25 suicides over the number expected, or 6.8%.

The table discloses two patterns, one familiar and one previously unsuspected. Because population declines with age, the number of suicides decreases markedly from age 20 to age 80. Superimposed on this pattern is another that is subtle, but very consistent: suicides show a remarkable tendency to peak at nearly all symbolic ages over the adult life span.

Table 1. Frequency of Suicides at Symbolic Ages, California, 1969–1985[a]

(1) Age	(2) Observed frequency	(3) Expected frequency	(4) Difference (2) − (3)	(5) % Difference [(4)/(3)]×100
20	1245	1218.75	26.25	2.15
25	1499	1495.75	3.25	.22
30	1359	1319.25	39.75	3.01
35	1057	1055.50	1.50	.14
40	977	947.50	29.50	3.11
45	975	942.50	32.50	3.45
50	1016	966.50	49.50	5.12
55	938	966.00	−28.00	−2.90
60	884	827.75	56.25	6.80
65	718	686.00	32.00	4.66
70	623	610.00	13.00	2.13
75	516	489.00	27.00	5.52
80	347	350.75	−3.75	−1.07

[a]See text for definition of method of calculation of expected frequency. Column 4, $t = 3.31$, $p = .003$ (one-tailed t-test for paired differences, 12 df); $p = .003$ randomization test for paired differences. The figures in column 4 show no evidence of autocorrelation or heteroscedasticity.

Table 2. Frequency of Motor Vehicle Passenger Deaths at Symbolic Ages, California, 1969–1985[a]

(1) Age	(2) Observed frequency	(3) Expected frequency	(4) Difference (2) − (3)	(5) % Difference [(4)/(3)]×100
20	912	869.50	42.50	4.89
25	456	438.00	18.00	4.11
30	238	257.75	−19.75	−7.66
35	137	164.25	−27.25	−16.59
40	117	120.00	−3.00	−2.50
45	131	106.00	25.00	23.58
50	96	107.25	−11.25	−10.49
55	101	97.75	3.25	3.32
60	90	93.25	−3.25	−3.49
65	95	92.75	2.25	2.43
70	85	92.00	−7.00	−7.61
75	83	80.00	3.00	3.75
80	77	60.50	16.50	27.27

[a]See text for definition of method of calculation of expected frequency. Column 4, $t = .57$, $p = .288$ (one-tailed t-test for paired differences, 12 *df*); $p = .297$ randomization test for paired differences.

It is interesting to note that mortality peaks at symbolic ages do not appear in the control group of motor vehicle passenger deaths (see Table 2). As noted above, this suggests that the suicide peaks at symbolic ages are not an artifact of reporting errors, because, if they were, these peaks should appear for passenger deaths as well.

It is important to determine whether the age-heaping effect exists in all major demographic groups or is concentrated in a few. If noticeable age-heaping appears in most demographic groups and at most ages, this would suggest that the phenomenon might have substantive importance to the population at large. On the other hand, if age-heaping is concentrated in a few demographic groups, this might shed light on the psychosocial processes that produced the phenomenon.

Table 3 shows that age-heaping of suicides on symbolic birthdays is not a uniform characteristic of the population at large. The "percent difference" column in this table is defined as in Tables 1 and 2, but, for brevity, separate data on observed and expected frequencies are not included. Table 3 presents strong evidence that age-heaping on symbolic birthdays is primarily a male phenomenon ($t = 3.26$; $p = .0035$; one-tailed test). With few exceptions the age-heaping appears to occur consistently over most of the male adult life span. In strong contrast, females do not display a statistically significant tendency to commit suicide in abnormal numbers at symbolic ages ($t = .34$; $p =$ n.s.; one-tailed test).

Although there are many patterns evident in Table 3, we have chosen to focus

Table 3. Percentage Increase/Decrease of Observed Suicides Compared to Expected Suicides at Symbolic Ages, by Sex, by Marital Status, California, 1969–1985[a]

(1)	(2)	(3)	(4)	(5)	(6)	(7)
			Male		Female	
Age	Male	Female	Married	Unmarried	Married	Unmarried
20	3.69	−2.61	−4.33	3.53	−4.11	−3.31
25	3.86	−10.14	−4.66	5.82	−15.57	−9.91
30	2.38	4.62	1.74	3.99	4.00	8.02
35	−.42	1.32	5.05	−4.84	8.12	−3.28
40	5.73	−1.54	14.67	−3.77	−4.76	4.35
45	4.99	1.18	3.91	4.07	.48	4.69
50	1.38	11.22	5.86	−3.32	6.60	20.98
55	−3.66	−1.64	−1.68	−4.86	1.75	−7.69
60	9.83	1.49	2.14	26.50	−9.03	11.45
65	6.06	1.94	14.18	−8.86	5.54	3.73
70	3.28	−.25	4.58	−1.62	−8.77	5.91
75	−2.95	28.09	−.93	−.70	59.29	22.49
80	9.34	−28.50	29.06	−4.76	−36.51	−24.58
t-test *p*	.004	.368	.014	.162	.490	.242
Randomization test *p*	.004	.360	.013	.169	.505	.234
n	40530	19125	17493	20421	8579	9155

[a]See text for definition of method of calculation of expected frequency. Both the randomization test and the *t*-test are based on the rawresidual = observed − expected number of deaths. The *t*-test is for paired differences, 12 *df*, one-tailed. Totals for columns (4) and (5) do not equal the total for column (2) and the totals for columns (6) and (7) do not equal the total for column (3) because columns (2) and (3) include unknown marital status.

on only a few. Male age-heaping appears throughout the life span, but it is stronger for some ages than others. Two of the most obvious instances are ages 40 and 65. These are traditional boundaries between youth and middle age, and middle age and old age. At these boundary ages a man may reflect on whether or not he has achieved his goals, has properly provided for his family, and has good prospects for the future. As with so many other topics, Shakespeare provided one of the best descriptions of the commonly felt distress at reaching 40: "When forty winters shall besiege thy brow, and dig deep trenches in thy beauty's field, thy youth's proud livery, so gazed on now, will be a tattered weed, of small worth held. . ." (Sonnet 2). Similarly, 65 has been frequently recognized as a boundary between two stages of life. For many men, the years of productive work are over, and the prospect of decaying health looms larger and larger on the horizon. Many persons passing this age anticipate a passage from active work to being a spectator on the sidelines, a passage from relative health to increasing helplessness and incapacitation. While some are able to enjoy an active and productive retirement, others can realistically expect to play a diminished role and to be a financial and emotional burden to their families.

It is important to note that the suicide peaks at ages 40 and 65 are evident only for married males and not for their unmarried counterparts. This is consistent with the following considerations that underlie much of the discussion in this chapter. While individual cases will obviously vary widely from the following simplified paradigm, it seems plausible that many people experience some or all of the following stages: (1) On various occasions people reflect (consciously or unconsciously) on whether they have met their own expectations or those of others. (2) In our society these periods of reflection often coincide with symbolic occasions, such as New Year or the birthday, particularly important birthdays like 40 and 65. (3) Because many people fail to meet expectations, they may feel pain and a deep sense of inadequacy. (4) Recently, females have dramatically expanded their financial contribution to the family, but during our study period males bore the principal responsibility for providing the family with income and a respectable position in society. (5) Thus, if a family does not achieve a respectable status, either in an absolute or in a relative sense, males are particularly likely to accept a sense of personal failure. (6) This sense of failure is likely to be stronger for married than for unmarried men, because the married man is striving to meet both his own expectations and those of the family that depends on him. (7) Given these considerations, suicide peaks at 40 and 65 should appear mainly among males, and particularly among married males. As women take an increasing central role in the marketplace, the male pattern observed in Table 3 may become a female pattern as well.

DISCUSSION

To our knowledge, this is the first large-sample, systematic study to provide evidence suggesting a peak in suicidal mortality at symbolic ages. Several alternative explanations for mortality peaks appear to be initially plausible, and these will be assessed below.

Misreporting on the Death-Certificate

As noted earlier, the age-heaping effect cannot be due to any putative tendency for survivors to misreport the decedent's age, because we are dealing here with the *calculated* rather than the reported age at death, determined by subtracting the reported birth date from the reported death date. Nonetheless, it is possible that the observed age-heaping is due to another type of misclassification: the misreporting of the birth year on the death certificate. This possibility is very small, for two reasons:

1. Misreporting of birth year would have to vary in a subtle and complex fashion in order to produce the observed age-heaping. For example, survivors of persons dying in 1981 would have to over-report birth years ending in 6 (to produce a peak in "mid-decadal" ages) and would have to over-report birth years ending in 1 (to produce a peak in "decadal" ages). A different pattern of misreporting would have to exist for persons dying in 1982. Survivors of these decedents would have to over-report birth years ending in 7 (to produce a peak in mid-decadal ages) and would have to over-report birth years ending in 2 (to produce a peak in decadal ages). Still another pattern of misreporting would have to obtain for persons dying in 1983, and so on. In short, there are a priori grounds for supposing that age-heaping at death is not caused by misreporting of the birth year.
2. There are also empirical grounds for this supposition. If this type of misreporting of the birth year did in fact exist, it would produce age-heaping, not only in male suicides, but also in female suicides, and indeed in motor vehicle passenger deaths as well. Because age-heaping is not found in these other causes of death, it seems very unlikely that our findings result from misreporting of year of birth.

   Misreporting of the year of *death* seems even less likely to produce the age-heaping under study. Almost all deaths are registered within a few days of the event, and it is very unlikely that officials would overlook a death date misreported by a year or more. In addition, the "misreported death year" explanation seems incapable of explaining why some causes of death display age-heaping while others do not.

Atypical Celebration of Symbolic Birthdays

Symbolic birthdays are likely to be celebrated with unusual fanfare. Perhaps it is the atypical celebration of these birthdays, or something associated with the celebration (such as increased drinking), which produces the age-heaping we have observed.

If this explanation were correct, the surge in deaths at symbolic ages should be most evident just after the birthday. Thus, one can test the "birthday celebration" explanation by examining the fine-scale distribution of deaths in the months following symbolic birthdays. Up to now, we have been examining mortality in relatively crude, 1-year age categories, e.g., 50 (= 50.00 to 50.99), 51 (= 51.00 to 51.99), 52 (= 52.00 to 52.99), and so on. Mortality can also be examined in finer 1-month age categories, e.g., 50.00 to just less than $50 + \frac{1}{12}$; $50 + \frac{1}{12}$ to just less than $50 + \frac{2}{12}$; $50 + \frac{2}{12}$ to just less than $50 + \frac{3}{12}$; and so on. When a detailed analysis of this sort is conducted, one finds that the surge in deaths at symbolic ages is *not* most evident just after the birthday. Instead, suicides are distributed rather evenly over the year following the symbolic birthday. This is inconsistent with the "birthday celebration" explanation.

Fluctuation of Birth Cohorts

Suppose, for the moment, that the presence investigation had examined mortality occurring in 1 year, 1970, rather than in the 17-year period (1969–1985) actually studied. Suppose further that there was a surge of births at 5-year intervals, in 1900, 1905, 1910, and so on. In 1970, this would imply an excess of persons whose ages were 70, 65, 60, and so on. Given this (hypothetical) excess of persons alive at symbolic ages, one would then expect, other things being equal, an excess of *deaths* at these ages, also.

The "birth-cohort explanation" might serve as an adequate account of the findings, if the situation were actually as described in the above simplified example (where there is a 5-year cycle in births and only 1 mortality year is studied). However, because a 17-year (1969-1985) period was studied, this explanation is inadequate: It is true that a surge in births in 1900 would imply an excess of 70-year-olds in 1970, but it would also imply an excess of 69-year-olds in 1969, an excess of 71-year-olds in 1971, of 72-year-olds in 1972, and so on. Thus, the effect of studying a 17-year period, rather than a 1-year period, is to spread the effect of a hypothetical cycle in birth cohorts onto nonsymbolic ages as well as symbolic ones.

A direct method for assessing the birth-cohort explanation is logically appealing but unfortunately not feasible. In the presence of an extremely large sample, one could subclassify the data into separate birth years, and examine the age-heaping effect for each birth cohort separately. Fortunately, there is a less direct but more feasible method for assessing this explanation: If this explanation were correct, age-heaping should be evident not only for suicides, but also for the control group under study. Because the control group did not display age-heaping, the birth-cohort explanation appears to be implausible.

Other Age Cycles in Mortality

It is conceivable that there is a peak in deaths, not only age ages ending in 0 and 5, but also at some other 5-year interval—perhaps at ages ending in 1 and 6; 2 and 7; 3 and 8; or 4 and 9. By definition, mortality cannot be abnormally high for all of these ages, but it is possible for deaths to display 5-year peaks at some of these nonsymbolic ages. If there are 5-year mortality peaks at nonsymbolic ages, this would undermine confidence in the symbolic age explanation, and suggest, instead, that age-heaping results from some type of subtle statistical artifact. To assess this possibility, we sought for age-heaping at ages ending in 1 and 6, 2 and 7, 3 and 8, and 4 and 9. No evidence of age-heaping for these nonsymbolic ages was found for suicides. This undermines the validity of the "artifact explanation."

The Effect of Autocorrelation and Heteroscedasticity

Significance levels are biased in the presence of these statistical phenomena, and thus it is possible that the apparently significant findings for column 4 in Table 1 are not actually significant at all. This explanation is implausible because autocorrelation and heteroscedasticity were tested for in column 4 in Table 1, and no evidence of these phenomena was found.

Tests for Autocorrelation. Column 4 in Table 1 presents the difference between the observed number of deaths at each symbolic age and the estimated number expected. We used Durbin's second method (Durbin, 1970) to test for first-order serial dependence among the estimates in this column. This test was originally developed for use when some of the regressors are lagged dependent variables, but it is not restricted to variables of this type. We found no statistically significant evidence of dependence for the figures in column 4 ($p = .0663$).

Tests for Heteroscedasticity. Glejser's test was used (Glejser, 1969) and no statistically significant evidence of heteroscedasticity was found for the suicide data in Table 1, column 4 ($p = .6469$).

These findings suggest that the statistically significant age-heaping found in Table 1 cannot plausibly be ascribed to autocorrelation or to heteroscedasticity.

We have now evaluated five alternative explanations for the observed age-heaping. At present, the best available explanation seems to be that reaching a symbolic age has a sufficiently severe effect on some people as to elicit an increase in suicides.

In this chapter we have discussed some negative psychological processes associated with symbolic ages. Although this discussion appears to be plausible and is empirically supported, it is nonetheless speculative; future research should attempt to identify empirically the detailed psychological mechanisms linking arrival at a symbolic age with a subsequent surge in deaths. For some, this link may be direct: Turning 65 may be a sufficient reminder of past failures and impending mortality to prompt suicidal thoughts. For others, the link may be less direct—arrival at a symbolic age may merely trigger a chain of circumstances that eventually leads to suicide. It will be interesting to elucidate the direct and indirect paths linking suicide and symbolic ages, and valuable to determine whether these paths differ for men versus women, married versus unmarried, and so on.

We have suggested that suicides increase at symbolic ages because these serve as "stocktaking occasions." One way to test this hypothesis would be to compare suicide notes written by persons at symbolic ages with notes written by a control group. In addition, it would be valuable to determine whether suicides increase during other stocktaking occasions. There is some fragmentary evidence suggesting that this may be so: suicides increase just after the New Year's holiday, which serves for many as a time of reflection and assessment (Phillips & Wills, 1987).

Future research should also seek to determine whether age-heaping is present, not only in suicides but also in other causes of death. Do deaths from accidental falls also display this phenomenon? If so, is there more age-heaping for falls from one level to another than for falls on the same level? In general, it may be possible to use the age-heaping phenomenon as a kind of litmus test, useful for systematically separating external causes of death into two categories: those that display age-heaping and those that don't. At present, our evidence suggests that the first category is more likely to have a suicidal component (whether conscious or unconscious) than the second.

In the long history of medical statistical research, compilers and users of mortality tables have almost always examined deaths classified into 5-year or 10-year age categories. The present study suggests that collapsing data in this fashion (though convenient and valuable in many respects) obscures some interesting patterns. It may be preferable for some types of future research to avoid age categorization as much as possible and to examine deaths for each age separately. Proceeding in this fashion will probably throw new light on psychosocial processes leading to suicide and to associated forms of death.

ACKNOWLEDGMENTS. We thank Dr. Ian Abramson, Mathematics Department; Dr. Jeff Miller, Psychology Department; Dr. Bennett Berger, Sociology Department; and Jim Rapp, Lucy Devan, Jerry Fitzsimmons, Computer Center (all at the University of California at San Diego); Dr. Cecil G. Sheps and Dr. Harry T. Phillips (School of Public Health, University of North Carolina at Chapel Hill); Dr. Mark Phillips, Carleton University, Ottawa; Dr. Eva J. Salber, Duke University Medical School; Dr. David Mechanic, Institute for Health, Health Care Policy, and Aging Research, Rutgers; and Dr. Otis Dudley Duncan, Sociology Department, University of California at Santa Barbara. Mortality data were provided by the California Department of Health Services.

REFERENCES

Beck, A. T., Steer, R. A., & Kovacs, M., Garrison, B. (1985). Hopelessness and eventual suicide: A ten-year prospective study of patients hospitalized with suicidal ideation. *American Journal of Psychiatry*, *142*, 559–563.

Birren, J. E. (1964). *The Psychology of aging*. Englewood Cliffs, NJ: Prentice-Hall.

Black, D. W., Winokur, G., & Nasrallah, A. (1987). Suicide in subtypes of major affective disorder. A comparison with general population suicide mortality. *Archives of General Psychiatry*, *44*, 878–880.
Colarusso, C. A., Nemiroff, R. A. (1981). *Adult development: A new dimension in psychodynamic theory and practice*, New York: Plenum.
Conover, W. J. (1971). *Practical nonparametric statistics*. New York: Wiley.
Durbin, J. (1970). Testing for serial correlation in least-squares regression when some of the regressors are lagged dependent variables. *Econometrica*, *38*, 410–421.
Dyer, J. A. T., & Kreitman, N. (1984). Hopelessness, depression and suicidal intent in parasuicide. *British Journal of Psychiatry*, *144*, 127–133.
Erikson, E. H. (1959). Identity and the life cycle—Selected papers. *Psychological Issues*, Vol. 1.
Falicov, C. J. (Ed.). (1988). *Continuity and change over the life cycle*. New York: Guilford.
Ganzeboom, H. B. G., & de Haan, D. (1982). Gepubliceerde zelfmoorden en verhoging van sterfte door zelfmoorden ongelukken in Nederland 1972–1980 (Publicized suicides and an increase in deaths from suicidal accidents in the Netherlands 1972–1980). *Mens en Maatschappij*, *57*, 55–69.
Glejser, H. (1969). A new test for heteroscedasticity. *Journal of American Statistical Association*, *64*, 316–323.
Kakar, S. (Ed.). (1979). *Identity and adulthood*. Delhi, India: Oxford.
Karp, D. A. (1988). A decade of reminders: Changing age consciousness between fifty and sixty years old. *The Gerontologist*, *28*, 727–738.
Levinson, D. J. (1978). *The seasons of a man's life*. Englewood Cliffs, NJ: Prentice-Hall.
Phillips, D. P. (1974). The influence of suggestion on suicide: Substantive and theoretical implications of the Werther effect. *American Sociological Review*, *39*, 340–354.
Phillips, D. P. (1977). Motor vehicle fatalities increase just after publicized suicide stories. *Science*, *196*, 1464–1465.
Phillips, D. P. (1979). Suicide, motor vehicle fatalities, and the mass media: Evidence toward a theory of suggestion. *American Journal of Sociology*, *84*, 1150–1174.
Phillips, D. P., & Carstensen, L. L. (1986). Clustering of teenage suicides after television news stories about suicide. *New England Journal of Medicine*, *315*, 685–689.
Phillips, D. P., & King, E. (1988). Death takes a holiday: Mortality surrounding major social occasions. *The Lancet*, (2): 728–732.
Phillips, D. P., & Paight, D. J. (1987). The impact of televised movies about suicide. A replicative study. *New England Journal of Medicine*, *317*, 809–811.
Phillips, D. P., & Wills, J. (1987). A drop in suicides around major national holidays. *Suicide Life Threatening Behavior*, *17*, 1–12.
Riley, M. W., Abeles, R. P., & Teitelbaum, M. S. (Eds.). (1982). *Aging from birth to death—Sociotemporal perspectives* (AAAS Selected Symposium). Boulder, CO: Westview Press.
Sampson, A. & Sampson, S. (Eds.). (1985). *The Oxford book of ages*. New York: Oxford.
Schmidtke, A., & Hafner, H. (1988). The Werther effect after television films: New evidence for an old hypothesis. *Psychological Medicine*, *18*, 665–676.
Sheehy, G. (1976). *Passages: Predictable crises of adult life*. New York: Dutton.
Tsuang, M. T. (1978). Suicides of schizophrenics, manics, depressives, and surgical controls. *Archives General Psychiatry*, *35*, 153–155.

III

Suicide by Time-Lines

Developmental ages (or time-lines) have their unique—despite commonalities—psychological issues. In line with the epidemiological findings that there are different rates of completed suicide across the life span, research shows that there may well be unique psychological issues at different ages for the suicidal person. Part III, though not intended to be reviews, presents five chapters: two addressing suicide in children and adolescents; a discussion of suicide in the young adult, utilizing their suicide notes as the source of data; a presentation of suicide in middle adulthood (with comment on mid-life); and a discussion of suicide in the elderly.

8

Suicide in the School-Age Child and Adolescent

Antoon A. Leenaars and Susanne Wenckstern

Both children and adolescents do commit suicide. Although suicide is rare in children younger than age 12, it occurs with greater frequency than most people imagine. The youngest child that we are aware of was 4. Suicide is also all too frequent in adolescents. Many countries saw a striking rise in suicide in this age group between the 1950s and the late 1970s. Australia, Canada, Great Britain, Holland, Israel, Japan, United States, West Germany, and others have all reported high rates by 1980, although the rate of suicide has leveled off in some countries (e.g., Canada, United States). Boys traditionally have a higher rate of completed suicide than girls in adolescence, but in childhood the reported rates are higher in girls. Lester and McIntosh elsewhere in this book have presented the demographic data.

Unlike the relatively low number of children who commit suicide, there is a much higher percentage of children who attempt suicide. What is even more alarming is the number of suicide attempts in teenagers. One recent study in the United States by Smith and Crawford (1986) reported that 8.4% of adolescents have attempted to kill themselves. Incidentally, unlike adolescents, the severity of suicidal behavior does not differ in boys and girls younger than 12 years (Pfeffer, 1986).

ANTOON A. LEENAARS • Private Practice, 880 Ouelette Avenue, Suite 702, Windsor, Ontario, Canada N9A 1C7. *SUSANNE WENCKSTERN* • The Board of Education for the City of Windsor, Windsor, Ontario, Canada N9A 6KI.

An even greater number of our youth think about suicide. Pfeffer, in her excellent book, *The Suicidal Child*, reported a study of elementary school children that found a high rate of 11.9%. In the Smith and Crawford (1986) study of high school students, 62.6% reported some degree of suicidal ideation (i.e., thoughts of suicide). Of course, it is not uncommon for people in general to have suicidal thoughts. Be that as it may, the current high rate of suicide, suicide attempts, and suicidal ideation in children and adolescents is of considerable concern worldwide.

If one attempts to understand this phenomenon psychologically, one becomes aware over time of its enormous complexity. This chapter should be seen as only one attempt to provide such understanding. It is divided into two major sections: The first discussion is on some important observations derived from our clinical experiences embedded in the current literature and the second is on some common clues to suicide, i.e., overt behaviors that the child or adolescent may exhibit. The observations in these sections are not derived from any a priori model of suicide but arose out of our need to understand such individuals in our clinical practice. The literature on suicide was enormously helpful in this task. We do wish to stress that these observations are not exhaustive (as the chapter by Berman verifies). In line with the tone of this book, these observations must be placed within a developmental context that has been previously outlined (Chapters 1 and 2, this volume).

THEORETICAL/CLINICAL OBSERVATIONS

This section consists of seven parts, all focused on clarifying suicide in children and adolescents: definition, concept of death, depression, learning disabilities, physical disabilities and illness, specific precipitating events, and the family system.

Definition

Defining suicide is a complex endeavor. Shneidman (1985) has provided the following definition:

> Currently in the Western world, suicide is a conscious act of self-induced annihilation, best understood as a multidimensional malaise in a needful individual who defines an issue for which suicide is perceived as the best solution. (p.203)

Pfeffer (1986) has suggested that the definition of suicide needs to be clarified somewhat for youth. She has provided the following comment:

> It is not necessary for a child to have an understanding of the finality of death but it is necessary to have a concept of death, regardless of how idiosyncratic it may be. Therefore, suicidal behavior in children can be defined as self-destructive behavior that has the intent to seriously damage oneself or cause death. (p.14)

Concept of Death

Do children understand death? Pfeffer's research (1986) suggests "yes," although ideas of death differ depending on the age of the child. Young children (approximately at age 7) see death as temporary; everything is alive and vulnerable to death. Children about 10 years of age see death as personified and temporary; an outside agent causes death. By the time a child—a young adolescent—is 13 years old, he or she sees death as final; internal biological processes cause death. Yet, even older adolescents may misunderstand the finality of death. For example, Jim, a 16-year-old suicidal individual, was referred to us because of a crisis at home. Jim wanted to punish his parents; he stated, "I'll teach my dad a lesson when I kill myself. Then, he'll learn a lesson." Of course, such reasoning is not logical. Jim cannot know his father's reaction. Jim's ideas here are based on a denial of death. Adolescents (and adults) often have an unrealistic concept of death (and also of life). Sometimes, people believe that somehow after they are dead they will *actually* continue to live in the hereafter. Thus, young people do have a concept of death, but it may be different than an adult's. Incidentally, Pfeffer has shown that intense fantasies about death may be an early warning sign of suicidal risk in youth.

Depression

First and foremost, it must be understood that not all suicidal youth are depressed, and that not all depressed youth are suicidal. Depression and suicide are *not* equivalent. Yet, Pfeffer (1986) has noted that depression distinguishes many suicidal children and adolescents from nonsuicidal groups. Depression can be noted in mood and behavior (ranging from feeling dejected and some hesitancy in social contacts, to difficult to contact, isolation, serious disturbance of appetite and sleep), verbal expression (ranging from talks about being disappointed, excluded, blamed, etc., to talks of suicide, being killed, abandoned, helpless), and fantasy (ranging from disappointed, excluded, mistreated, etc., to suicide, mutilation, loss of a significant person). Behaviors such as excessive aggressiveness, sleep disturbance, change in school performance, decreased socialization, somatic complaints, loss of energy, unusual change in appetite and weight have all been associated with depression (Pfeffer, 1986). However, not all depression is overt. Some children and especially teenagers exhibit what has been termed *masked depression*. Anorexia, promiscuity, drug abuse, for example, have been associated with depression. It is important to remember, however, that depression does not equal suicide in a simple one to one fashion. Most suicides experience *unbearable pain*, but not necessarily depression (Shneidman, 1985). The unbearable emotion might be hostility, despair, shame, guilt, dependency, hopelessness, or helplessness. What is critical is that the emotion—pain—is unbearable. *Unendurable psychological pain is the common stimulus in suicide* (Shneidman, 1985).

Learning Disabilities and Suicidal Youth

The importance of brain dysfunction in children and its relation to learning disabilities is well documented. The relation of brain dysfunction and socio-emotional problems is, however, a more neglected topic in the literature. Peck (1985) has observed that, although about 5% of children are diagnosed as learning disabled in the general population, in a sample of suicidal youngsters, 50% had been so labeled. He noted:

> it is clear that learning disabled youngsters may suffer from loss of esteem, and in those cases where youngsters experience both pressure from parents to be "normal" and pressure from peers deriding their disability, their feelings of frustrations and hurt may be so great as to place a very young child in an at-risk category for suicide. (p. 116)

Although Peck's observations are important for understanding the development of suicidal behavior, he does not take note of the observation that there are particular subtypes of learning disabilities and that these different subtypes may result in different levels of risk. Rourke and Fisk (1981) have documented that different patterns of cerebral dysfunction and their resulting learning disability(ies) render a child at risk for different types of socio-emotional disturbances. They report three major subgroups: The first group has a right brain dysfunction. These children are prone to learning problems with nonverbal, visual information. They may show the following socio-emotional problems: not paying attention to visual objects including other people in the classroom, playground, and so on; rarely expressing emotions appropriately in their facial expressions; having a voice that can be expressionless; being very talkative; talking to self; having flow problems in their speech; and being awkward socially. The second group has a left brain dysfunction. These children are prone to learning problems with verbal information. They may show the following socio-emotional problems: rarely initiating conversations; having problems paying attention, for example, in conversation; being brief and often concrete in their remarks; often stating "I don't know" to questions; and some are very impulsive, not thinking before they act. The third group has both left and right brain dysfunction and exhibit a conglomerate of symptoms.

Other more specific cerebral deficits render people at risk for other specific problems such as planning, sequencing social events, and so on. Although further empirical studies need to be conducted in the neuropsychology of youth suicides, these observations clearly warrant attention. Indeed, Rourke, Young, and Leenaars (1989) have shown that one possible adolescent and adult outcome of childhood central processing deficiencies is suicidal behavior as well as other socio-emotional problems. They have suggested that it is especially the first pattern associated with right brain dysfunction that predisposes those afflicted to adolescent (and adult) suicide risk.

Physical Disabilities and Illness

We would be remiss if we did not, at least, note the importance of physical problems in suicidal behavior in *some* youth. Physical illness interacts with an individual's emotional functioning; indeed, some illnesses affect one's emotions. Empirical study regarding illness and suicide in children and adolescents is urgently needed, although some physical illnesses that have been associated, according to Barraclough (1986), with suicidal behavior (although he does not differentiate for what age) are anorexia, bulimia, diabetes, epilepsy, traumatic brain injury, and muscular dystrophia. Some individuals with physical disabilities who are at risk are those with limb amputations or spinal injuries resulting in quadriplegia. Individuals with terminal illness such as AIDS (often at the early stages of this disease) appear also to be at high risk (Fryer, 1986; Marzuk, 1989). We also recall a case of a young male who had a genital malformation, which contributed significantly to his suicidal solution. Even acne may be too much in some vulnerable individual. However, it is important to realize that not all such youth are suicidal and that research is needed to substantiate these views.

Specific Environmental Precipitating Events

A current popular formulation regarding suicide is that suicide is simply due to an external event; for example, a rejection, the influence of the music of a pop singer, whatever. Although precipitating events (e.g., deprivation of love, sexual abuse, death of parent, divorce, a rejection) do occur in the suicides of adolescents, this is less frequent in children. We are here reminded of a clinical example, which is quite similar to one reported by Menninger (1938): A 16-year-old was found dead in a car, having died of carbon monoxide poisoning. People were perplexed, "Why did this young person from an upper middle class family kill himself?" The parents found out that his girlfriend rejected him the day of his suicide. That was *the* reason: when a young person gets rejected and is so in love, he may kill himself. A few friends and his teachers knew that he had been having problems in school. *That* was the reason. A few others knew that his father was an alcoholic and abusive. *That* was the reason. His physician knew that he had been adopted and had been recently upset about that. She knew *the* real reason. And others knew. . . .

Shneidman (1985) has noted that the common consistency in suicide is not the precipitating event but *life-long coping patterns*. Even in youth, one can see a continuity despite developmental changes. Children and adolescents who kill themselves experience a steady toll of threat, stress, failure, challenge, and loss that gradually undermines their adjustment process. One merely has to reflect on the frequent statement that Sally killed herself because her boyfriend rejected her. *Most of us do not, why Sally*? The answer here is not what kind of person Sally is but what such youth have in common, that is, the commonalities in suicide.

One event, however, that has frequently been identified as a possible precipitating event is the death of a parent (Pfeffer, 1986). Indeed, when the death occurs by suicide, everyone in the family is at risk.

This discussion also raises the issues of the contagion (copycat) effect. A few years ago in Japan, an 18-year-old pop idol, Yukiko Okada, after a fight with her lover, leaped to her death from the building that housed her recording company in Tokyo. In the 17 days following her suicide, the suicide toll reached 33 young people. Phillips (1986) has recently documented that teenage clusters do exist and that such an effect is much higher for teenagers than adults. Brenner (1988) has, however, shown that a contagion effect in boys (5–14 years old) may not exist. Phillips, in his studies of adolescents has, however, noted that if a suicide is sensationalized by the media, there is an increase (especially for girls) in suicide. The greater the publicity, the greater the rate of suicide. Obviously, this raises the issue of how to expose our children and adolescents to information about suicide effectively. Recent research (Smith & Crawford, 1986) has shown that suicide is a personal concern for most high school students; yet, many—especially boys—deny or distance the problem. It is our belief that professionals, teachers, and parents need to work together in developing suicide prevention and postvention programs in their community, especially in the schools. The latter are, in part, attempts to address the contagion effect (Leenaars, 1985, 1986; Leenaars & Wenckstern, 1990).

Suicidal Youth and their Families

A review of the literature (e.g., Corder & Haizlip, 1984; Corder, Parker, & Corder, 1974; Leenaars, 1988; Maris, 1985; Pfeffer, 1981a, 1981b, 1986; Toolan, 1981; Seidan, 1984) suggests that the family system and its functioning is a central factor associated with suicide and suicidal behavior in children and adolescents, although by no means do *all* families show these characteristics. There are no universals in suicide. A few common observations of families will be provided, and then a few specific additional observations for teenagers:

1. There is, at times, a lack of generational boundaries in suicidal families. There is an insufficient separation of the parent from his or her family of origin. Often grandparents, for example, take over the parenting role.
2. The family system is often inflexible. Any change is seen as a threat to the survival of the family. Denial, secretiveness, and especially a *lack of communication* are seen in the family. One 8-year-old boy once reported to us, "If I try to kill myself, maybe my dad will listen." Additionally in teenagers, such families have stringent discipline patterns and limit setting, which bind the individual in his or her identity development,

which is critical at this time of a person's life. At times, love affairs are stopped by parents, even in 18-year-olds.

3. At times, there is a symbiotic parent-child relationship. A parent, usually the mother, is too attached to the youth. Not only is such a relation disturbing, but the parent also does not provide the emotional protection and support that a parent usually provides intuitively to a youth as he or she grows. Sometimes the parent treats the child as an "adult." One such teenager tried to break this bond by attempting to kill herself in her mother's prized car, while another—a straight A student—intentionally obtained a B resulting in a parental conflict and a suicide attempt by the youth. Additionally, it has been noted over and over in children that if such a parent dies, the child may kill himself to be magically reunited with that same parent.

4. Long-term disorganization (malfunctioning) has been noted in these families, for example, mother or father absence, divorce, alcoholism, mental illness. In teenage girls there is a very high rate, compared with the general population, of incest.

In addition, three differentiating observations about the families of suicidal teenagers have been made: First, adolescents in such families often feel a lack of control over their environment stemming from rigid family rules or symbiotic relationships. Second, adolescence is a time of stress and turmoil. It is not, as some believe, a time of simple joy and peace. Often, parents do not allow any conflict, turmoil, and development to occur. Third, recent family disorganization, for example, recent moves, unemployment in the home, physical or mental illness, parental conflict, have been noted in the family.

Berman (1986), by way of critique of some of this literature, has argued that much of the current research is not empirical enough; for example, the research study has not used control groups, that is, comparing suicidal youth and their families with other troubled or nontroubled youth and their families. Thus, the conclusions may be too premature. It may well be that our information is about families at risk for perturbation. We do not know how the suicidal family differentiates from other families with other problems, for example, promiscuity, drug abuse, delinquency, and learning problems. Be that as it may, we do know that suicide in young people is often related to disturbances in the family and, at times, other systems, especially schools (Leenaars, 1986).

We wish to strongly state our opinion that we need to know what suicidal families have in common, *not* what kind of parent causes the suicide. There are no evil, weak parents, only perturbed parents or, more accurately, perturbed and suicide-enhancing *families*.

BEHAVIORAL OBSERVATIONS

In understanding suicide in children and adolescents, we need to be aware of behaviors that are potentially predictive of suicide. However, there is no *one* or *the* definitive behavior. Two concepts that may be helpful here are *lethality* and *perturbation*. Lethality refers to the probability of a person killing himself or herself, ranging from low to moderate to high. Perturbation refers to subjective distress, also ranging from low to moderate to high. Both have to be evaluated. It is important to note that one can be perturbed and not suicidal. Lethality kills, not perturbation. Perturbation is often relatively easy to evaluate; lethality is not. Our own experience with parents, teachers, clergy, family physicians, and others is that lethality is best assessed by a professional (e.g., psychiatrist, psychologist, social worker) *with* experience in this area; yet, it is important that everyone be aware of these concepts to understand the clues. The clues here are ones that are equally applicable to other age groups and not just children and adolescents (although the mode of expression may differ depending on age).

Previous Attempts

Although it is obvious that one has to "attempt" suicide in order to commit it, it is equally clear that the event of "attempting suicide" need not have death as its objective. It is useful to think of the "attempter," now often referred to as parasuicide, and the "completor," as two sets of overlapping populations: (a) a group of those who attempt suicide, a few of whom go on to commit it, and (b) a group of those who commit suicide, a few who previously attempted it. A good deal has to do with the lethality of the event. The ratio between suicide attempts and completions in the general population is about 8:1—one committed suicide for every eight attempts; however, in teenagers some studies report a rate of 50:1, even 100:1. No such data are yet available for children.

A previous attempt is a good clue to future attempts, especially if no assistance is obtained after the first attempt. However, not all previous attempters go on to attempt again (or kill themselves). All too frequently such behavior is not taken seriously. We recall an 11-year-old (very depressed) girl who cut her wrists at school and the principal's response was merely, "She is just trying to get attention." What an extreme way to get attention! The girl was moderately lethal and highly perturbed, requiring considerable intervention.

Verbal Statements

As with behavior, the attitude toward individuals making verbal threats is too frequently negative. Statements are seen as *just for attention*. This attitude results in the writing off or ignoring the behavior of a person who is genuinely perturbed and potentially suicidal. The important question is, "Why this way of getting attention when there are so many other constructive ways?"

Examples of verbal statements from young people are the following: "I'm going to kill myself" or "I want to die," both being very direct. Other more indirect examples are the following: "I am going to see my (deceased) mother" or "I know that I'll die at an early age."

Cognitive Clues

The single most frequent state of mind of the suicidal person is *constriction*. There is a tunnel vision, a narrowing of the mind's eye. There is a narrowing of the range of perception or opinions or options that occur to the mind. Frequently, the person uses words like "only," "always," "never," and "forever." Examples of young people are the following: "No one will ever love me. Only mom loved me"; "John was the only one who loved me"; "Dad will always be that way"; and "Either I'll kill my brother or myself."

Emotional Clues

The child or teenager who is suicidal is often highly perturbed; he or she is disturbed, anxious, perhaps agitated. Depression, as already noted, is frequently evident. Teenagers are often very angry and hostile—in fact, these may well be, based on our clinical experience, more predictive of suicide than depression in youth—and they may feel boxed in, rejected, harassed, and unsuccessful. A common emotional state in most suicidal people is *hopelessness-helplessness*. The hopelessness goes something like this, "Nothing will change. It will always be this way." The helplessness goes something like this, "There is nothing I can do. There is nothing my parents can do."

Sudden Behavioral Changes

Changes in behavior are also suspect, both the outgoing individual who suddenly becomes withdrawn and isolated and the normally reserved individual who starts being outgoing and seeking thrills may be at risk. Such changes are of particular concern when a precipitating painful event is apparent. Performance in school, such as sudden failure, may be an important clue. Making final arrangements such as giving away a record collection, a favorite watch, or other possessions may be ominous and often not responded to by the receiver; the receiver is simply too pleased to get the "gift." A sudden preoccupation with death, such as reading and talking about death, may be a clue. Nonetheless, constructive discussion of this topic as a class project may be helpful for the individual and his or her classmates. We remember a 16-year-old girl who asked us for help with a class project after the suicide of a 12-year-old boy she had known as a babysitter. It seemed to be a very constructive task for her.

Life-Threatening Behavior

We recall a 9-year-old boy who killed himself who had previously been seen leaning out of an open window in his apartment as well as, at another time, playing with a gun. We also know about a 17-year-old teenager who died in a single car accident on an isolated road after having had several similar accidents following his mother's death. *Self-destruction is not rare.* Often alcoholism, drug addiction, mismanagement of medical treatment and automobile accidents can be seen in this light. Farberow (1980) has called this "the many faces of suicide." Here are a number of questions:

Why did the young child, knowing that the gun was loaded and warned by his parents, play with it?

Why did the teenager drive so fast on a slippery wet road when he knew for the last 3 months that his brakes were bad?

Why did a person, knowing what cocaine can do to you, get hooked?

We are not suggesting that these young people intentionally want to die; yet, their behavior made them as "good as dead."

Suicide Notes

Like previous attempts and verbal statements, suicide notes are important clues; however, they are often read but not listened to by the reader. Notes are very rarely written by children, but not by adolescents. Although most adolescents who kill themselves do not leave a note, Michel (1988) has documented that notes are more frequently written by teenagers than by adults. Art work, diaries, music, and other personal documents can be seen as similar expressive behavioral manifestations. We remember one suicide note stating, "I finally completed something I've always wanted to do. I removed the guilt from every person. . . p.s. Happy Father's Day." Figure 1 presents a number of other *genuine* suicide notes. They are presented here to allow the reader to better understand the subjective frame of mind of our young people who actually kill themselves.

We would also like to offer one final note here that is a "suicidal" note, not a suicide note. It was written by an 11-year-old girl (of high perturbation, but low lethality) who was contemplating suicide. She wrote the following to her teacher:

1. Single, age 13, male

I know what I am doing. Annette I found out. Ask Carol. I love you all.

Bill

2. Single, age 16, female

Dear Mother & Dad

Please forgive me. I have tried to be good to you both. I love you both very much and wanted to get along with you both. I have tried.

I have wanted to go out with you & Dad but I was always afraid to ask for I always felt that the answer would be no.

And about Bill, I want to dismiss every idea about him. I don't like any more than a comparison, for a while I though I did not no more, in fact, I am quite tired of him, as you know, I get tired of everyone after a while.

And mother, I wish you hadn't called me a liar, and said I was just like Hap. as I'm not. It is just that I am afraid of you both at times, but I love you both very much.

So long,
Your loving daughter
That will always
love you
Mary

P.S. Please forgive me. I want you to, and don't think for one minute that I haven't appreciated everything you've done.

3. Single, age 18, male

My life would have been a failure anyway. I guess I could have changed, but I just didn't have the will power. I'm sick of suffering and sick of seeing you suffer. Tell ________, Aunt ________, & ________ I love them and am sorry but this is the best way. Return my 2 library books & give my literature books back to school. Demand a refund of $15 tuition & $15 class dues. Bury me in my blue suit & new shoes. Pallbearer ________ ________ ________ ________.

You will find me in the garage.

Figure 1. A sample of suicide notes.

Hi hows your day going? I hope fine. I've been trying hard in french real hard Mrs. T. I know what im going to say isnt your problem but I just needed to tell someone my feelings I can't keep it in. I hate living I want to die noone understands why I cant explain why. I wish I wasn't born why did it hapen to me why did God make me. I'm frightened to get my tests signed even when good ones. I'm scared of failing. No-one really cares any way your a nice friend, special. I hope you have a nice future. The best I really like you and sometimes im afraid to live scared—I want to kill myself but I can't do it cause its against the law. Ill go to the oppisite of heaven. I really like you and want to say your a great friend. I love my family alot also. I love you. Other kids think im a baby writing notes. If it weren't for my stupid eyes I wouldn't be as ugly. I don't understand why im so ugly. I'm not feeling sorry for myself I'm just telling you how i feel inside. I don't want to pass cause i want to stay here with you. Sorry if I buged you or took up your time.
I hate life
P.S. you probably can't read my writing

What is important here is that the teacher, the parents, and the professionals did something. People understood the significance of the behavioral manifestations.

CONCLUDING REMARK

Suicide and suicidal behavior in children and adolescents does occur. We all need to increase our understanding. This chapter should be seen as an introduction to some of the theoretical/clinical and behavioral aspects of a *multidimensional malaise* in school-age children and adolescents. It is apparent to us that this chapter has a number of limitations. Some of it is idiosyncratic, being what we have learned to be important. Some of it is too abstract, lacking empirical data. Even where there is research, it is limited. For example, are we discussing suicide? Parasuicide? We need, as the chapter by Benjafield suggests, to *develop* our understanding. However, our chapter, we hope, will be heuristic at this time in understanding a child or adolescent who defines an issue for which suicide is perceived as the best solution.

ACKNOWLEDGMENTS. We would like to thank E. Shneidman, C. Pfeffer, and the American Association of Suicidology for their contributions; many of the ideas in this chapter were gleaned from them. Appreciation is expressed to the Suicide Prevention/Awareness Committee, Windsor, for cooperation in gathering some of the data.

REFERENCES

Barraclough, B. (1986). The relation between mental illness, physical illness and suicide. In J. Morgan (Ed.), *Suicide: Helping those at risk.* London: King's College.

Berman, A. (1986, April). *Suicidal youth.* Paper presented at the conference of the American Association of Suicidology, Atlanta, GA.

Brenner, M. (1988, April). *Economic and behavioral risk factors. Accounting for suicide over the life cycle.* Paper presented at the conference of the American Association of Suicidology, Washington, DC.

Corder, B., & Haizlip, T. (1984). Environmental and personality similarities in case histories of suicide and self-poisoning in children under ten. *Suicide and Life-Threatening Behavior, 14,* 59–66.

Corder, B., Parker, P., & Corder, R. (1974). Parental history, family communication and interaction patterns in adolescent suicide. *Family Therapy, 3,* 185–190.

Farberow, N. (Ed.). (1980). *The many faces of suicide.* New York: McGraw-Hill.

Fryer, J. (1986). Aids and suicide. In J. Morgan (Ed.), *Suicide: Helping those at risk.* London: King's College.

Leenaars, A. (1985). Suicide postvention in a school system. *Canada's Mental Health, 33-4,* 29–30.

Leenaars, A. (1986, June). *Suicide prevention in school systems.* Workshop presented at the Canadian Psychological Association. Toronto, Ontario, Canada.

Leenaars, A. (1988). Preventing youth suicide: Education is the key. *Dimensions in Health Service,* October, 22–24.

Leenaars, A., & Wenckstern, S. (Eds.). (1990). *Suicide prevention in schools.* Washington, DC: Hemisphere Publishing.

Maris, R. (1985). The adolescent suicide problem. *Suicide and Life-Threatening Behavior, 15,* 91–109.

Marzuk, P. (1989, April). Aids-related suicides. Paper presented at the conference of the American Association of Suicidology, San Diego, CA.

Menninger, K. (1938). *Man against himself.* New York: Harcourt.

Michel, K. (1988). Suicide in young people is different. *Crisis, 9,* 135–145.

Peck, M. (1985). Crisis intervention treatment with chronically and acutely suicidal adolescents. In M. Peck, N. Farberow, & R. Litman (Eds.), *Youth suicide.* New York: Springer.

Pfeffer, C. (1986). *The suicidal child.* New York: Guilford.

Pfeffer, C. (1981a). Suicidal behavior of children: A review with implications for research and practice. *American Journal of Psychiatry, 138,* 154–160.

Pfeffer, C. (1981b). The family system of suicidal children. *American Journal of Psychotherapy, 35,* 330–341.

Phillips, D. (1986, April). *Effect of the media.* Paper presented at the conference of the American Association of Suicidology, Atlanta, GA.

Rourke, B., & Fisk, J. (1981). Socio-emotional disturbances of learning disabled children: The role of central processing deficits. *Bulletin of the Orthopsychiatry Society, 31,* 77–88.

Rourke, B., Young, G., & Leenaars, A. (1989). A childhood learning disability that predisposes those afflicted to adolescent and adult depression and suicide risk. *Journal of Learning Disabilities, 22,* 169–175.

Seiden, R. (1984). The youthful suicide epidemic. *Public Affairs Report.* Los Angeles: Regents of the University of California.

Shneidman, E. (1985). *Definition of suicide.* New York: Wiley.

Smith, K., & Crawford, S. (1986). Suicidal behavior among "normal" high school students. *Suicide and Life-Threatening Behavior, 16,* 313–325.

Toolan, J. (1981). Depression and suicide in children: An overview. *American Journal of Psychotherapy, 35,* 311–322.

9

Child and Adolescent Suicide
From the Nomothetic to the Idiographic

Alan L. Berman

AND THE WALLS CAME TUMBLING DOWN

Penny (she liked that much better than Penelope), a black female, was only 12 years old, but already she had lived a lifetime. Her cocaine-addicted father walked out when she was 5, only weeks after her brother was born and was diagnosed as having cerebral palsy. Her father was never to be seen again. As a single parent, Penny's mother was overwhelmed with the demands of attending to her brother's needs. Penny frequently was thrust into a surrogate parent role in order to help her mother merely cope. Yet, Penny was still a child and when her mother could afford them, babysitters were hired to alleviate the stress on both Penny and her mom. That was the good news. The bad news was that one babysitter, a middle-aged woman, had a teenage son who, whenever he could, sexually abused Penny. As is common to scripts like this, Penny was "sworn to secrecy" lest some more intolerable fate were to befall her or her brother. So the walls went up.

Penny withdrew into herself. A bright student at first, her school performance faltered. For the past 6 months (now in the 3rd year of abuse), she had difficulty concentrating. She complained of dysmenorrhea. She increasingly threw temper tantrums and was oppositional toward her mother and her teachers. More often, she simply would avoid her teachers, her work, and her peers; she missed 15 days of school in one recent 30-day period. Twice, unbeknownst to anyone, she tried a different kind of withdrawal, toying with some of her mother's sleeping pills, taking "a few to test out how long [she] would sleep."

Three days prior to her death, Penny watched a television movie about sexual abuse . . .

ALAN L. BERMAN • Department of Psychology, American University, Washington, D.C. 20016.

and the walls came tumbling down. Penny's rage, fear, and sense of worthlessness tearfully poured out to her mother, along with her story of abuse. With her mother's disbelief, there now emerged in Penny a panic that her abuser's threats now would be enacted. No one had a chance to console her or help her. Her anxiety simply overwhelmed her; and death must have looked inviting as relief. And it became immediately possible when she found the .22 caliber handgun her mother had hidden in the rear of her nightstand. Now she had peace in her grasp. Now she became a statistic.

THE NOMOTHETIC NET

Cases such as Penny's, taken collectively, have provided researchers with an epidemiological snapshot of youth suicide. Cases additively contribute to estimates of prevalence and incidence (rates per 100,000 population) that, in turn, allow for temporal comparisons (e.g., changes in rates over time) and to subgroup comparisons (e.g., males vs. females, whites vs. blacks, young vs. old, etc.). Differences in the distribution of cases in different populations or at different times suggest general explanatory factors and theories that may define risk variables. Once validated, knowledge of risk factors may lead to the early detection of and intervention with defined at-risk youth as well as larger scale preventive efforts, thus lowering the prevalence and incidence of suicide and suicidal behavior among youth in the future.

Much has been learned, to date, from this nomothetic approach. Among the generally validated findings regarding youth suicide in the United States, for example, are that suicide completions increase with age into the early 20s, are four to five times as frequent among males as among females, are most common and occur at about twice the rate among white males as among nonwhite males, and are most likely to occur by use of firearms by both males and females.

It is neither the intent nor purpose of this chapter to summarize these large-scale research findings as several reasonably current reviews and their implications for prevention are available to the reader (cf. Berman, 1986a; Shaffer, 1988; Shaffer, Garland, Gould, Fisher, & Trautman, 1988).

As valuable and important as these studies are, they typically paint with such a broad brush that the caregiver is potentially and inadvertently misled; additionally, they obscure significant discriminations necessary for their translation into clinically relevant tools. Take, for example, the demographic profile outlined above, one that frequently is most cited in establishing risk profiles, that is, suicide is most frequent among older white males. Of what value would that risk profile have been were the reader-clinician confronted with interviewing Penny (a black female, aged 12) in the last 2 days of her life? Demography has little use in our understanding and assessment of the individual case who may be atypical of at-risk suicides on one level, yet greatly at risk for suicide on another.

Perhaps nowhere is this complication more apparent than in the study of differences between youthful suicide completers and parasuicides. In contrast to the former group, adolescent parasuicides are predominantly females who ingest drugs at home in front of others with, therefore, questionable intent to die. Estimates of lethality for the typical parasuicide appropriately would be low. Yet, one of the generally agreed-upon risk factors for suicide completion is a prior suicide attempt, particularly if there are multiple attempts even when some of these behaviors are of low lethality. Thus, clinicians and gatekeepers must be able to transcend profiles established by means of the nomothetic brush to define more clinically pertinent profiles of risk of use to the individual case.

There are a number of observations regarding youth suicide that often appear in the professional literature and in material distributed for gatekeeper education (e.g., lists of "warning signs") that through repetition have become adopted practically as universal truths. The quality of research (Berman & Carroll, 1984) and the sophistication of research strategies to date (Smith & Maris, 1986) should make us wary of what we believe and considerably more questioning of what we know about youth at risk. There, indeed, is much that we can agree on and much we yet need to discern. What follows is the author's admittedly selective, gun and camera safari through the research literature and some observational caveats.

Suicide as a Rank-Ordered Cause of Death Among Youth

It has little meaning to note that suicide is the third leading cause of death among adolescents aged 15 to 24. First, suicide is a *manner* of death, not a cause. Second, there are essentially only four determinations of manner of death available to the coroner and medical examiner, excluding undeterminable deaths: natural, accidental, suicidal, and homicidal. Natural deaths (illnesses and diseases) are rare at young ages. More than three fourths of mortalities among 15- to 24-year-olds are due to injuries (Baker, O'Neill, & Karpf, 1984), with the overwhelming majority of these being unintentional and resulting from motor vehicle accidents. That leaves suicide and homicide, with almost equal numbers annually such that in 1985 suicide ranked second and homicide third, but their positions were reversed in both 1984 and 1986. Third, the 15 to 24 age group is too broad. There are different trends evident when smaller age ranges are compared, for example, 15 to 19, and 20 to 24 (cf. Fingerhut & Kleinman, 1988).

Youth Suicide and Demographics

As noted above, it is necessary that we focus increasingly on subgroup demographics in order to have clinical utility. Most studies of suicidal youth have been conducted in urban settings; little is known empirically about those youth living and dying in rural settings. Blacks undoubtedly are different from whites, but most of what is written about black youth suicide is theoretical and lacking in discrimination (no pun intended), that is, applies to all blacks and insufficiently attends to black suicides as different from black nonsuicides no less from white suicides.

One noteworthy example of the state of the art with regard to race and ethnicity as risk variables is that of Native American youth, an often defined high-risk group. Reported rates of completed suicides among Native American youth vary from a low of 0 per 100,000 to well over 100 per 100,000 annually depending on tribe, blood type, or reservation (Berman, 1980; Shore, 1975). To talk about Native Americans as one homogeneous group blurs important distinctions necessary to understand self-destructive patterns among some and health-promoting patterns among others, the latter of which has received practically no research attention whatsoever. It is probable that similar distinctions need to be made among whites, blacks, males, females, and so forth.

Predisposing Conditions versus Precipitating Events

The same lack of discrimination is evident in the excessive interest shown in precipitating events, none of which appears profoundly helpful to our understanding of the when or why of suicidal behaviors among youth. Shaffer et al. (1988), for example, note that many teens complete suicide "in the context of an acute disciplinary crisis or shortly after a rejection or humiliation." These observers then correctly note that these observations have no useful implication for prevention or intervention because these are events (stresses) common to all youth, they are not readily avoided, and there typically is too short an interval between event and suicidal response to allow for preventive intervention.

What is inestimably more important for us to understand are those conditions that predispose a youth to be vulnerable to everyday negative life events in such a way that suicidal behavior is the observed response. Here there are both some singular faults and some exciting trends in the empirical literature on youth suicide literature.

Despite the trend in the more general literature to not describe suicidal youth as mentally disordered, the empirical literature overwhelmingly has documented a variety of diagnosable conditions as risk factors. It is true that the transient thought of suicide is not pathologic (in contrast to existential), but enacting some active behavior toward self-harm or self-destruction, regardless of intent, reflects some breakdown in the drive toward self-preservation, in defensive structure and in adaptational flexibility. Suicidal behavior is not simply "problem-solving." It reflects the inoperability of problem-solving thinking, aggression, poor or inadequate control over impulsivity, an inability to effectively use available resources and psychological supplies (or the unavailability of same). These are reflections of psychopathology.

Elsewhere (Berman, in press) I have suggested that there appear to be eight discernible "types" of adolescent suicides, all but one of which (and that being typically the least lethal) are related to diagnostic labels: depressed, substance abusing, personality disordered (borderline and/or schizotypal), antisocial (conduct disordered), isolated loner (schizoid), rigid perfectionist (obsessive-compulsive), psychotic, and crisis-responder impulsive.

Still, this focus is far too cloudy. The great majority of even these types are not suicidal in their behavior. Shaffer and Bacon (1986), for example, have estimated that the ratio of depressed to depressed suicidal adolescents is approximately 660:1 (for males).

Depression is the most frequently cited form of pathology underlying suicide; the symptoms of depression most often comprising the majority of those proferred "warning signs" of suicide. However, the relationship between depression and suicidality is complex. Depression appears most directly related to suicide ideation (Pfeffer, Zuckerman, Plutchik, & Mizruchi, 1984; Velez & Cohen, 1988); and ideators with depression have been differentiated from depressives without ideation primarily in terms of the former having more disturbed intrafamilial relationships (Kosky, Silburn, & Zubrick, 1986).

Among suicide completers, however, a more complicated picture emerges. Although bipolar symptoms have been found to be common to completers (Brent, Perper, Goldstein, Kolko, Allan, Allman, & Zelenak, 1988; Shafii, Carrigan, Whittinghill, & Derrick, 1985), conduct disorders and substance abuse disorders appear to predominate in samples of adolescent completers (Shaffer & Gould, 1987; Shafii et al., 1985). The relationship between depression and suicide attempts is not all that clear (Carlson & Cantwell, 1982) and may be mediated by both deficits in cognitive coping strategies (Asaranow, Carlson, & Guthrie, 1987) and hopelessness (Kazdin, Rodgers, & Colbus, 1986). Even here, however, there appear to be differences noted in the role hopelessness plays in suicidal attempts among adolescents in contrast to its clear mediational role found among adult populations (Rotheram-Borus & Trautman, 1988).

Among children, although no particular diagnosis stands out as associated with suicidal tendencies (Pfeffer, Lipkins, Plutchik, & Mizruchi, 1988), there is almost universal agreement that suicidality signals pathology and, most probably, pathology in the family as well (Orbach, 1986; Pfeffer, 1986; Rosenthal, Rosenthal, Doherty, & Santora, 1986).

It has been well documented among adults that psychopathology, in general, is associated with higher rates of early mortality, particularly violent death, but long-term follow-up studies of younger populations have yet to be reported. Among adolescents, the variety of associated pathologies noted above await significant subgroup-controlled research studies to distinguish which high achieving, perfectionistic youngsters are at risk, who among borderlines are more lethal, and so on (cf. Eaton & Reynolds, 1985).

Similarly, among adults there is a developing zeitgeist, paralleling the biologic movement in psychiatry, to pinpoint biologic markers of later suicidality. These studies have focused primarily on serotonergic neurotransmission, particularly of the metabolite CSF 5-HIAA, and variables associated with certain neuroendocrine functions (Asberg, Nordstrom, & Traskman-Bendz, 1986) and genetics (Kety, 1986); however, there is little data as yet to support these as accounting for a significant amount of the variance in suicidal behavior observed in adolescence.

Two related areas of inquiry do appear to be promising, that of the influence of co-morbidity and that pertaining to the role of substance abuse.

Co-morbidity Increasingly, research is recognizing that the co-occurrence of pathologies or multiple symptoms describe the suicidal youngster. In particular, depression and various presentations of anxiety or panic appear corelated among samples of suicidal individuals (Bernstein & Garfinkel, 1984; Mattison, 1988; Miller, 1986; Pospiszyl, 1985). As well, depression and conduct disorders (Alessi, McManus, Brickman, & Grapentine, 1984) and depression and substance abuse (Crumley, 1979) are frequently noted as co-morbid diagnoses among adolescent suicide attempters.

Substance Abuse A number of studies have found substance abuse to be more common among samples of adolescent attempters than among samples of controls (Garfinkel, Froese, & Hood, 1982; Riggs, Alvario, McHorney, DeChristopher, & Crombie, 1986; Slap, 1988). Similarly, substance abuse histories have been found in 15% to 33% of adolescent completers (Hoberman & Garfinkel, 1988; Poteet, 1987; Thompson, 1987), with case-control comparisons again documenting significant differences (Shaffer et al., 1987; Shafii et al., 1985).

To date, however, there has been little research focused on differentiating which substance abusers may be at risk. In addition to conduct disorders, as noted above, those factors that may serve as concurrent or intervening risk variables are co-morbid depression (Berman & Schwartz, 1990; Stefanis & Kokkevi, 1987), recent interpersonal disruptions (Rich, Fowler, Fogarty, & Young, 1988), and parental drug abuse (Berman & Schwartz, 1990).

THE IDIOGRAPHIC UNDERSTANDING OF YOUTH SUICIDE

As we refine our profiles of at-risk youth through more sophisticated research methodologies and study, we may develop sufficient clinical tools to apply to the assessment of the suicidal youngster. With a focus on risk profiles particular to black females, with a clearer understanding of the role of co-morbid symptom presentations of depression, oppositional behavior, and intense anxiety, we may have been more alert to Penny's suicidal risk and have been able to intervene before she effected her death.

Ultimately, the true understanding of suicidal behavior must rest on more idiographic methods, through intensive study of unique and individual suicidal cases such as that of Penny. Here the *meaning* of suicidal behavior becomes clearer, both as it relates to the adolescent and to those charged with developing preventive interventions. Consider the following case of Kathy, whose unique story has some clear parallels with that of Penny.

Kathy's father walked out on her mother when Kathy was in utero. In response, and since it was too late to abort her pregnancy, Kathy's mother purposely tried but failed to miscarry.

Upon hearing her mother later relate this story, Kathy began to understand why she felt she had to prove herself "worthy just to exist." As a single parent, Kathy's mother had to work to support Kathy and her older sister. In order to facilitate this, Kathy and her sister were delivered to their maternal grandmother for parenting. Kathy grew clingingly close to her grandmother over the next several years, later describing her grandmother as "the only person who ever loved me."

When Kathy was 10, her father, whom she had never seen, kidnapped both girls from their grandmother's house. During the next 2½ years during which Kathy and her sister lived in hiding with their father, Kathy was frequently and severely abused physically by him. As if that were not enough, twice she was almost killed by her sister who years later would be diagnosed and institutionalized as a paranoid schizophrenic. Kathy reported that she was convinced she was going to die by the hands of one or the other of these family members. In addition, Kathy cried herself to sleep every night because she so missed her grandmother.

Somehow, Kathy endured. Reunited with her mother, whom Kathy believed neither loved nor wanted her; still suffering the uncounted effects of years of abuse and violence; Kathy, now at the age of 13, suffered the precipitous death of her grandmother from a heart attack. Deeply mourning the loss of the one person from whom she had incorporated any sense of self-worth, Kathy wished both to die and to lie side by side with her grandmother. On her 14th birthday, Kathy ingested a drug cocktail amounting to some 85 different pills culled from her mother's medicine chest. To her dismay, she was inadvertently discovered by her mother, hospitalized, and consequently involved in the first of several short-lived attempts at therapeutic intervention.

For the next several years, Kathy ambivalently chose life. Diagnosed as having co-morbid affective and borderline personality disorders, Kathy struggled, unsuccessfully, to find a stable and healthier sense of herself. She was bright and attempted to prove her worth through her academics, at which she was reasonably successful. Interpersonally, however, she was understandably unable to trust, so she formed few significant friendships. At best, she managed a fragile alliance with an older female teacher, no doubt a symbolic replacement for her grandmother. This alliance, however, was insufficient to thwart her second serious suicide attempt at the age of 17.

During her senior year in high school, Kathy had her first significant heterosexual relationship. She dated Carl for 3 months and had her first sexual experience with him. But Carl increasingly began to show *his* instability. As arguments and coercion replaced the blush of first love, Kathy attempted to break off the relationship. Carl's response was to severely beat and rape her. Kathy, in turn, responded by entering her mother's car at 2 a.m. and in the closed garage ran the engine until the carbon monoxide fumes could bring her the peace of death. Her mother, awakened by the smell of gas, once again intervened and rushed Kathy to the emergency room. Initially, Kathy was given but a 20% chance of survival. But, she beat the odds, recovering after a lengthy hospitalization with but a slight memory loss—a loss we might have wished for her had it been selective, only for the abuse and trauma of her life.

Kathy felt that her life lacked value. She was the way she had been treated, and her death was compelled by an urgent and intense need to end her pain. Although both of her suicide attempts were death intentioned, this attempt had a very different motivation than did her first. This attempt was a desperate, rageful protest; a rejection of what her life had been and of a future predicted to have only more of the same. The *meaning* of her second attempt was defined by goals of escape and relief, profoundly influenced by hopelessness and rage.

Suicide is inherently motivated and controlled by feelings of pain, entrapment, and hopelessness. When the British psychiatrist Hawton (1987) asked parasuicidal patients to explain their overdose attempts, the most frequently expressed "reason" given was, "The situation was so unbearable that [I] had to do something and [I] didn't know what else to do." Next most frequently cited was "to get relief from a terrible state of mind," followed by "to escape [for a while] an impossible situation." In these patients' words we hear echoed these themes: painful affect, entrapment, unendurability, cognitive constriction, hopelessness, helplessness, and solutions of escape and relief. Embedded in these statements are 7 of the 10 "common characteristics" of suicide elucidated by Shneidman (1985) in his psychological model of suicide (see Chapter 4, this volume).

Kathy's third near-death experience was not an overt suicide attempt. About a year after her carbon monoxide attempt, still depressed and feeling devalued, but, nevertheless, functional, she was driving home from work late one night. She had taken an antihistamine for some cold symptoms and remembered fighting drowsiness. She lost that fight, awakening to great pain and profuse bleeding after her car had crossed the highway median, striking another car head-on. Miraculously, both drivers survived. As Kathy later reported, "I believed at that moment I could have just let myself die . . . But, I couldn't let myself . . . not this way . . . This was not *my* decision . . . *I* wanted to be in control of my death . . . I fought to live."

Kathy's words convey a powerful reminder about another important understanding of suicidal behaviors. Whereas the operational definition of suicide must be culture-free, its *meaning* cannot be free of a sociocultural context. For Kathy, suicide represented some semblance of *control* in (and perhaps *of*) a pathologic environment. Had she merely wanted death, it was within her grasp on that highway. When life feels outside of one's control, suicide appears as the ultimate existential answer, as the only true form of mastery and control. It is this premise that fuels the arguments of those who propose that there can be a "rational suicide." But, this logic is irrational. As suicide appears to be the ultimate statement of autonomy, of free-will and choice, it can only seriously be considered by one who feels no free-will, but, rather, trapped and controlled by unbearable forces with which one otherwise cannot cope.

An 18-year-old patient of mine, referred on discharge from a hospitalization necessitated because he had slashed his wrists and smeared blood all over his apartment walls in a fit of rage, described his now relative calm with the phrase, "It's now more blue than red." I first thought he was telling me that the crisis had abated, that he now was out of suicidal danger. Had I not intuitively distrusted that message, I might not have asked to know more. What he told me he *meant* was that he now felt no anxiety about hurting himself, that his wrist cutting had served as a successful dress rehearsal, defusing his stage fright about being self-destructive. Now he had a way out, a hope, posed by the option of suicide. He now no longer felt only hopelessness and rage. Instead, he had peace and direction.

Increasingly, I believe, this sense of suicidal death as a form of control in an uncontrollable world defines what appears to be a more normative "acceptability" of suicidal behavior as a solution to painful problems prevalent among today's youth. Mack (1986) refers to this in a discussion about suicide with his 18-year-old son who remarked, "It's an option that's opened up" (p.57); and at least one Canadian study (Boldt, 1982) has documented cross-generationally the great acceptability of suicide to youth. In part, it is this context that may help explain increased frequencies of suicide among modern day youth in societies marked by greater instability and rapidly changing value systems.

Today's sociocultural context provides dramatic and provocative testament to the different world of today's child and adolescent. In the United States, rates of divorce have doubled over the last two decades, leaving significantly more children in single-parent living situations. Teen pregnancies and births have increased threefold since the early 1960s; rates of arrests and juvenile court cases have doubled; and homicides have increased at about the same rate, with the character of urban homicides increasingly occurring in a drug-related context (Berman & Cohen-Sandler, 1982). As well, we can document dramatic increases in the availability of and accessibility to means of violence and self-destruction (Brent et al., 1988) and a greater exposure to violent stimuli in the media (Berman, 1986b). As but one example, 1 in 10 of today's movies depicts a suicide attempt or completion of a major character, three times the frequency of exposure of 40 years ago (Berman, 1986c).

This is the sociocultural frame within which individual lives and deaths are played out. Youthful deaths that *collectively* are too frequently violent and self-inflicted. Youthful lives that must be attended to *individually* in order to significantly lessen the tragedy of child and adolescent suicide.

REFERENCES

Alessi, N. E., McManus, M., Brickman, A., & Grapentine, L. (1984). Suicidal behavior among serious juvenile offenders. *American Journal of Psychiatry, 141*, 286–287.

Asaranow, J. R., Carlson, G., & Guthrie, D. (1987). Coping strategies, self-perceptions, hopelessness and perceived family environments in depressed and suicidal children. *Journal of Consulting and Clinical Psychology, 55*, 361–366.

Asberg, M., Nordstrom, P., & Traskman-Bendz, L. (1986). Biological factors in suicide. In A. Roy (Ed.), *Suicide*. Baltimore: Williams and Wilkins.

Baker, S. P., O'Neill, B., & Karpf, R. (1984). *The injury fact book*. Lexington, MA: Lexington, Books.

Berman, A. L. (1980). Indian suicides: The Duck Valley Reservation. *Nevada Public Affairs Review*, No. 1, 24–31.

Berman, A. L. (1986a). Adolescent suicide: Issues and challenges, *Seminars in Adolescent Medicine, 2*, 269–277.

Berman, A. L. (1986b, June). *Mass media and youth suicide prevention*. Paper presented at the National Conference on Prevention and Intervention in Youth Suicide, Oakland, CA.

Berman, A. L. (1986c, April). *Suicide and the American film*. Paper presented at the American Association of Suicidology convention, Atlanta, GA.

Berman, A. L. (in press). Child and adolescent suicide: Research findings. In J. McIntosh & J. Santos (Eds.), *Suicide across the life cycle*. New York: Springer-Verlag.

Berman, A. L., & Carroll, T. A. (1984). Adolescent suicide: A critical review. *Death education, 8* (Suppl.), 53–64.

Berman, A. L., & Cohen-Sandler, R. (1982). Childhood and adolescent suicide research: A critique. *Crisis, 3*, 3–15.

Berman, A. L., & Schwartz, R. (1990). Suicide attempts among adolescent drug users. *American Journal of Diseases of Children, 144*, 310–314.

Bernstein, G. A., & Garfinkel, B. D. (1984). School phobia: The overlap of affective disorders and anxiety disorders. *Journal of the American Academy of Child and Adolescent Psychiatry, 25*, 235–241.

Boldt, M. (1982). Normative evaluations of suicide and death: A cross-generational study. *Omega, 13*, 145–157.

Brent, D. A., Perper, J. A., Goldstein, G. E., Kolko, D. J., Allan, M. J., Allman, C. J., & Zelenak, J. P. (1988). Risk factors for adolescent suicide: A comparison of adolescent suicide victims with suicidal inpatients. *Archives of General Psychiatry, 45*, 581–588.

Carlson, G. A., & Cantwell, D. P. (1982). Suicidal behavior and depression in children and adolescents. *Journal of the American Academy of Child Psychiatry, 21*, 361–368.

Crumley, F. E. (1979). Adolescent suicide attempts. *Journal of the American Medical Association, 241*, 2404–2407.

Eaton, P., & Reynolds, P. (1984). Suicide attempters presenting at an emergency department. *Canadian Journal of Psychiatry, 30*, 582–585.

Fingerhut, L. A., & Kleinman, J. D. (1988). Suicide rates for young people [letter]. *Journal of the American Medical Association, 259*, 356.

Garfinkel, B. D., Froese, A., & Hood, J. (1982). Suicide attempts in children and adolescents. *American Journal of Psychiatry, 139*, 1257–1261.

Hawton, K. (1987). *Attempted suicide*. New York: Oxford.

Hoberman, H. M., & Garfinkel, B. D. (1988). Completed suicide in children and adolescents. *Journal of the American Academy of Child and Adolescent Psychiatry, 27*, 689–695.

Kazdin, A. E., Rodgers, A., & Colbus, D. (1986). The hopelessness scale for children. *Journal of Consulting and Clinical Psychology, 54*, 241–245.

Kety, S. S. (1986). Genetic factors in suicide. In A. Roy (Ed.), *Suicide*. Baltimore: Williams and Wilkins.

Kosky, R., Silburn, S., & Zubrick, S. (1986). Symptomatic depression and suicidal ideation: A comparative study with children. *Journal of Nervous and Mental Disease, 174*, 523–528.

Mack, J. (1986). Adolescent suicide: An architectural model. In G. L. Klerman (Ed.), *Suicide and depression among adolescents and young adults*. Washington, DC: American Psychiatric Press.

Mattison, R. E. (1988). Suicide and other consequences of childhood and adolescent anxiety disorders. *Journal of Clinical Psychiatry, 49* (Suppl 10), 9–11.

Miller, D. (1986). Affective disorders and violence in adolescents. *Hospital and Community Psychiatry, 37*, 591–596.

Orbach, I. (1986). The "insolvable problem" as a determinant in the dynamics of suicidal behavior in children. *American Journal of Psychotherapy, 40*, 511–520.

Pfeffer, C. R. (1986). *The suicidal child*. New York: Guilford.

Pfeffer, C. R., Lipkins, R., Plutchik, R., & Mizurchi, M. (1988). Normal children at risk for suicidal behavior: A 2-year follow-up study. *Journal of the American Academy of Child and Adolescent Psychiatry, 27*, 34–41.

Pfeffer, C. R., Zuckerman, S., Plutchik, R., & Mizruchi, M. (1984). Suicidal behavior in normal school children: A comparison with child psychiatric inpatients. *Journal of the American Academy of Child and Adolescent Psychiatry, 23*, 416–423.

Pospiszyl, K. (1985). Extraversion, neuroticism and anxiety in self-injurers and suicide attempters. *Polish Psychological Bulletin, 16*, 109–112.

Poteet, D. J. (1987). Adolescent suicide: A review of 87 cases of completed suicide in Shelby county, TN. *American Journal of Forensic Medicine and Pathology, 8*, 12–17.

Rich, G. L., Fowler, R. C., Fogarty, L. A., & Young, D. (1988). San Diego suicide study: III. Relationship between diagnoses and stressors. *Archives of General Psychiatry, 45*, 589–592.

Riggs, S., Alario, A., McHorney, C., De Christopher, J., & Crombie, P. (1986). Abuse and health related risk-taking behaviors in high school students who have attempted suicide. *Journal of Developmental-Behavioral Pediatrics, 7*, 205–206.

Rosenthal, P., Rosenthal, S., Doherty, M. B., & Santora, D. (1986). Suicidal thoughts and behaviors in depressed hospitalized preschoolers. *American Journal of Psychotherapy, 40*, 201–212.

Rotheran-Borus, M. J., & Trautman, P. D. (1988). Hopelessness, depression and suicidal intent among adolescent suicide attempters. *Journal of the American Academy of Child and Adolescent Psychiatry, 27*, 700–704.

Shaffer, D. (1988). The epidemiology of teen suicide: An examination of risk factors. *Journal of Clinical Psychiatry, 49* (Suppl 9), 36–39.

Shaffer, C., & Bacon, K. (1986). *A critical review of prevention intervention efforts in suicide with particular reference to youth suicide*. Paper presented at the national conference on prevention and intervention in youth suicide, Oakland, CA.

Shaffer, C., Garland, A., Gould, M., Fisher, P., & Trautman, P. (1988). Preventing teenage suicide: A critical review. *Journal of the American Academy of Child and Adolescent Psychiatry, 27*, 675–687.

Shaffer, D., & Gould, M. (1987). A study of completed and attempted suicide in adolescents (Grant No. MH 38198). Progress Report. Rockville, MD: NIMH.

Shafii, M., Carrigan, S., Whittinghill, J. R., & Derrick, A. (1985). Psychological autopsy of completed suicide in children and adolescents. *American Journal of Psychiatry*, 142, 1061–1064.

Shneidman, E. S. (1985). *The definition of suicide*. New York: Wiley.

Shore, J. H. (1975). American Indian suicide—Fact and fantasy. *Psychiatry*, *38*, 86–91.

Slap, G. B. (1988, April). *Risk factors for adolescent suicide attempts*. Paper presented at the American Association of Suicidology convention, Washington, DC.

Smith, K., & Maris, R. (1986). Suggested recommendations for the study of suicide and other life-threatening behaviors. *Suicide and Life-Threatening Behaviors*, *16*, 67–69.

Stefanis, C. N., & Kokkevi, A. (1987). Depression and drug use. *Psychopathology*, *19* (Suppl 2), 124–131.

Thompson, T. R. (1987). Childhood and adolescent suicide in Manitoba. *Canadian Journal of Psychiatry*, *142*, 1061–1064.

Velez, C. N., & Cohen, P. (1988). Suicidal behavior and ideation in a community sample of children: Maternal and youth reports. *Journal of the American Academy of Child and Adolescent Psychiatry*, *27*, 349–356.

10

Suicide in the Young Adult

Antoon A. Leenaars

In recent years, a great deal of attention has been focused on suicide in the young. However, by expanding one's view of "young," it becomes immediately obvious that young adults are more at risk than other groups of young people. Indeed, one of the most concerning trends in suicide today is the alarming rate of suicide—and parasuicide—for young adults. Very recent research, including research on the *suicide notes* they leave, demonstrates a very important observation on this at-risk group: *the suicide of young adults is different from that of other adults.*

A difficult problem in suicide research is the matter of obtaining suitable data. Shneidman and Farberow (1957), Maris (1981), and others have suggested the following possible data sources: statistics, third party interviews, the study of nonfatal suicide attempters, and documents (including suicide notes). Each of these sources has its limitations, yet each has proven valuable in expanding our understanding of suicide. Suicide notes are an especially rewarding source of data. For example, with respect to life-span issues, the very earliest research on suicide notes clearly indicated that age is important in understanding suicide.

Though published studies on age as a significant variable in the writings of individuals who killed themselves date from Shneidman and Farberow's work (1957), few subsequent studies of suicide notes have examined this variable. The few studies published on age (Darbonne, 1969; Leenaars, 1987; Leenaars & Balance, 1984c; Lester & Hummel, 1980; Lester & Reeve, 1982; Tuckman,

ANTOON A. LEENAARS • Private Practice, 880 Ouelette Avenue, Suite 702, Windsor, Ontario, Canada N9A 1C7.

Kleiner, & Lavell, 1959) indicate the following: (1) suicidal ideation varies with age; (2) inwardly directed aggression is more prevalent in younger adults; (3) younger adults are more harsh, self-critical, and self-depreciating; and (4) older adults exhibit a greater wish to die. In recent studies on suicide notes, Leenaars (1987, 1988a, 1989a,b) showed that young adults may differ significantly from other adults in their suicide.

CLASSIFICATION OF AGE: A DEVELOPMENTAL SCHEMA

Various students of suicide notes have divided their age samples differently; this makes direct comparison among studies difficult. Various definitions of young, old, and so on cloud the literature. This problem reflects in part the difficulty of obtaining adequate samples of notes themselves. Given a current archive of over 1,200 suicide notes, we have proposed an a priori classification of age in the hope of bringing some clarity into this difficult area (Leenaars, 1987, 1988a). Our schema has been influenced by our knowledge of adult development (Colarusso & Nemiroff, 1981; Kalish, 1975; Kimmel, 1974; Troll, 1975) and by Erikson's theoretical model on the stages (time-lines) of such development (Erikson, 1963, 1968). The three groups are young adulthood, middle adulthood, and late adulthood. The three groups with characteristics and age ranges, are shown in Table 1.

We shall recapitulate previous studies here (Leenaars, 1987, 1988a, 1989a,b), hoping to demonstrate how young adults' suicide notes and, by implication, their suicides are psychologically different from other adults. This observation is important not only to understand the suicides of young adults, but also because most previous studies of suicide notes have utilized Shneidman and Farberow's 1957 sample. The age range for that sample was 25 to 59, being generally consistent with only middle adulthood. We must ask, therefore, if the previously published findings from suicide notes are generalizable across the adult life span. Our previous understanding of suicide, based on previous studies of suicide notes, may not apply to young adults or late adults but to middle adults only.

Table 1. The Three-Group Classifications of Adulthood

Group	Classification	Erikson's stage	Chronological age
1	Young adulthood	Intimacy versus isolation	18–25
2	Middle adulthood	Generativity versus stagnation	25–55
3	Late adulthood	Integrity versus despair	55 and older

SUICIDE BY SPECIFIC TIME-LINES

That there are different rates of completed suicide across the life span is a well-established fact. Young, middle, and late adults show discrete different rates of suicide in the United States and elsewhere (see Chapters 5 and 6, this volume).

A consideration of annual suicide rates by specified age (time-line) groups illustrates the different rates of suicide across the adult life span. Table 2 presents the rates of U.S. suicide by specified age groups, 1980 to 1985. The rates, at least over the 6 years, i.e., 1980 to 1985, suggest that adults in late adulthood have consistently the age range with the highest rate. The average of the rates (per 100,000) over the 6 years for each group is as follows: young adults, 14.74; middle adults, 15.61; late adults, 17.78. Figure 1 presents the same data graphically.

Young adults in the United States have the lowest suicide rate of all adults, but the same trend is not evident in other countries such as Canada. In Canada, young adults exhibit one of the highest rates of suicide across the life span (Health and Welfare, 1987; Leenaars & Lester, 1990). Further, McGinnis of the U.S. Department of Health and Welfare Services (1987) has provided, in light of his understanding of the rates and trends, the following statement: "by far the most profound and disturbing trend in the last decade is the increase in suicide rates among young adult(s)." (p.23)

McGinnis (1987) and Leenaars and Lester (1989) also emphasize that it is the young adult *males* who are most affected—the rate of completed suicide in males to females in this age group is, at least, 5:1; that is, 5 males to 1 female (compared to the general ratio of 3:1). Furthermore, much of the popular and professional concern about suicide in young people in both United States and Canada centers on young adults; their rate of suicide is much higher than that of adolescents.

YOUNG ADULTHOOD

Young adulthood is a distinct time-line in development (Frager & Fadiman, 1984; Kimmel, 1974; Troll, 1975). It has its unique—despite commonalities—psychological issues as well as biological, sociological, anthropological, and other differences from other stages of life (see Chapters 13, 14, and 15, this volume). As we have already suggested, there is a consistent controversy regarding what should be the range of the chronological age for this time-line. We tentatively supported Kimmel's (1974) position in limiting this time-line from 18 to 25. This division is consistent with the views of other researchers (e.g., Neugarten, Moore, & Lowe, 1965) but not all (e.g., Colarusso & Nemiroff, 1981). Sometimes, this time-line has been treated as a transition, not a true phase (Levinson, 1978, 1986). Of course, no developmental period can be rigidly defined chronologically, and at best the 18 to

Table 2. U.S. Suicide by Specific Age Groups, 1980 to 1985[a]

	18–25 yr			26–54 yr			55 yr and older		
		Suicide			Suicide			Suicide	
Year	Population	Number	Rate	Population	Number	Rate	Population	Number	Rate
1980	34,228	5,202	15.20	81,868	12,772	15.60	47,465	7,993	16.84
1981	34,373	5,128	14.92	83,789	13,473	16.08	48,191	8,067	16.74
1982	34,379	5,052	14.70	85,725	13,606	15.87	48,940	8,660	17.70
1983	34,074	4,759	13.97	87,770	13,610	15.51	49,661	8,957	18.04
1984	33,522	4,919	14.67	89,895	13,971	15.54	50,289	9,367	18.63
1985	32,862	4,926	15.00	92,017	13,846	15.05	50,871	9,513	18.70

[a]Compiled by John L. McIntosh, Ph.D., Associate Professor of Psychology, Indiana University at South Bend. Suicide data were extrapolated from annual mortality detail computer tapes prepared by the National Center for Health Statistics and purchased from the National Technical Information Service. Population data are from the U.S. Bureau of Census (1987), *Current Population Reports*, Series P-25, No. 1000. The suicide rates are per 100,000.

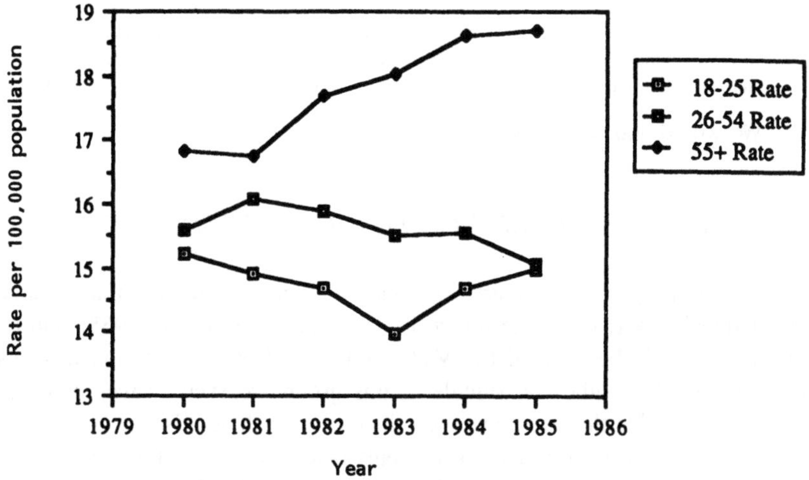

Figure 1. U.S. suicide rates by specified age groups, 1980 to 1985.

25 range approximates what can only be defined developmentally. Some people mature earlier, others later than the mean.

It is important to note that this phase of development is relatively uncharted, not only regarding suicide. It is the time-line after adolescence. Adolescence is a stage marked by the development of a sense of identity. The young adult continues to develop his sense of identity, evolving a finer and more discrete sense of who he is in relation to others. Kimmel (1974) notes, "perhaps the central issues in this later stage of identity would primarily concern the relation between the individual and the social system. 'How do I fit the sense of who I am into my sense of what my society is about?' "(p.90)

Not distinct from this process, the demand to master the challenge of intimacy emerges as the central crisis of young adulthood. Interaction with others within a social context leads toward an exploration of intimate relationships for their own sake, not merely to identify oneself (i.e., Identity Confusion).

Erikson (1963, 1968) was one of the first to pioneer work on intimacy (Intimacy vs. Isolation) in young adulthood. Although the capacity to relate to others emerges in adolescence, "the individual does not come capable of a fully intimate relationship until the identity crisis is fairly well resolved" (Kimmel, 1976, p.23). One must have a sense of who one is before one can appreciate the uniqueness of another. Often, before such development, the individual can only avoid genuine closeness or engage in fantasy, sexual, or narcissistic relationships.

Mutuality of commitment in love with another person is a developmental achievement that typically occurs in young adulthood. The psychosocial strength or virtue is *love*. As Frager and Fadiman (1984) note:

> Without a sense of intimacy and commitment, one may become isolated and be unable to sustain intimate relationships. If one's sense of identity is weak and threatened by intimacy, the individual may turn away from or attack whatever encroaches. (p.152)

We would add, even oneself!

PREVIOUS RESEARCH ON SUICIDE IN YOUNG ADULTS

Research regarding any area of young adulthood is scarce. Early studies included foci on sexuality (Thornberg, 1971), alienation (Keniston, 1965), political activities (largely because of the Vietnam War) (Flacks, 1967), and drug use (Kimmel, 1974). Studies on suicide in this group are even scarcer. Even the volumes on suicide that are apparently directed to include this age group (e.g., Klerman, 1986), disappoint us, for they only take note of our lack of knowledge about this group of individuals. Insights are often generated from general developmental issues, but we do not find specific information about suicide (see Levinson, 1986). Often young adults are classed together with adolescents (e.g., Araki & Murata, 1986; Berger, 1986; Freidman, 1987; Holinger, Offer, & Ostrov, 1987; Michel, 1988), a taxonomic maneuver both theoretically and empirically unsound. We do not mean to suggest that such information is not useful, only that it clouds our understanding. Michel (1988), in fact, in an excellent paper on the aforementioned research, reminds us that suicide in young people is different from suicide in adults. He notes the following about young people compared to other adults: that fewer were living alone; that fewer made previous attempts; that clearer depressive symptoms were evident; that higher levels of lethality were evident; that fewer exhibited warning signs before the act; and that suicide notes were left behind much more often (although Posener, LaHaye, and Cheifetz [1989] report no such trend). Holinger, Offer, and Ostrov's (1987) study is also noteworthy; they concluded (based on U.S. data) that there is a significant correlation between suicide and homicide in the 15 to 24 age group, but a negative correlation for older groups. It is important for the reader to be reminded, however, that Michel's and Holinger's studies included adolescents, not only young adults. Young people were defined as adolescents and young adults by these authors. These very beginnings of research on young adulthood, however, allow one to conclude that further investigations will likely be most fruitful. Suicide in young adults is likely different from other adults and, we would add, adolescents.

SUICIDE NOTES: THE METHOD

Early research (e.g., Wolff, 1931) on suicide notes largely utilized an anecdotal approach that incorporated descriptive information. Subsequent methods of study have primarily included classification analysis and content analysis. There are currently more than 70 published articles on suicide notes; an extensive review with an annotated bibliography has been presented elsewhere (Leenaars, 1988a). Only a very few of these studies have utilized a theoretical-conceptual analysis despite the assertion in the first formal study of suicide notes, that such an approach offered much promise (Shneidman & Farberow, 1957). In a series of studies spanning the last 12 years (e.g., Leenaars, 1979, 1985, 1986, 1987, 1988a,b, 1989a,b; Leenaars & Balance, 1981, 1984a,b; Leenaars, Balance, Wenckstern, & Rudzinski, 1985), the author and his colleagues have applied a logical, empirical analysis to suicide notes. Our method permits a theoretical analysis of suicide notes and augments the effectiveness of controls.

Our method has been previously described in detail (Leenaars, 1988a; Leenaars & Balance, 1984a). It treats the notes as an archival source. This source is subjected to the scrutiny of control hypotheses, following an ex post facto research design (Kerlinger, 1964). Suicide notes are recast in different theoretical contexts (hypotheses, theories, models) for which lines of evidence of each of these positions can then be pursued in the data, utilizing Carnap's logical and empirical procedures (1931/1959) for such investigations. These positivistic procedures call for the translating of theoretical formulations into observable (specific) *protocol sentences* in order to test the formulations. The protocol sentences express the meaning of a given theory as they are matched empirically, by independent judges, with the actual data. Next, conclusions are developed from the verified protocol sentences. To date, the theories of 10 suicidologists have been investigated (Leenaars, 1988a, 1989a,b). Specifically, studies of A. Adler, L. Binswanger, S. Freud, C.G. Jung, K.A. Menninger, G. Kelly, H.A. Murray, E.S. Shneidman, H.S. Sullivan, and G. Zilboorg have been undertaken. The results of these studies regarding specific investigations of young adults will be presented next.

THE SUICIDE NOTES OF YOUNG ADULTS: THE NOMOTHETIC FINDINGS

Our research (Leenaars, 1987, 1988a, 1989a,b) has indicated that it is, indeed, the age group from 18 to 25 that differs most from other adults in their suicide notes and, by implication, their suicides. Young adults differ from other adults in several essential characteristics. These differences are quantitative ones; the characteristics of suicide are largely the same across the entire life span. The following observations have been made:

Perturbation

The suicidal person is highly perturbed (Shneidman, 1980, 1985). The pain is unbearable. The anguish is unendurable. The emotion is intolerable. Our research showed that perturbation is evident in the individual's heightened emotions and constricted cognition in what they write in their suicide note (although less so in late adults than young adults). We believe that it is noteworthy that young adults often write in their notes about a life (or world) that is not going well in terms of felt pressures. Life is too painful—they often see themselves, given the level of perturbation, as not able to handle those pressures, mostly pressures of intimacy.

Intimacy

Previous research on suicide notes (Bjerg, 1967; Darbonne, 1969; Leenaars, 1988a,b, 1989a,b; Leenaars & Balance, 1984b) has shown that suicidal people have problems in establishing or maintaining relationships across the entire life span. Suicide is often related to unsatisfied or frustrated (attachment) affiliation needs although other thwarted needs may be detected; e.g., needs for achievement, autonomy, dominance, perfection. Even more than other adults, young adults describe disturbed, unbearable interpersonal situations in their suicide notes.

It is, indeed, the pain of isolation (i.e., Erikson's crisis of Intimacy vs. Isolation) in these young adults that is critical in understanding their suicide. Erikson (1968) stated:

> Where a youth does not accomplish such intimate relationships with others—and I would add, with his own inner resources—in late adolescence or early adulthood, he may settle for highly stereotyped relations and come to retain a deep sense of isolation. (pp.135–136)

What is critical, during young adulthood, is that these adults develop intimacy, attachment, affiliation, partnership. It is "mutuality of devotion" that allows young adults, according to Erikson, the increased capacity to function (or adjust) effectively (see below). Without intimacy, one becomes isolated and unable to establish or maintain relationships. Loss or rejection, as suggested by several authors (Freud 1920/1974; Leenaars, 1988a; Shneidman, 1985) often provokes a specific crisis for young adults (at least more often than middle adults in our research). Our results have indicated that young adults often write about a sense of total rejection in their notes. The individual, however, may not only turn away from others as a sequel to the rejection, but turn his anger to whatever else approaches. Holinger et al.'s (1987) observation of the positive correlation between suicide and homicide for young individuals may well be very important here. It appears that some young adults may not just settle for a deep sense of isolation but instead choose death as a solution to their unbearable interpersonal pain.

Identification–Egression

Freud (1917/1974, 1920/1974) hypothesized that an intense identification (or bond) with a lost or rejecting person or, as Zilboorg (1936) showed, to any ideal (e.g., health, young age, employment, freedom) is critical in understanding the suicidal person. If this loss goes uncompensated, the suicidal person experiences a deep discomfort (pain) and he wants to be gone, to be elsewhere, to exit—to egress. Such phenomena are more evident in young adulthood than late adulthood and obviously relate to the crisis of Intimacy versus Isolation. It is, however, for these people more than a loss of a relation. The loss precipitates an ego regression in which everything, including the self, is repudiated and the person gives up on life. It is loss of everything, *all* of one's attachment . . . and there is no reason to live, only to egress.

Identity

A critical aspect of a young adults' suicide appears to be their cognitions regarding themselves, issues of Identity. Erikson (1968) has, in fact, observed that frequent inability to adjust at this age "is explained by the fact that often only an attempt to engage in intimate fellowship and competition or in sexual intimacy reveals the latent weakness of identity" (p.134).

Young adults are extremely self-depreciating in their notes. They appear to see themselves as not effective. More frequently than other adults, they communicate a sense of shame, loss of face, disgrace, or sense of dereliction of duty. These results can be interpreted to signify that inwardly directed aggression is more frequently evident in young adults than other adults. They rage mercilessly against themselves.

Two specific findings regarding Identity also emerged in our research about young adults. Their self-perceptions and their perceptions of others are black or white, excessively dichotomous. They compartmentalize. It is either everything or nothing, all or none. We believe that this goes deeper than the cognitive surfaces and expresses a disturbed relation to (value of) self. There is a *totalistic* characteristic to their identity—"either everyone loves me or I am unlovable."

Young adults also more often than other adults confuse aspects of their identity. They confuse the *personal self* and *social self*. The self as it is experienced by the individual himself and the self as the individual is experienced by others. There is a lack of certainty about who one is, the role one is playing in the scheme of life. Worse yet, many of these people have never developed a personal self. It may well be that the crises of identity (Erikson, 1963, 1968) provokes a role confusion that is very much an issue for the young adult who kills himself.

Indirect Expressions

Complications, ambivalence, redirected aggression, unconscious implications, and other indirect expressions (or behavior) are often evident in suicidal people. The suicidal person, according to Tripodes (1976), may even confuse what is real and not real, objective and subjective, and so on. The observation of dynamic unconscious implications is especially important here. Such processes, by clinical judgments and operational definitions, have been identified to be more often present in genuine suicide notes than simulated ones (i.e., control data) (Leenaars, 1986; McLister & Leenaars, 1988). We have shown (Leenaars, 1986) that the unconscious processes in suicide are intimately related to the interpersonal aspects of suicide. Repressed unconscious dynamics (e.g., wishes, needs) may well be the driving force for an individual who defines an issue for which suicide is perceived as the best solution. Such characteristics are more evident in the suicide notes and, by implication, suicides of young (and middle) adults than late adults. Very often these adults are confused and likely unaware of significant processes, often connected to difficulties with intimacy that lead to their deaths.

Inability to Adjust

Erikson (1968) has noted that with isolation, the young individual becomes increasingly unable to function (or adjust) effectively. Our research has, indeed, suggested that even more than other adults, young adults are diagnosable (if one wishes to use such labels) as exhibiting a psychiatric disorder. Although the majority of suicides do not fit best into any specific nosological classification, the "down phase" of manic-depressive disorders, hysterical disorders, depressive disorders, obsessive-compulsive disorders, schizophrenic disorders, psychopathic disorders, and other disorders have been related to some suicides (Leenaars, 1988a; see also Sullivan, 1962, 1964). All these disorders suggest a maladjustment; the suicidal person himself states in the note that he is unable to adjust. These young adults, considering themselves too weak to function effectively, reject everything except death—they cannot survive *life's* difficulties.

Long-Term Instability

Young adults who kill themselves are not only unable to adjust to their current isolation but exhibit long-term problems. Young adults (and late adults), in fact, often see their suicide themselves as related to long-term instability. Their suicide had a tragic history.

Ego

The person himself is a critical common aspect in the suicidal act. Shneidman (1985) has, correctly from our view, noted the common consistency in suicide is with life-long coping patterns. People have enormous lifetime consistency in their ego. The suicidal person consistently has failed to function and adapt effectively.

This is especially true of young adults; young adults (compared to middle and late adults) more frequently exhibit in their suicide note a relative weakness in their capacity to develop constructive tendencies (e.g., love and work) and to overcome their personal difficulties. Their egos have been weakened by a steady toll of trauma.

A DEVELOPMENTAL VIEW OF YOUNG ADULTS' SUICIDES

When one is attempting to understand the suicide of adults, developmental age (time-line) is a significant variable to be accounted for in that perspective model. The suicide notes and, by implication, suicides of young adults are psychologically different from other adults. There appear to be differences on such psychological issues as "I love you"; "This is me"; "I am caving-in"; "I want to be gone"; "I am weakened"; and "This is the only thing I can do."

A life-span developmental perspective is essential in understanding suicidal phenomena. It is also important to know that although there may be no overall sex differences on important psychological variables in suicide notes (Leenaars, 1987, 1988a,b, 1989a,b), there are age by sex interactions on the characteristics discussed. Specifically, regarding young adults, the following variations have been noted: (1) young (and middle) adult females appear to exhibit a greater concern about their relations (Intimacy) than their male counterparts (although the reverse pattern is evident in late adults); (2) young (and middle) adult females appear to exhibit greater confusion regarding their self cognitions (Identity) than their male counterparts; (3) young adult males (compared to their female counterparts) appear—but only at a borderline level of significance—to be more frequently judged from their notes to have a definable disorder (Inability to Adjust); and (4) young adult females appear to be more preoccupied in their notes about their lack of constructive tendencies (Ego) than male counterparts. These observations suggest that one should understand young adults' suicides from the perspective of both their time-line and their sex; that is, *an age by sex perspective*. Hopefully, these observations can be expanded to allow us to understand why in young adulthood, suicide is such a severe problem for males.

The current formulation about young adults should not be construed to mean that development is simply discontinuous—development across the life span is both *discontinuous* and *continuous* (Piaget, 1970). Adult development is dynamic, ongoing, and serial. The suicidal person does not respond anew to each crisis—with a small *c*—in his adult life, but his reactions are consistent in many ways with that individual's previous reaction to loss, threat, impotence, and so on. There is an *elliptical* nature to his development (Shneidman, 1985) as well as change. Our point here is simply that, within the adult life span, young adults' suicides are psychologically different from other adults, despite enormous commonalities across the life span.

SUICIDE NOTES OF YOUNG ADULTS: IDIOGRAPHIC SUMMARY

To summarize, a number of genuine suicide notes of young adults are presented. They allow us, from an idiographic point of view, to know what it was really like for these individuals as they engaged in the penultimate act:

1. *Male*

NO NEED TO WORY ANY MOOR I'M OUT OF YOUR LIFE

SO MUCH TO SAY
SO LITTLE TIME

2. *Female*

Dear Bill: I am sorry for causing you so much trouble. I really didn't want to and if you would have told me at the first time the truth probably both of us would be very happy now. Bill I am sorry but I can't take the life any more, I don't think there is any goodness in the world. I love you very very much and I want you to be as happy in your life as I wanted to make you. Tell your parents I am very sorry and please if you can do it don't ever let my parents know what happened.
Please, don't hate me Bill, I love you.

Mary

3. *Female*

Dear Mom,

I wanted to make it out here, and save you the embarassment of my cominghome. I want you to know that I love Heather. No one can explain why. I was only tired, I felt cornered with the only ways out, the ways I didn't want.
I Love You

Mary

Forgive Me
Mom I want Heather to have everything, this is my dying wish.
I was only tired, cornered, unwilling to get up and fight.

4. Male

Dear Mary,

I am writing these last few words to you because these are the last ones. I really thought you and Little Bill were going to come back into my life, but you didn't. I know you found some body else who's better than me. I hope the son of a bitch dies. I've made love to five girls but they werent as good as you. I love you very much and Bill to. I hope you get some were one of these days. If you ever have a little girl please name her Lindsey. I've always wanted a little girl. It really hurts me alot that you and I didn't make it. I had a lot of dreams for all of us. But they were only dreams. I always thought dreams would come true, but I guess not. You'll never see me again or hear from me because what I'm going to do is that I'm never coming back. I hope I go to heaven but in case I'll probley go to hell. I want you to have every thing I own. My vacation money I want you to have. Please take care of Little Bill because I love him with all my heart. Take my bike and sell it or keep it for Little Bill I wrote my mom & Dad a letter to. I told them not give the car to Bill, I told them to save it for Little Bill for when he grow's up. They will to. He's going to need it. I didn't throw any of your belongings away. Their all in the same place where you and I put them with this letter they can't hold you back from taking anything. Every time you came over it made me feel so good I really thought we were going to get back together. I guess all you wanted from me was my money. That's way you could make love to me was because of my money it wasn't because you loved me. Well I know that's why I have to do what I have to do. Please don't tell Little Bill what happen tell him I went some where far and that I'll come back one of these days. Tell him you don't know when. I really thought I was going to make with out you but I guess wrong. Please take Little Bill to my mom & Dad every other weekend because they love him so much it pitiful. He's there live it once again if you know what I mean. There's no way I can live with out you so that's why I'm do it Bring him up well and try to give him every thing he wants. Tell I love him very much. When he get's to the point that he under stands tell him what I did. I know I'm running away from rasopablity but you did to. just remember take care of my little boy. Well I guess that's all. Take care of your self.

P.S. to bad I didn't get to see you and hold you and to make your life better. I know we would have made it but you didn't want to because you wanted to get fucked by some body else well you got it. I can't really say that I hate you or love you. You'll never know.

Yours Truly
Your husband

Bill ______

P.S.S. belive me I'm going to do the job right this time. You made me do it. No body else but you. keep your fucked friends they'll never give you what I've could of given you.

ACKNOWLEDGMENTS. The author acknowledges the cooperation and assistance of Dr. E. Shneidman, Dr. J. Maltsberger, Dr. J. McIntosh, Dr. W. Balance, and the American Association of Suicidology.

REFERENCES

Araki, S., & Murata, K. (1986). Factors affecting suicide in young, middle-aged and elderly men. *Journal of Biosocial Science, 18*, 103–108.

Berger, P. (1986). Suicide in young adult literature. *High School Journal, 70*, 14–19.

Bjerg, K. (1967). The suicidal life span: Attempts at a reconstruction from suicide notes. In E. Shneidman (Ed.), *Essays in self-destruction*. New York: Science House.

Carnap, R. (1959). Psychology in physical language. In A. Ayer (Ed.), *Logical Positivism*. New York: Free Press. (Original work published 1931)

Colarusso, C., & Nemiroff, R. (1981). *Adult development*. New York: Plenum.

Darbonne, A. (1969). Suicide and age: A suicide note analysis. *Journal of Consulting and Clinical Psychology, 33*, 46–50.

Erikson, E. (1963). *Childhood and society*, (2nd ed). New York: W.W. Norton.

Erikson, E. (1968). *Identity: Youth and crisis*. New York: W.W. Norton.

Flacks, R. (1967). The liberated generation: An exploration of the roots of student protest. *Journal of Social Issues, 23*, 52–75.

Frager, R., & Fadiman, J. (1984). *Personality and personal growth* (2nd ed.). New York: Harper & Row.

Freidman, R. (1987). Suicide and borderline depressed adolescent and young adult. *Journal of the American Academy of Psychoanalysis, 15*, 429–448.

Freud, S. (1974). Mourning and melancholia. In J. Strachey (Ed. and Trans.), *The standard edition of the complete psychological works of Sigmund Freud* (Vol. 14). London: Hogarth Press. (Original work published 1917)

Freud, S. (1974). A case of homosexuality in a woman. In J. Strachey (Ed. and Trans.), *The standard edition of the complete psychological works of Sigmund Freud* (Vol. 18). London: Hogarth Press. (Original work published 1920)

Health and Welfare, Canada. (1987). *Suicide in Canada*. Ottawa: Department of National Health and Welfare.

Holinger, P., Offer, P., & Ostrov, E. (1987). Suicide and homocide in the United States: An epidemiological study of violent deaths, population changes, and the potential for prediction. *American Journal of Psychiatry, 144*, 215–219.

Kalish, R. (1975). Late adulthood: Perspectives in human development. Monterey, CA: Brooks/Cole.

Keniston, K. (1965). *The uncommitted: Alienated young in American society*. New York: Harcourt, Brace and World.

Kerlinger, F. (1964). *Foundations of behavioral research*. New York: Holt, Rinehart & Winston.

Kimmel, D. (1974). *Adulthood and aging*. New York: Wiley.

Klerman, G. (Ed.) (1986). *Suicide and depression among adolescents and young adults*. Washington, DC: American Psychiatric Press.

Leenaars, A. (1979). *A study of the manifest content of suicide notes from three different theoretical perspectives: L. Binswanger, S. Freud, and G. Kelly*. Unpublished doctoral dissertation, University of Windsor, Canada.

Leenaars, A. (1985). Freud's and Shneidman's formulations of suicide investigated through suicide notes. In E. Shneidman (Chair), *Suicide Notes and Other Personal Documents in Psychological Science*. Symposium conducted at the meeting of the American Psychological Association, Los Angeles, CA.

Leenaars, A. (1986). A brief note on the latent content in suicide notes. *Psychological Reports, 59*, 640–642.

Leenaars, A. (1987). An empirical investigation of Shneidman's formulations regarding suicide: age and sex. *Suicide and Life-Threatening Behavior, 17*, 233–250.

Leenaars, A. (1988a). *Suicide notes*. New York: Human Sciences Press.

Leenaars, A. (1988b). Are women's suicides really different from men's? *Women & Health, 18*, 17–33.

Leenaars, A. (1989a). Are young adults' suicides psychologically different from those of other adults? (The Shneidman lecture) *Suicide and Life-Threatening Behavior, 19*.

Leenaars, A. (1989b). Suicide across the adult life-span: An archival study. *Crisis, 10*.

Leenaars, A., & Balance, W. (1981). A predictive approach to the study of manifest content in suicide notes. *Journal of Clinical Psychology, 37*, 50–52.

Leenaars, A., & Balance, W. (1984a). A logical empirical approach to the study of the manifest content in suicide notes. *Canadian Journal of Behavioral Science, 16*, 248–256.

Leenaars, A., & Balance, W. (1984b). A predictive approach to Freud's formulations regarding suicide. *Suicide and Life-Threatening Behavior, 14*, 275–283.

Leenaars, A., & Balance, W. (1984c). A predictive approach to suicide notes of young and old people from Freud's formulations regarding suicide. *Journal of Clinical Psychology, 40*, 1362–1364.

Leenaars, A., Balance, W., Wenckstern, S., & Rudzinski, D. (1985). An empirical investigation of Shneidman's formulations regarding suicide. *Suicide and Life-Threatening Behavior, 15*, 184–195.

Leenaars, A., & Lester, D. (1990). A comparison of rates and patterns of suicide for Canada and the United States, 1960–1985. Paper submitted for publication.

Lester, D., & Hummel, H. (1980). Motives for suicide in elderly people. *Psychological Reports, 47*, 870.

Lester, D., & Reeve, C. (1982). The suicide notes of young and old people. *Psychological Reports, 50*, 334.

Levinson, D. (1978). *The season's of a man's life*. New York: Knopf.

Levinson, D. (1986). Development in the novice phase of early development. In G. Klerman (Ed.), *Suicide and depression among adolescents and young adults*. Washington, DC: American Psychiatric Press.

Maris, R. (1981). Pathways to suicide: A survey of self-destructive behaviors. Baltimore: Johns Hopkins University Press.

McGinnis, J. (1987). Suicide in America—moving up the public health agenda. *Suicide and Life-Threatening Behavior, 17*, 18–32.

McLister, B., & Leenaars, A. (1988). An empirical investigation of the latent content in suicide notes. *Psychological Reports, 63*, 238.

Michel, K. (1988). Suicide in young people is different. *Crisis, 9*, 135–145.

Neugarten, B., Moore, J., & Lowe, J. (1965). Age norms, age constraints, and adult socialization. *American Journal of Sociology, 70*, 710–717.

Piaget, J. (1970). *Structuralism* (C. Maschler, Trans.). New York: Harper & Row.

Posener, J., LaHaye, A., & Cheifetz, P. (1989). Suicide notes in adolescence. *Canadian Journal of Psychiatry, 34*, 171–176.

Shneidman, E. (1980). *Voices of death*. New York: Harper & Row.

Shneidman, E. (1985). *Definition of suicide*. New York: Wiley.

Shneidman, E., & Farberow, N. (1957). *Clues to suicide*. New York: McGraw-Hill.

Sullivan, H. (1962). Schizophrenia as a human process. In H. Perry, N. Gorvell, & M. Gibbens (Eds.), *The collected works of Harry Stack Sullivan* (Vol. 2). New York: W.W. Norton.

Sullivan, H. (1964). The fusion of psychiatry and social sciences. In H. Perry, N. Gorvell, & M. Gibbens (Eds.), *The collected works of Harry Stack Sullivan (Vol. 2)*. New York: W.W. Norton.

Thornberg, H. (1971). Student assessment of contemporary issues. In H. Thornberg (Ed.), *Contemporary adolescents: Readings*. Belmont, CA: Brooks/Cole.

Tripodes, P. (1976). Reasoning patterns in suicide notes. In E. Shneidman (Ed.), *Suicidology: Contemporary developments*. New York: Grune and Stratton.

Troll, L. (1975). *Early and middle adulthood*. Monterey, CA: Brooks/Cole.

Tuckman, J., Kleiner, R., & Lavell, M. (1959). Emotional content of suicide notes. *American Journal of Psychiatry*, *116*, 59–63.

Wolff, H. (1931). Suicide notes. *American Mercury*, *24*, 264–272.

Zilboorg, G. (1936). Suicide among civilized primitive races. *American Journal of Psychiatry*, *92*, 1347–1369.

11

Suicide in Middle Adulthood

W. D. G. Balance and Antoon A. Leenaars

Much attention of late has been drawn to the tragedy of suicide among the young, and this kind of event is truly tragic, because life expectancy is then greatest in terms of both the interval of years and the diversity of experience that should await them. Shocking descriptive statistics, as suicide is a major cause of death in the early 20s and is the second or third major cause of death in adolescence, are truly appalling. Nonetheless, the relative neglect of suicide during the midlife period appears unwarranted. For example, Maris (1987) has raised the spectral worry that the high suicide rates of the baby boomers during adolescence and early adulthood are likely to carry over to the midlife period. This would result in truly alarming suicide rates for this generation as it moves into the latter half of life.

Moreover, if one sketches the average life expectancy like a line across a page and fixes a point at its middle, some facts readily emerge that also have major impact on our thoughts and feelings. First of all, just where does this point fall? Common usage describes the term middle age as a period falling just before old age and the age range estimates for this period tend to shift in the direction of the age of any given speaker. Still, most people are given more than somewhat of a start upon realizing the objectively quite obvious fact that the midpoint of most people's lives falls somewhere between 35 and 40 years of age. For our purposes, midlife can be thought of as the period 40 plus or minus 15 years or if you prefer 25 to 55 or 60 years, which corresponds roughly to Eriksen's (1968) stage of adulthood. The

W. D. G. BALANCE • 813 Pemberton, Grosse Pointe Park, Michigan 48230. *ANTOON A. LEENAARS* • Private Practice, 880 Ouelette Avenue, Suite 702, Windsor, Ontario, Canada N9A 1C7.

majority of midlife suicides occur during the latter part of this period after a decade and a half of declining rates.

RATES OF SUICIDE

Although individuals in middle adulthood are typically not perceived as having one of the highest rates of suicide in the life span (Leenaars, 1989), for women a peak occurs in middle age (Leenaars & Lester, 1990). A computation of the annual suicide rates for people in middle adulthood over the 6 years 1980 to 1985, revealed an average rate per 100,000 of 15.61, compared with a rate of 14.74 in young adulthood (18-25 age group) and a rate of 17.78 in late adulthood (55 and older age group). Table 1, derived from Leenaars (1989), presents the rates of suicide in the United States for middle adulthood.

Other countries, such as Canada, show a similar pattern. Lester, elsewhere in this volume, has presented some international rates of suicide, including those for middle adulthood.

Table 2, derived from Leenaars and Lester (1990), presents the rates of suicide

Table 1. U.S. Suicide Rates for Individuals in Middle Adulthood[a]

Year	Middle adult population	Number of suicides	Rate per 100,000
1980	81,868,000	12,772	15.60
1981	83,789,000	13,473	16.08
1982	85,725,000	13,606	15.87
1983	87,770,000	13,610	15.51
1984	89,895,000	13,971	15.54
1985	92,017,000	13,846	15.05

[a]Data were obtained from the National Center for Health Statistics.

Table 2. Suicide Rates per 100,000 for before and after Age 40[a]

Year	Before	After
1980	14.5	16.3
1981	15.1	17.2
1982	14.5	17.4
1983	14.5	16.7
1984	14.5	17.5
1985	14.0	17.3

[a]The rates of those younger than 10 years of age were not included. The rates were averaged for rates presented for males and females by Leenaars and Lester (1990). Median scores for each group were used. The data were obtained from the National Center for Health Statistics.

in the United States before and after age 40. The data in Table 2 show that the rate of suicide increases moderately after midlife. However, Leenaars and Lester (1990) suggest that the difference is lessening, mainly because of the recent increase of suicide in young adult males and the concomitant decrease of suicide rates in older adults (McIntosh, 1988–1989). Leenaars and Lester (1990) noted that a similar pattern regarding suicide rates before and after the midlife point does not exist in Canada; in fact, they showed that the suicide rates before and after age 40 were almost identical in that country; Leenaars and Lester (1990) questioned whether the traditional pattern of higher suicide after midlife is changing in both countries.

PERSPECTIVES ON MIDLIFE

We thought it would be useful to consider some of the major writers who have studied this period before proceeding to our more focused study of the contents of suicide notes from a midlife sample, which we did primarily from a Freudian perspective. Generally, scholars have taken issue with the common plateau-like image of the midlife period and tend instead to portray midlife in terms of important milestones along a path that is by no means flat.

Based on studies of biographies and autobiographies conducted in Vienna during the 1930s, Buhler (1968) described the 25- to 45-year period as a time when vitality is still high and self-direction and specification have replaced the shifting attitudes and uncertainties of youth. This period is often experienced subjectively as the culmination of life. She then observed that the transition to the 45- to 65-year period is often introduced by a crisis. The unfolding of one's individual powers comes to a standstill, and all that depends on physical abilities and needs enters a period of decline. Weighing against this biologic down slope are new and increasing interests in the results and productivity of life.

Kuhlen (1964), citing a number of studies, offered an even starker view of midlife events. He suggested that there is a shift from active direct efforts at gratification to indirect and vicarious methods. Moreover, the second half of life is marked by increases in the importance of anxiety and threat as sources of motivation.

Both Buhler and Kuhlen viewed life's midpoint as a marker for major stressful shifts. Both regarded the relative success in making these shifts as crucial for subsequent adjustment.

Jung (1933/1971) viewed the early part of midlife as a continuation of the "period of youth," which extends from puberty to age 35 to 40. He indicated that the major tasks during youth are giving up childhood dreams, dealing with sexual drives, and feelings of inferiority. This phase is characterized by a widening of the horizon of life. He believed that disturbances during this period are usually indications of attempts to continue the program of childhood into the period of youth. He pointed out that the 35- to 40-year period calls for major changes in that

". . .we cannot live the afternoon of life according to the program of life's morning. . ." (p. 17). He maintained that it is "fatal" to look back and viewed neurotic disturbance during this period as a sign of attempts to cling to what was meaningful during youth. The major challenge is to find purpose for the latter half of life. Essential to this endeavor is the acceptance of death as a goal, which in turn is dependent on the discovery of meaning and wholeness in life through an inward turning of attention and self-exploration.

According to Kimmel (1980), the term *midlife crisis* was probably coined by Jaques (1965). He, like Buhler, studied biographical material. He chose for his subjects 310 artists, who were painters, sculptors, composers, poets, and writers. Jaques reported a higher than expected death rate between 35 and 39 followed by a lower than expected death rate between 40 and 44. He also claimed a progression in their works from "lyrical and descriptive" in early adulthood to "tragic and philosophical" content during the crisis years to greater "serenity" in their productions after this period. He regarded a growing awareness of mortality as the main theme of the midlife crisis.

For Eriksen, three principal dialectics mark his period of adulthood that we are calling midlife. At the early boundary of this period, the opposing tendencies are between seeking intimate relationships as opposed to a sense of isolation. By intimacy, Erikson means mutually close and committed relationships, which may well involve feelings of fusion and self-abandonment. Only a person with a strong sense of personal identity can be secure enough to risk such closeness. Those still afflicted with confusion about their identities feel forced to stand well back from such intimacy and to endure a sense of profound isolation; their interpersonal relationships, sexual and otherwise, are promiscuous in nature and their behavior is role-like and stereotypic. In the healthy course of events, this dialectic is ending as midlife is beginning. The healthy solution is through compromise and synthesis rather than by siding with either of the polarities. The enduring legacy of a successful synthesis is the ability, or virtue, or strength to love in a committed way.

Early in midlife the striving for intimacy and expressions of love are supplanted or perhaps expanded by a more general caring and striving for a sense of generativity, which is a wish to do and produce in ways that have enduring value. This can be expressed in child rearing, but broader communal concerns and the world of ideas are certainly included as well. Failure at this stage results in a sense of stagnation, the feeling that one is going nowhere.

Toward the end of midlife as one approaches age 60, increasing concern about the finitude of life and the approaching nearness of death lead into the next and final stage in Erikson's system. The dialectic marking the close of midlife is one of integrity versus despair. The crucial task is the recollective one of evaluating and accepting one's own life as unique and meaningful. Such self-accepting individuals tend to be accepting of the life-styles of others: even those that are widely discrepant from their own. On the other hand, those who are dissatisfied and sense that life is too short to begin again are subject to feelings of despair and self-disgust. The strength that grows out of the integrity versus despair dialectic is that of wisdom, which is characterized by a sense of wholeness and meaning. Such people are truly sage models to look to as patterns to follow as well as representing successful solutions for the ending of midlife and the beginning of life's last phase.

It is perhaps ironic that Erikson, who is so associated in popular thinking with the term *midlife crisis*, has not really described life's midpoint as a time particularly prone to crisis. In this he stands in contrast to the other writers discussed so far. Although he viewed a crisis as possible at any time, one is more likely to occur in his view at the boundaries of life spans. Thus, in the case of midlife, one would expect more difficulty at about 25 to 30 years and again at 55 to 60 years (see Phillips and Smith).

If one looks at recent literature, considerable disagreement is found about whether the years immediately surrounding life's midpoint are particularly prone to crisis.

Ciernia (1985) noted that his middle-aged sample engaged in less alcohol abuse, was divorced less than younger males, and was less likely to commit suicide than either younger or older age groups. On the other hand, Fernando and Storson (1984) reported that their sample of psychiatric patients evidenced a higher vulnerability to suicide among middle-aged compared with younger or older subjects. They included midlife crisis along with other factors as suggesting a particularly high suicide risk during psychiatric treatment. Black, Warrack, and Winoker (1985) found that being middle aged significantly increased the risk of accidental death among formerly hospitalized psychiatric patients. No significant relationship with suicide was found, however. Dorsch and Roder (1983) reported that middle-aged Australians generally had higher rates of suicide than did 20- to 29-year-olds. Humphrey and Palmer (1987) in a very ambitious study did find differences in frequency of suicide between parts of midlife. However, the interactions reported for race, sex, marital status, and age are very complicated indeed. Sorting out this state of affairs probably cannot be done at present. Even comprehensively reviewing the empirical literature on suicide during midlife would turn this chapter into a book and a perplexing one at that. Nonetheless, it is thought that a meta-analysis of this literature might well be a useful undertaking, particularly with those many studies that appear to have only incidentally included subjects who are in some part of midlife.

Generally, looking at the relationships of suicide to the parts of midlife has been the subject largely of neglect as if midlife and its suicides could really be understood in terms of the plateau of popular thinking.

FREUD'S FORMULATIONS

Although the major theoretical frameworks within which Freud described and speculated about suicidal events underwent major shifts during his lifetime, particularly with the formulation of his death instinct, these shifts pertain largely to his efforts to assimilate his views on suicide into a general dynamic or energy flow model of human personality. Litman (1987) has provided us with a thoroughly interesting account of the relationships between Freud's specific formulations regarding suicide and the evolution of the abstract aspects of his model. We, in fact, in the beginning wanted to contrast Freud's early statements about suicide with his post-death instinct formulations in terms of their ability to predict the content of suicide notes. When we went to his collected works (1974) to extract specific observable statements, we made an interesting and perhaps important discovery. We could not do this study, because early on Freud had made all of his specific comments about suicide; only the broad frameworks changed. Thus, his specific statements about suicide represent collectively a major continuity in his life work. For our purposes, we have grouped Freud's specific observations and beliefs under six headings.

Conscious-Unconscious Processes

Although suicide is by definition an intentional act and thus at least in part a conscious one, Freud thought that the motivations were largely unconscious. One chooses the time and means or opportunity quite consciously; the intentions are unconscious as appears to be the case in many accidents and cases of self-injury as well.

Loss-Rejection

In "Mourning and Melancholia" (1917) Freud examined the developmental history of suicidal tendencies. These he thought originated in experiences of loss or rejection involving a significant person. The lost or rejecting person becomes the object of a vexing preoccupation. The feelings aroused are ambivalent consisting of both love and anger.

Identification Processes

Freud (1920) has stated:

> Probably no one finds the mental energy to kill himself unless, in the first place, in doing so he is at the same time killing an object with whom he has identified himself and, in the second place, is turning against himself a death wish which had been directed against someone else.

Through the process of identification the wounding sense of rejection by another becomes a personal feeling. One rejects oneself: By hurting oneself, one acts on this rejection and seems to hurt the rejecting person, who is now reacted to as a part of oneself.

Aggressive Processes

Anger is directed against the lost or rejecting person, who is also loved. Through identification this anger is turned against oneself and through self-damage the lost person seems to be hurt. Vengeance is sought.

Superego Processes

The superego is that part of Freud's structural model that deals with values and guilt feelings. Developmentally, this structure also results from identification processes. So, when one identifies with the perceived rejection of an important person, one becomes morally umbraged and burdened with feelings of guilt and worthlessness. Thus, self-punishment attempts to assuage these guilt feelings. Penitence is sought.

Ego Processes

The ego is that part of Freud's structural model that is burdened with finding rational or at least effective ways to satisfy the often conflicting demands of one's physical needs, the demands of the superego, and the requirements of the external world. The ego is implicated when suicide is a defensive act, that is, an attempt to reduce stress or satisfy a need. The ego is also implicated when there is a breakdown of its coordinating and need-satisfying capacities.

Protocol Sentences

Twenty-five protocol sentences were derived from Freud's formulations regarding suicide. For this chapter we have grouped these protocol sentences into the six theoretical classifications outlined above (Table 3).

STUDIES

We shall recapitulate previous studies here (Leenaars, 1988; Leenaars & Balance, 1984a,b), which sought to verify Freud's formulation regarding suicide through an analysis of suicide notes. The protocol sentences presented above were subjected to a theoretical-empirical analysis that has been outlined in detail elsewhere (Leenaars, 1988). Independent judges were asked to verify whether the

Table 3. Protocol Sentences about Suicide

I. Conscious-Unconscious Processes
  1. In the suicide note, the person communicated that he had consciously chosen the time, means, or opportunity to kill himself.
  2. . . . the person communicated that he had consciously planned to kill himself, however, the act appeared to be motivated by unconscious intentions.

II. Loss-Rejection
  3. . . . the person communicated that he had experienced the loss or rejection of a significant person.
  4. . . . the person communicated that he was preoccupied with a person that he had lost or who had rejected him.
  5. . . . the person communicated that he was feeling quite ambivalent, i.e., affectionate and hostile toward a lost or rejecting person.

III. Identification Processes
  6. . . . the person communicated that he was in some direct or indirect fashion identifying himself with a rejecting or lost person.
  7. . . . the person communicated that he was treating himself as if he were reacting to another person.
  17. . . . the person communicated that by killing himself he would be destroying someone else with whom he had identified.

IV. Aggressive Processes
  8. . . . the person communicated feelings or ideas of vengefulness and aggression toward another person.
  9. . . . the person communicated feelings or ideas of vengefulness and aggression toward himself.
  10. . . . the person communicated feelings or ideas of vengefulness and aggression toward himself; however, he appeared to be angry toward someone else.
  11. . . . the person communicated that he wanted to kill himself to strike a single blow at himself and at a "loved-hated" person.
  12. . . . the person communicated that by killing himself he had gotten rid of another person.
  13. . . . the person communicated that his suicide would be an act of sadism directed toward himself.
  14. . . . the person communicated that he was turning back on himself murderous impulses that he had been directed against someone else.
  16. . . . the person communicated that his suicide was a fulfillment of a wish.
  18. . . . the person communicated that he was turning against himself a death wish that had been directed toward someone else.

V. Superego Processes
  15. . . . the person communicated that his suicide was a filfillment of punishment, that is, self-punishment.
  19. . . . the person communicated that he was experiencing a sense of guilt or rather criticism.
  20. . . . the person communicated prohibitions of extraordinary harshness and severity toward himself.
  21. . . . the person communicated that he must kill himself for he deserved no better.

[a]Derived from S. Freud.

classes of content described by the individual protocol sentences did, in fact, occur in each of 33 genuine and 33 simulated notes (Shneidman & Farberow, 1957). What is important to know about Shneidman and Farberow's set of notes is that the age range of the author is roughly synonymous with middle adulthood. All notes were written by individuals between the ages of 25 and 59.

Our research indicated the following results: A Mann-Whitney *U* test (Siegel, 1956) was used to assess overall differences in verification instances between genuine and simulated notes for the set of 25 protocol sentences. The protocol set derived from Freud's theory was significantly more often verified in the genuine notes (U [25,25] = 216; $p < .05$).

Chi-square tests for two independent samples (Siegel, 1956) were performed to assess the significance of differences in verification instances for each of the protocol statements. No sentences were verified significantly more often in the simulated notes.

The protocol sentences that were verified significantly more often within the genuine notes were the following: (3) the reported experience of the loss or rejection of a significant person ($x2 = 5.52$; $df = 1$; $p < .05$); (4) the reported preoccupation with a person that she/he had lost or who had rejected her/him ($x2 = 8.68$; $df = 1$; $p < .01$); (5) the reported feeling of ambivalence, that is, affectionate and hostile, toward a lost or rejecting person ($x2 = 4.47$; $df = 1$; $p < .05$); (6) the reported identification, directly or indirectly, with a rejecting or lost person ($x = 6.67$; $df = 1$; $p < 0.01$); (10) the person communicated feelings or ideas of vengefulness and aggression toward him/herself; however, appeared to be angry toward someone else ($x = 6.13$; $df = 1$; $p < .05$); (14) the person communicated that he/she was turning back upon him/herself murderous impulses that had been directed against someone else ($x = 10.97$; $df = 1$; $p < .01$); (15) suicide was seen as fulfillment of punishment, that is, self-punishment ($x = 6.67$; $df = 1$; $p < .01$); and (18) the person communicated that he/she was turning against him/herself a death wish that had been directed toward someone else ($x = 5.78$; $df = 1$; $p < .05$). One other sentence approached significance as more frequent in the genuine notes: (7) The person communicated that he/she was treating him/herself as if he/she were reacting to another person ($x2 = 3.74$; $df = 1$; $p < .06$).

These results, placed within our theoretical framework, can be interpreted as follows:

No specific sentence classified under Conscious/Unconscious Processes was observed more frequently in the genuine notes. We do not mean to suggest that such processes do not occur in suicidal individuals. It may well be that the individual does not write them down. Furthermore, Leenaars (1986) and McLister and Leenaars (1988) were able to demonstrate utilizing blind clinical judgments and structured operational definitions that unconscious psychodynamic forces are more frequently observed in genuine suicide notes than simulated ones. There may well be more communicated in the note than what the person consciously thinks.

Loss-Rejection is important in understanding the suicide. Freud noted that the suicidal person often describes the root cause of his suicide as a loss or rejection. This is often related to a highly cathected person ("object"). Our results verified that suicidal individuals in middle adulthood more frequently than those who only imagine being suicidal describe in their notes the loss or rejection of a significant person. All three protocol sentences within our Loss-Rejection category were, in fact, more frequently verified in the genuine notes. Suicidal individuals communicate in their notes that they are singly preoccupied with a person that they have lost or who had rejected them. They further have noted that they feel quite ambivalent, that is, affectionate and hostile toward this lost or rejecting person. We believe that these findings in suicide notes begin to give voice to Freud's (1920) "deeper interpretation" that the suicide turns against himself a death wish originally directed at someone else.

Our results of the comparison between genuine and simulated notes significantly verified some sentences classified under Identification Process. It seems that the suicidal person has developed a strong direct or indirect identification with a lost or rejecting person. Here identification is defined as an attachment or bond, based on an important emotional tie with an "object" (Freud, 1920/1974). The suicidal person is deeply bonded to the "object" (such as a person or other ideal) that he has lost or who has rejected him. Our results suggest that he may well, in fact, treat himself as an object, that is, as if he were reacting to someone else. Freud has termed such an identification as "narcissistic" and, according to Shneidman and Farberow (1957), this process aids in allowing one to kill oneself. One kills only an "object," not the personal self.

According to Freud (1917/1974), the person turns back on himself "all the acts of aggression and expressions of revengefulness which had been aimed at the object." Our results of the comparison of genuine and simulated suicide notes of individuals in middle adulthood indicate that Aggressive Processes occur in some suicides. The person appears to be turning back upon himself murderous impulses or a death wish that had been directed toward someone else. The person communicated feelings or ideas of vengefulness and aggression toward himself; however, he appeared to be angry toward someone else.

Only one protocol sentence classified under Superego Processes was verified more frequently in the genuine notes. This result suggests that the suicide of some adults in middle adulthood may be a form of punishment. Suicide may be self-punishment.

None of the statements related to Ego Processes attained significance. This as well as the other negative findings may suggest that such processes do not occur. Alternately, given Freud's view of the unconscious as dynamic, we wonder if a suicidal person is always able to express such processes in a final letter.

In a second study, we analyzed suicide notes that were written by individuals before or after midlife. The question raised here is as follows: Are the suicide notes written by individuals before midlife different from those written after midlife?

Two independent judges were asked to verify whether the classes of content described by the specific protocol sentences did occur in a sample of 52 suicide notes. The note writer's mean age was 42 years; the standard deviation was 17 years and the range 18 to 74 years. The mean of 42—which is roughly synonymous with our midlife point—was used to divide the set into two samples: Before and after midlife.

The results were as follows: A Mann Whitney *U* test (Siegel, 1956) was used to assess overall differences in verification instances between the notes of those younger than the mean and those older than the mean for the set of 25 protocol sentences. The protocol set was significantly more often verified in the notes of those before midlife (U [25, 25] = 81.5, p <.01). Chi-square tests for two independent samples (Siegel, 1956) were performed to assess the significance of differences in verification instances for each of the protocol sentences. The protocol sentences that were verified significantly more often within the notes of those before midlife were the following: (19) the person communicated that he was experiencing a sense of guilt or self-criticism ($x2$ [1, N = 52] = 8.21, p .01); (20) the person communicated prohibitions of extraordinary harshness and severity towards himself ($x2$ [1, N = 52] = 6.13, p <.05); and (21) the person communicated that he must kill himself for he deserved no better ($x2$ [1, N = 52] = 4.74, p <.05). One other sentence approached significance as more frequent with the notes of those before midlife: (7) The person communicated that he was treating himself as if he were reacting to another person ($x2$ [1, N = 52] = 3.72, p <.06).

Our results indicated that the set of protocol sentences derived from Freud's theory discriminated in favor of the notes of people who were before midlife. Our results further suggest specifically that people before midlife differ in terms of superego processes from those who kill themselves after midlife. The younger adults more often described a sense of guilt. They were more often extremely self-critical, and they more often prescribed prohibitions of extraordinary harshness and severity for themselves. They, in fact, more often stated that they must kill themselves for they deserved no better.

Only one other finding and that at a borderline level of significance was found: namely, that people before midlife treat themselves more like an "object," an observation that would not be theoretically distinct from the Superego Processes. One has to be an "object," perhaps, to rate so mercilessly upon oneself.

These results raise, at least, the following question: Why should people after midlife commit suicide more often than those before? Although the characteristics of suicide are largely the same across the entire life span, our results indicate that individuals in the younger half of midlife differ in terms of statements that were classified under Superego Processes. It may well be that the greater rates of the older group are attributable to sociological (see Chapter 14, this volume), biological (see Chapter 13, this volume), anthropological (see Chapter 15, this volume) or some other factor(s) including possible psychological ones such as those described early in this chapter (also see Chapters 3, 4, and 12, this volume).

CONCLUDING REMARKS

Certainly we are not the first to have found Freud more effective for describing the events of early adulthood than for the later parts of midlife. Still, it is meaningful that in the latter part of midlife suicides appear less distanced from and less angry at themselves, and during the first half of midlife the converse tendencies toward more self-distance and more intense self-rejection are evidenced. Taken together, the data reported in this chapter point to a shift in the frequency of suicide before and after midlife and indicate some shifts in the meanings of these suicides as well, which is broadly in accord with the consensus of scholarly thinkers that midlife is a period of important and frequently stressful personality changes.

We believe that it would surely be a mistake to conclude that values play a less crucial role in late midlife suicides, because the protocol sentences from Freud indict Superego Processes more often among the younger suicides. Freud's statements may have simply been more accurate at describing the superego problems experienced by young adult suicides and can probably be most meaningfully related to this age group. In fact, his theory of suicide in general was more applicable to this age group.

It is possible that values or superego concerns are even more crucial to the understanding of suicide in late midlife. To address this issue and indeed the whole problem of the special meanings of suicide in this age group, we need among other things to apply the formulations of midlife theorists for whom the stressful shifts during this life span have been a central focus.

A SAMPLE OF SUICIDE NOTES

In closing, a number of genuine suicide notes of middle adults are presented for you to experience directly.

1. *All hope is gone. No recourse except this.*
I have taken enough alcohol to give me courage to
die. Children—please finish school and be a
comfort to your mother. Everything to Mary my
dear wife. I have tried to live and make a come
back but the world offers no encouragement for someone
like me. I have malice toward no one.
Insurance and other data in my alligator pocket-
fold. You all will be infinitely better off without
me. Have me cremated and forget me please. My death
will be a blessing to me and to all of you. I am
trying to escape having to drag you down to my absymal

level. All of you are still able to make a new life and certainly will improve over the status to which I have sunk.

William Smith

2. *Please tell Bill's folks I love them very much but my heart breaks when I see or hear from them. Also all our friends especially Betty and Joe and Ella I love them also. Forgive me for not seeing them.*

   Every one seems so happy and I am so alone. Amy. I wanted to visit you but am going around in a dream. Alice I wanted to help you paint but how could I with a broken heart. And my head aches so much any more my nerves are ready to break and what would happen if they did.

   You will say I am crazy and I cant go on this way just half living.

   I loved this house once but now it is so full of memories I cant stay here. I have tried to think of some way to go on but cant. Am so nervous all the time—I loved Bill too much but is that a sin, with him gone I have nothing Oh I have the girls and family but they dont fill the vacant spot left in my heart. . .

   Xmas is coming I cant go on I'm afraid I would break down. Ive thot of this so many times. I love every one but I cant be one of you any more. Please think kindly of me and forgive me. I only hope this is fatal then I can rest and no more trouble to any one. Do with Ann whats best I know she has been a lot of worry to mama and I'm sorry. I tried to keep the yard up that seemed to be the only comfort I had. I loved it but that wasnt any thing. I've lost every thing so why go on. I worshipped Bill and when he went I lost my whole world and everything.

   I'm so tired and lonely.

   There goes a siren. Oh how can I stand being left. I need to go to a Dr. but I am afraid. Im so cold.

Mother Love Mary

3. *Mother,*

I was intending to comet suicide like it was an accident, see, but so you could colect the 10,000 insurance, by acting like I got drunk and started to throw up out through the window, but since God told me I don't have to act like that. I can tell you that God let me go like I wanted to in a dream. God said to tell you that he would forgive all. Mother, I have a disease of the nose, and I can't get over it so I just as well die now or better now than later. I don't know if I got it overseas or before.

Mother, it is actualy easy to go. You might not think so, but it is the only reason I stoped to rite this letter is because God told me to and I knew you'd feel better, because you're the swellest mother any one ever had. Goodbye.

4. *I Turn to God and to you, to some of you to forgive me. I cannot live any longer, I do not wish to live any longer. Death is better than living. Sometimes it is the best. Such is life worth living in a miserable existence to gain in the end the sublime privilege of dying.*

Bill, what did I do bad? Wanting you? No, I could not have done it for that reason. Because for wanting you, was I born. So now you can be happy.

Pray to God for me, I who did not know how to love you.

REFERENCES

Black, D., Warrack, G., & Winoker, G. (1985). Suicide and accidental deaths among psychiatric patients. *Archives of General Psychiatry*, *42*, 71–75.

Buhler, C. (1968). The developmental structure of goal setting in group and individual studies. In C. Buhler & F. Massarik (Eds.), *The course of human life*. New York: Springer.

Ciernia, J. (1985). Myths about midlife crisis. *Psychological Reports*, *56*, 1003–1007.

Dorsch, M., & Roder, D. (1983). A comparison of Australian suicide rates in 1969–75 and 1976–80. *Australian and New Zealand Journal of Psychiatry*, *17* (3).

Erikson, E. (1968). *Identity: Youth and crisis*. New York: W.W. Norton.

Fernando, S., & Storson, V. (1984). Suicide among psychiatric patients of a district general hospital. *Psychological Medicine*, *14*, 661–672.

Freud, S. (1974). Mourning and melancholia. In J. Strachey (Ed. and Trans.), *The standard edition of the complete psychological works of Sigmund Freud* (Vol. 14). London: Hogarth Press. (Original work published 1917)

Freud, S. (1974). A case of homosexuality in a woman. In J. Strachey (Ed. and Trans.), *The standard edition of the complete psychological works of Sigmund Freud* (Vol. 18). London: Hogarth Press. (Original work published 1920)

Freud, S. (1974). Group psychology on the analyses of the Ego. In J. Strachey (Ed. and Trans.), *The standard edition of the complete psychological works of Sigmund Freud* (Vol. 28). London: Hogarth Press. (Original work published 1921)

Humphrey, J., & Palmer, S. (1987). *Mid-life suicide*. Paper presented at the Annual Conference of the American Association of Suicidology, San Francisco, CA.

Jaques, E. (1965). Death and the mid-life crisis. *International Journal of Psychoanalysis*, *46*, 502–514.

Jung, C. (1971). The stages of life. (R. F. C. Hull, Trans.). In J. Campbell (Ed.), *The portable Jung*. New York: Viking. (Original work published 1933)

Kimmel, D. (1980). *Adulthood and aging* (2nd ed.). New York: Wiley.

Kuhlen, R. G. (1964). Developmental changes in motivation during the adult years. In J. E. Birren (Ed.), *Relations of development and aging*. Springfield, IL: Charles C Thomas.

Leenaars, A. (1986). A brief note on the latent content in suicide notes. *Psychological Reports*, *59*, 640–642.

Leenaars, A. (1988). *Suicide notes*. New York: Human Sciences Press.

Leenaars, A. (1989). Are young adults' suicides psychologically different from those of other adults? (The Shneidman Lecture). *Suicide and Life-Threatening Behavior*, *19*, 249–263.

Leenaars, A. & Balance, W. (1984a). A predictive approach to Freud's formulations regarding suicide. *Suicide and Life-Threatening Behavior*, *14*, 275–283.

Leenaars, A., & Balance, W. (1984b). A predictive approach to suicide notes of young and old people from Freud's familiarities with regard to suicide. *Journal of Clinical Psychology*, *40*, 1362–1364.

Leenaars, A., & Lester, D., (1990). *A comparison of rates and patterns of suicide in Canada and the United States, 1960–1985*. Paper submitted for publication.

Litman, R. (1987). Sigmund Freud on suicide. In E. Shneidman (Ed.), *Essays in self-destruction*. New York: Jason Aronson.

Maris, R. (1987). *Mid-life male suicides*. Paper presented at the Annual Conference of the American Association of Suicidology, San Francisco, CA.

McIntosh, S. (1988–1989). Official U. S. elderly suicide data; Bases, levels, availability, omissions. *Omega*, *19*, 337–350.

McLister, B., & Leenaars, A. (1988). An empirical investigation of the latent content of suicide notes. *Psychological Reports*, *63*, 238.

Shneidman, E., & Farberow, N. (1957). *Clues to suicide*. New York: McGraw-Hill.

Siegel, S. (1956). *Nonparametric statistics*. New York: McGraw-Hill.

12

Suicide and the Elderly

Joseph Richman

The reasons for suicide in the elderly are not as self-evident as they seem to some persons who attribute the event primarily or even solely to being old. For most of those so "afflicted," old age is a very pleasing time, one of high morale and high life satisfaction.

Many of the elderly do, nevertheless, succumb to despair and suicide. Older persons are consistently the winners in the undesirable race to have the highest suicide rates, and there is evidence that the rate is increasing. Some of the increase is attributed to medical progress, leading to some elderly people living—or dying—longer. Medical progress, however, can be seen as a blessing too, making the lives of the elderly a period of greater joy and satisfaction. It may be reflective of our times that less than 20 years ago the literature was discussing reasons for the decline in elderly suicides since 1950 (Resnik & Cantor, 1970).

My clinical experiences in the treatment of the suicidal elderly, and intensive discussions with family survivors, indicate that the vast majority of these suicides are preventable. These despairing elderly need not choose death, but instead can go on to live enjoyable lives, no matter how much or how little time is left. My work in couple's therapy with the seriously or terminally ill (Richman, 1981) indicates that the last months or even days can be among the most satisfactory and meaningful. Those who emphasize the right of the elderly to die do not address that issue. Why there is so much unquestioning acceptance as well as ignorance regarding

JOSEPH RICHMAN • Professor Emeritus, Albert Einstein College of Medicine, New York, New York 10461.

suicide in the elderly is a social phenomenon that deserves a more intensive inquiry.

It is the thesis of this chapter that knowledge about elderly suicide, and good will by both the professional community and the public, can save lives and increase happiness. The remainder of this chapter will explore some of the major variables associated with elderly suicide, explore some of the strengths and assets of the elderly, and discuss some implications for theory and practice.

THE BASIC PRINCIPLES OF ELDERLY SUICIDE

Contributions to the theory and understanding of suicide and the elderly are to be found in every field of endeavor concerning the human condition; from sociology and demography, psychology and education, biology and medicine, and even literature and the arts, such as Tolstoy's *Anna Karenina* and Flaubert's *Madame Bovary*—perhaps especially the arts.

Basic contributions to the study of suicide were made by Freud (1917/1957) and Durkheim (1951). Freud covered the individual, interpersonal, and drive aspects, while Durkheim's demographic and social studies dealt with society and the suicide rate, especially the centrality of social integration or else alienation in the prevention or etiology of suicide. The more recent study of suicide in the elderly has been enriched by Miller (1979), whose scholarly survey was brought up to date by Osgood and McIntosh (1986). Both these volumes are required reading for everyone interested in elderly suicide.

One of the more influential theories was presented by Menninger in *Man Against Himself* (1938), a title that might seem sexist today. I recall that early in my involvement with suicide prevention, I saw young suicidal men walking around the clinic and hospital corridors carrying copies of that book. Menninger hypothesized that suicides could be classified along three major motives or reasons: the wish to kill, the wish to be killed, and the wish to die.

Farberow and Shneidman (1957), in a study of suicide notes, classified the content into Menninger's triad of the wishes to kill, be killed, or die. They reported that the wishes to kill or be killed decreased with age, while the wishes to die increased. They reported, too, that interpersonal motives decreased with age.

Based on my experiences with the suicidal elderly, I suspect that the interpersonal motives may be concealed, rather than decreased. The recommendations made by Farberow and Shneidman were for dynamic psychotherapy and restoration or continuation of functioning for the suicidal young, and supportive therapy, milieu manipulation, and psychological crutches for the suicidal old.

I also suspect that with the added wisdom of age, both authors may have modified their views in the succeeding 32 years. Shneidman (1971) conducted a blind psychological autopsy based on life history factors in five men who had committed suicide, in middle age, compared with a closely matched group. He found that using the guiding concepts of perturbation and lethality, there was a highly significant rate of success in his blind identification of those who had committed suicide. He concluded that suicide in a person of 50 could be predicted by age 30. The concept of "suicidal careers" (Maris, 1981) has analogous conceptual ramifications. Shneidman emphasized the role of significant others, the burning out of affect, and suicide as the outcome of a destructive life-style.

Suicide in old age is best understood as the multidetermined outcome of many factors. The tasks and crises that accompany or threaten these goals in the elderly are best understood through Erikson's (1950) description of the ages of man, especially the last two, of generativity versus stagnation and ego integrity versus disgust and despair; and the more detailed elaboration of these tasks by such investigators as Peck (1975).

Successful aging does require an ability to be flexible and adapt to changing circumstances. With increasing age, for example, a greater dependence often becomes necessary. Some might consider that as part of man's humanity to man, which has made countless millions grateful. However, that is so unacceptable to some as to be seen as the essence of psychopathological misery and development.

Similar to the rejection of dependency, there is a form of bias that might be called "useless-ism," as a materialistic charge against the elderly. Chesser (1967) considered it "rational" for an old man to commit suicide; presenting no other reason than age. Portwood (1978) advocates suicide for the elderly because they are of no use to anyone and not productive. Pollinger-Haas and Hendin (1983) predicted an increase in elderly suicide because of the self-destructive proclivities of the current cohort of young people.

Despite some distinguished exceptions, in sum, the literature presents suicide in old age as based on the irrevocable loss of what makes life worth while and the loss of the energies and skills needed to cope and function. The eventual suicide, then, is only a postponement of built-in or intrinsic death drives. The picture begins to resemble Freud's (1920/1955, 1923/1961) theory of the death instinct. I am thankful for the exceptions to these views that are present in the literature, and hope that this chapter will serve as a further antidote to discouraging and despairing attitudes.

RECOGNITION AND EVALUATION OF THE SUICIDAL ELDERLY

This section discusses the major social, biological, situational, and psychological conditions associated with elderly suicide, at both conscious and unconscious, overt and covert levels. Table 1 summarizes the major indices of suicidal potential in old age, derived from all these areas.

Table 1. Recognition of the Elderly Suicidal Person: The 21 Most Frequent Signs

1.	Depression
2.	Paranoia or a paranoid attitude
3.	Rejection of help; a suspicious and hostile attitude toward helpers and society
4.	A major loss such as the death of a spouse
5.	A major mental, physical, or neurologic illness
6.	Major crises or transitions such as retirement or imminent entry into a nursing home
7.	Major crises or changes in others, especially among family members
8.	Typical age-related blows to self-esteem such as loss of income or loss of meaningful activities
9.	Loss of independence when dependency is unacceptable
10.	Expressions of feeling unnecesary, useless, and devalued
11.	Increased irritability and poor judgment, especially following a loss or some other crisis
12.	Alcoholism or increased drinking
13.	Social isolation: Living alone; having few friends. The social isolation of a couple is also associated with suicide
14.	Expression of the belief that one is in the way, a burden, or harmful to others
15.	Expression of the belief that one is in an insoluble and hopeless situation
16.	Communication of suicidal intent: The direct or indirect expression of suicidal ideation or impulses. Included, too, are symptomatic acts such as giving away valued possessions, storing up medication, or buying a gun. In this area is the presence of previous suicide attempts and a family history of suicide
17.	Intractable, unremitting pain, mental or physical, that is not responding to treatment
18.	Feelings of hopelessness and helplessness in the family and social network
19.	Feelings of hopelessness in the therapist or other helpers, or a desire to be rid of the patient
20.	Expression of a belief in ageism, especially that the aged should not be
21.	Acceptance of suicide as a solution

Depression

Depression is one of the more frequent conditions associated with suicide. As is true of most of the significant variables, depression is a biopsychosocial condition. It is characterized by an unhappy state, with a low mood, vegetative signs such as insomnia, early morning awakening, gastrointestinal upsets, fatigue, withdrawal, and an inability to perform one's usual activities or meet one's ordinary social role demands.

According to psychoanalytic theory (Freud, 1917/1957), depression is based on a return to earlier or infantile mechanisms of introjection and identification, instead of the more mature object or interpersonal relationships. (See the comparison with paranoia, which follows.)

In the elderly, the signs of depression are often disregarded or seen as the manifestations of old age and dementia. They may even be ridiculed.

Old Silas P., for example, was laughed at for his preoccupation with his bowels. The laughter ceased, permanently, when he jumped out the window to his death.

Fortunately, there are other reactions to a suicidal despair that are more realistic and appropriate, and these have saved many lives. Depression and its accompanying symptoms are communications, just as all other recognition signs are communications, of a situation or condition that needs alleviation.

Paranoia

According to a psychoanalytic theory, in paranoia a part of one's self, especially one's own thoughts and feelings, is attributed to or projected onto others. Depression, in contrast, is based on introjection, the process of identification with someone at a very elemental level. The other is swallowed, as it were, and reproaches regarding that person and the love/hate relationship continues, but is turned against the self.

In my experiences with severely suicidal persons, the processes of both introjection and projection exist alternately or together. Especially in suicidal psychotic persons, in whom the potential for suicide may be very high, reproaches and complaints are both internalized against the self and projected onto enemies or others, such as an ill-defined "they."

Anna B., for example, was depressed, withdrawn, and suicidal. She regularly heard voices telling her she was no good and deserved to die, and she alternated between denying the charges and agreeing with them.

On a less extreme and more frequent level, most suicidal persons are excessively preoccupied with what the neighbors and others might think. The phenomenon has been studied as an outcome of "role narcissism," where one's self and social role is excessively determined by internalized and then externalized outside appraisals (Richman, 1986).

Projection is also an essential component of blaming. Sometimes, an entire family attributes all its ills to one person within the family. Such scapegoating is frequent after any death, but occurs with even greater frequency when the death is due to suicide.

For example, Vilma C.'s brother committed suicide, leaving a wife and five children. The entire rest of the family, including her remaining brother and sisters, and their children, wives, and husbands, as well as more remote cousins, uncles, and aunts all declared it was Vilma's fault, because she had publicly betrayed a secret involving illicit sexual behavior in the past of the family. The blaming was a projection, to absolve everyone else in the family from all guilt or shame, and the painful but ultimately satisfying process of self-examination, and genuine grieving.

I have been saying more about paranoia and projection than most of the other variables because their contribution to suicide is large but relatively ignored. Fortunately, however, the role of paranoia in suicide, as well as in other emotional disturbances, is receiving increased attention. Allen (1967) saw paranoia as a last ditch defense against suicide. Zigler and Glick (1988) recognized the affective and dynamic roots of projection and other paranoid mechanisms. They postulated that the diagnostic category of paranoid schizophrenia is most often a form of camouflaged depression. My clinical experience is consistent with both Allen and Ziegler. Paranoid reactions and symptoms are as frequent as depressive ones in the suicidal elderly.

Help Rejection

Help rejection consists of a refusal to obtain vital professional help, to accept such help when it is offered, or to deny that one is dysfunctional or ill, at a time when the person is in a highly vulnerable state. It is particularly prevalent among those elderly who are at a very high risk for suicide.

Similar help-rejecting attitudes are present in other irrationally stigmatized conditions, such as schizophrenia. In a major study of suicides among hospitalized schizophrenics, Farberow, Shneidman, and Leonard (1965) found that a large group of such suicides were what they called "the unaccepting." Despite their severe and manifest symptoms, they insisted they were not ill or suicidal, and refused to enter or cooperate with the treatment program. Their pattern was very similar to that of the help-rejecting suicidal persons, even though the latter were not psychotic or delusional.

A second factor is the presence of parallel attitudes in the suicidal person's family and social network. Attached to such stigmatization is an identification of the person at risk with a supposedly deranged or suicidal ancestor. Similar stigmatizing attitudes are prominent in society, especially within the organized euthanasia movement.

A third factor is the inadequate response of the helping professions when someone does go for help. Haggerty (1973) presented a harrowing account of a 70-year-old man who came to a physician complaining of depression, physical complaints, sleeplessness, and suicidal feelings. He was given a prescription for sleeping medication, which he promptly used to take an overdose. Thus began a series of meetings with medical and mental health professionals, none of whom was sufficiently interested or knowledgeable to provide competent treatment.

Help rejection, in sum, is a social disease, not only an individual problem. It is not only the suicidal elderly who are rejecting help, but society, the professionals, and others who reject helping the suicidal elderly.

A series of events, associated with life-threatening crises, are major danger signs of a high suicidal potential. These include the following.

Loss of Important Others

Separation and loss are implicated in all suicides, at every age. A frequent major loss in the elderly is the death of a spouse or other emotionally close figures. The losses may begin at a very early age and continue throughout life, with an escalation of such events shortly preceding the suicide.

The question of loss and separation is the most important of all factors in my experience. It is discussed in more detail under "Family Determinants."

Role Change and Loss

Every major developmental and situational change in life requires a change and re-evaluation of one's status, activities, and obligations. In the elderly, these include widowhood, retirement, loss of job, of income, and the effects of mental and physical illness. When these requisite role changes are not negotiated properly, the result is a loss of self-esteem, feelings of being useless, unwanted, and unnecessary. Despair and hopelessness follow almost inevitably.

A Major Illness

Major illness is a hazardous event that may precipitate a crisis. Early senility, for example, can pose a threat of suicide, especially in someone who had been functioning well, is still aware of what is happening, and cannot tolerate the implication for future functioning.

Other Major Crises in the Self

These cannot be separated from the reactions of the family, as well as of the medical professions and other support systems.

An example is Fernando M., who was forced to retire at the age of 70. Neither he nor his wife could tolerate his being at home and underfoot, day and night. He attempted suicide, and, as his wife said, "It was either him or me." He attempted suicide because there was too much closeness with his wife. Ironically, he completed the job because of the separation from his wife. He killed himself 10 years later, following her death.

Blows to Self-Esteem

These result from a variety of circumstances, some of which have been touched upon as a function of necessary role changes. An illness can destroy a self, the spiritual even more than the physical.

Major Crises in Others

More frequently than we realize, an illness, an unresolved problem, the necessity of making an undesired change, or a suicidal state in one person can lead to a suicidal act in another.

Social Isolation

In the elderly, this phenomenon can be seen as the geriatric analogue of "the expendable child," described by Sabbath (1969). These are people estranged from their families, who display no discernible role in the lives of their relatives, or whose role is primarily negative.

Clinical Portents and Communications

These include all the signs and messages that can alert an available and perceptive other to the possibility of a suicidal act. Most relevant are a variety of verbal and nonverbal messages, made by the person at risk. Examples include various changes in behavior and personality, increased drinking, and statements that one is a burden, in a hopeless and insoluble situation, and others will soon not have to worry about them. Nonverbal messages include giving away valued possessions, hoarding pills, buying a gun, and indicating the presence of a specific plan to commit suicide.

Table 1 can be used as a check list of suicidal potential, accompanied by other guides such as the training manual of the Los Angeles Suicide Prevention Center (Farberow, Heilig, & Litman, 1970). The greater the number of indices, and the greater their intensity, the greater the suicidal risk. Their effects and quality can be best understood in the context of the social networks and support systems, especially the family.

THE FAMILY

Elderly suicide rests on a foundation of pervasive despair, failure, and hopelessness. Nevertheless, the conditions associated with suicide in the elderly are also present in a large proportion of the nonsuicidal elderly population. The differences between suicide and life, ill being and well being, lie in two major factors; the acceptability of suicide as a solution to the person at risk and the availability of support systems consisting of people who value the person's existence. The family is the major social system and resource of the suicidal elderly, and, fortunately, they can be helped to help (Richman, 1986).

The importance of family relationships for the person at risk for suicide is true at all ages. I once conducted a study comparing the motives and precipitants of attempted suicide or ideation in younger and older suicidal persons (Richman, 1975). Age differences were found. Most striking, however, was the pervasiveness of family conflicts and dissension at all ages. These were apparent in 90% of the younger subjects and 70% of the older subjects.

The major features of the family at the time of a suicidal attempt are summarized in Table 2. There is a dramatic correspondence between family characteristics, as seen in Table 2, and the most frequent danger signs as summarized in Table 1. Both demographic and family studies highlight the central significance of separation and loss, incomplete or failed mourning, role problems, and unresolved crises. These are present at all ages. The specific forms they assume in the elderly include the following.

1. With age, there is inevitably a greater number of losses of all kinds. In the suicidal elderly, the loss of a spouse and other important persons and an accumulation of such losses are prominent experiences.

There is a difference between the separation dynamics of the older and younger suicidal person. The younger is struggling for greater autonomy. The older is striving toward a return to his or her roots and traditions. The family members of the suicidal older persons are more often striving to separate from them, sometimes in the false belief that they are preserving their autonomy.

2. The separation is from a person or social system with whom there is an intense symbiotic relationship. The problem is not only separation, but the wish to merge, to become one with the person that is lost or unavailable. The increased suicidal risk among widowers occurs in these close relationships.

In psychotherapy with suicidal elderly couples, suicidal pact ideation is not uncommon, in analogy to the suicidal ideation of individuals. One reason is that with long-term relationships, there is a greater tendency toward symbiosis. Like individual ideation, dual-pact ideation can be responded to as valuable communications and major steps toward recovery from the suicidal state.

3. The separation or loss is often associated with early experiences and attachments. In the family with an older suicidal member who becomes suicidal, especially a parent, early influences assume the form of a rearousal of earlier family and parent-child relationships. The unresolved childhood conflicts and resentments are activated and played out once again.

Fred E., for example, attempted suicide at age 73. He had abandoned his wife and three children 25 years before when he had run away with the next-door neighbor's wife, thus ruining her life and that of her family as well as his own. His act could be understood as part of a middle-age crisis at its most intense.

In therapy, frequent telephone contacts with the betrayed wife, as well as his children, led to fruitful family sessions with Mr. E., his children, and sons-in-law. His ex-wife refused to attend, but understood and accepted the therapeutic need for

Table 2. Characteristics of Families with an Elderly Suicidal Member[a]

- An inability to accept necessary change
  - An intolerance for separation
  - An association of change with separation
  - An association of development with separation
  - An association of separation with death
  - A symbiosis without empathy
  - A rearousal of earlier parent-child conflicts and relationships
  - An inability to mourn
- Role and interpersonal conflicts, failures, and fixations
  - An intolerance for failure
  - A fear of success
  - A fusion of self and social role
  - Age associated with loss of role and status
- A disturbed family structure
  - A closed family system
  - An association of the open family with loss
  - A prohibition against intimacy outside the family
  - An isolation of the potentially suicidal person within the family
  - Fragility of a key family member
- Unbalanced or one-sided intrafamilial relationships
  - A specific kind of scapegoating
  - Double-binding relationships
  - Sadomasochistic relationships
  - Ambivalent relationships
  - An association of relationships outside the home with loss
- Affective difficulties
  - A one-sided pattern of aggression
  - An association of aggression with death
  - A family depression
  - An intolerance for autonomous emotions, especially those involving mourning and loss
- Transactional difficulties
  - Communication disturbances
  - An excessive secretiveness
  - Open communication associated with danger
- An intolerance for crises
  - An association of crisis with separation
  - An association of crisis with preventing separation

[a]Adapted from Richman, J. (1986). *Family therapy for suicidal people*. New York: Springer.

such family sessions. Although she did not attend, she insisted that her son and daughters describe every detail of the family sessions.

The rearousal of early conflicts helps explain the persistence and seriousness of elderly suicide. Bringing in the family may be life saving. Such a step may be problematic when the family is resistant, but persistence and frequent telephone contacts can overcome such resistances. Stanton, Todd, and Associates (1982) have described noble and successful efforts along these lines with drug addicts and their families.

4. An inability of the family to deal with mourning. The failure to grieve is arguably the major stumbling block to growth and well-being in the family. The elderly, potentially suicidal person is often the recipient of the family's inability to deal with mourning. The process includes a turning away from the elderly woman or man who has lost a spouse, and the aforementioned rearousal of unfinished business or old resentments with the surviving spouse. Similarly, a serious illness in the potentially suicidal older person may be reacted to by an upsurge of rage by other family members over past misdeeds or related events.

5. A closed family system is one of the more serious danger signs in someone who has evidenced a high suicide risk. It assumes various forms. In the depressed and suicidal elderly, there is a strong tendency by the patients to keep their family members from contact with the therapists. "They have their own problems" is the most frequent reason. The closing off may be even more prominent in the paranoid suicidal person, where there may be efforts to protect the family from the dangers that are perceived.

The closing off may include other family members, such as spouses, when it is someone from the family of origin who is at risk. It is as though the unresolved early conflicts are kept encapsulated, and therefore unresolved, except by suicide.

One man had a talk with his father who had been remaining in his room. That night the elderly father killed himself. The man said nothing to his wife. However, he called his mother-in-law and ordered her to take her daughter home because she was mentally ill and a drug addict. She was, in truth, a chronically depressed, borderline personality, who was addicted to Valium. She was hospitalized following this incident, and expressed wonder to her therapist about the reasons or events behind her father-in-law's self-imposed isolation in his room (where he lived with her and her husband), and suicide.

6. The variety of role disturbances in the elderly, which are such a major part of the demographic and clinical danger signs, contain a major family component. A role assignment in one person is part of a pattern of roles in the family. Conversely, a change in the role of one person in the family impacts on the roles of others.

There is one global change of role that is potentially one of the most positive aspects of aging, depending on how it is met by others in the family and society. The elderly, that is, represent the traditions of the family and society, and their roots in the past. Thus do the elderly make a major contribution to the basic real and symbolic meaning of the family in time. The elderly do so by virtue of their existence, not because they are productive in a material sense. The family and the social system that does not realize this role of the elderly are suffering a greater loss, with more serious implications for the future than it realizes.

7. A vulnerability to crises combined with an inability to handle them. A crisis is a call for change, but as Pittman (1987) pointed out, it can also be utilized

to prevent change. In the family vulnerable to suicide, a crisis may be utilized to prevent separation. At the same time, the crisis communicates the presence of an untenable situation, where neither separation nor remaining together is possible. That is why a crisis precipitated by a real or threatened separation is both a danger and an opportunity.

Although the family is heavily involved in the conditions and tensions leading to suicide, it is rarely intentionally destructive. More often the family members are frustrated or feel trapped, with their resources exhausted, and they are unable to deal with the vicissitudes of their own lives and of the suicidal old person. When the family members are helped and part of their burdens are lifted, the elderly, despairing, suicidal member is helped; and when the suicidal old person is helped, so too is the family.

THE ASSETS OF THE ELDERLY: OLD AGE AS A TIME OF STRENGTH AND RENEWAL

More has been written about the ills of growing old than about the wells. Old age is described almost purely as a period of loss and decline and the escalating presence of many ailments, both acute and chronic.

This negative and implicitly hopeless picture is presented in even graver terms with the suicidal elderly. Considering the accumulated evidence from biology, sociology, and psychology there is some validity to this picture, even though different conclusions and interpretations are possible. The majority of the elderly persons who are vulnerable to suicide present with a variety of ailments and vicissitudes. Many of these are also present in younger suicidal persons. However, they are more severe and of a longer duration in the suicidal elderly. To quote from the title of one popular book, "aging is not for sissies" (Schuckman, 1975). It takes strength to age successfully, but these strengths have been overlooked by many writers.

Gitelson (1975), for example, describes the elderly in the following terms:

> The elders are being left behind by life. They as individuals can experience this only as a desertion . . . there is increasing sensitiveness to slights . . . increasing querulousness . . . his own powers become atrophied . . . the process of introversion which characterizes old age involves what we refer to as a regression of the emotions.

On the other hand, Erikson (1950), also a psychoanalyst, saw the problems of the elderly as based on how the individual has succeeded or failed at the age-related developmental tasks and crises that continue throughout the life span. Gitelson's application of psychoanalysis became a source of negative judgments about aging, while Erikson's formulations led to a major expansion of psychoanalytic developmental theory. This chapter accepts the insights of Erikson, whose life-span approach to aging combines fruitfully with both Freud and Durkheim.

Many elderly persons whose morale and life satisfaction remain high are subject to the same biologic, social, and personal ills and do not succumb to despair and suicide.

Ida C., for example, an 85-year-old woman, her body disabled by a stroke and confined to a wheelchair, was bemoaning her fate. She lives now in a nursing home and had to give up a beautiful home. She is a widow who misses her husband, and her children who live hundreds and thousands of miles away were rarely able to visit her.

"Do you think you might be better off dead?" I asked.

She looked at me with an astonished, "The very idea!" look. "What, be buried in the ground," she said. "I have time for that."

I met Ida when visiting a cousin in the same nursing home. Ida would wheel herself over and we would chat. Recognizing my interest and positive response to humor, she usually greeted me with a joke from her extensive repertoire.

The person who retains his or her sense of humor is not ready for death and certainly not for suicide. That is true, even on one's deathbed. Humor is the major asset of the elderly.

The positive qualities become most evident in group situations, including group psychotherapy. Get a group of depressed and suicidal old people together to discuss and share their situation with each other. They will talk about their ailments, complain about their husbands, wives, or children, and the general condition of the world. Soon, they will come up with advice and suggestions. They will become more relaxed and at ease with each other. They will talk about their hopelessness and suicidal feelings. The others will respond in a more insightful, productive, and therapeutic manner than the most accomplished professional. And thus, a community of caring and concern arises. Similar positive developments arise in family therapy and other forms of counseling. They are all based, in essence, on activating the positive qualities of the emotionally distressed elderly. Add to these, the availability of a supportive family and other available support systems, including medical and other professional resources, and the picture of aging becomes more realistically positive and hopeful.

The treatment process requires the recognition and respect for these positive forces, even when they are not clinically evident. Working with the elderly suicide may then open up another world for the therapist. With the discovery of how much the elderly have to offer, the therapist, too, grows in wisdom, knowledge, understanding, and strength.

CONCLUSION

The 1989 Conference of the World Federation for Mental Health in Luxor, Egypt, drafted a "Declaration of Human Rights for the Mentally Ill." They accepted the definition of health of the World Health Organization. Health is defined as "a state of complete physical, mental, social and moral well-being." That comprehensive definition is the one accepted here and that is the goal of our therapeutic efforts with the elderly suicidal person.

Ours is a world where violence is in the ascendance and terrorism against the innocent is part of social policy. At the same time, this is an age of medical and biologic miracles, as a result of which people can live longer, more fulfilled, and richer lives than ever before. It is within these two forces, the life expanding and the life destructive that a movement to permit and encourage suicide, especially in the elderly, has grown. That is a misplaced use of energies. Rather, we must exert greater efforts to deal with the destructive forces in the world. I consider the struggle to prevent suicide in the elderly part of the goal to prevent all self-inflicted and other inflicted man-made disasters that are being unleashed today.

REFERENCES

Allen, T. E. (1967). Suicidal impulse in depression and paranoia. *International Journal of Psycho-Analysis*, *46*, 433–438.

Chesser, E. (1967). *Living with suicide*. London: Hutchinson.

De Vos, G. A. (1968). Suicide in cross-cultural perspective. In H. L. P. Resnik (Ed.), *Suicidal behaviors: Diagnosis and management*. Boston: Little, Brown.

Durkheim, E. (1951). *Suicide: A sociological and statistical study*. New York: Ronald.

Erikson, E. (1950). *Childhood and society*. New York: W.W. Norton.

Farberow, N. L., & Shneidman, E. S. (1957). Suicide and age. In E. S. Shneidman, & R. L. Farberow (Eds.), *Clues to suicide* pp. 41–49. New York: McGraw-Hill.

Farberow, N. L., Shneidman, E. S., & Leonard, C. V. (1965). Suicide among schizophrenic hospital patients. In E. S. Shneidman, & N. L. Farberow (Eds.), *The cry for help* (pp. 78–109). New York: McGraw-Hill. Reprinted in Shneidman, E. S., Farberow, N. L., & Litman, R. E. (Eds.). (1970). *The psychology of suicide*. New York: Science House.

Farberow, N. L., Heilig, S. M., & Litman, R. E. (1970). Evaluation and management of suicidal persons. In E. S. Shneidman, N. L. Farberow, & R. E. Litman (Eds.), *The psychology of suicide* (pp. 273–291). New York: Science House.

Freud, S. (1955). Beyond the pleasure principle. In J. Strachey (Ed. and Trans.), *The standard edition of the complete psychological works of Sigmund Freud* (Vol. 18, pp. 3–64). (Original work published 1920)

Freud, S. (1957). Mourning and melancholia. In J. Strachey (Ed. and Trans.), *The standard edition of the complete psychological works of Sigmund Freud* (Vol. 14, pp. 243–258). London: Hogarth Press. (Original work published 1917)

Freud, S. (1961). The ego and the id. In J. Strachey (Ed. and Trans.), *The standard edition of the complete psychological works of Sigmund Freud* (Vol. 19, pp. 12–66). London: Hogarth Press. (Original work published 1923)

Gitelson, M. (1975). The emotional problems of elderly people. In W. C. Sze (Ed.), *Human life cycle* (pp. 575–587). New York: Jason Aronson.

Haggerty, J. (1973). Suicidal behavior in a 70-year-old man: A case report. *Journal of Geriatric Psychiatry*, *6*, 43–51.

Maris, R. W. (1981). *Pathways to suicide: A survey of self-destructive behavior*. Baltimore: Johns Hopkins University Press.

Menninger, K. (1938). *Man against himself*. New York: Harcourt, Brace & World.

Miller, M. (1979). *Suicide after sixty*. New York: Springer.

Osgood, N. J., & McIntosh, J. L. (1986). *Suicide and the elderly. An annotated bibliography and review*. Westport, CT: Greenwood Press.

Peck, R. (1975). Psychological developments in the second half of life. In W. C. Sze (Ed.), *Human life cycle* (pp. 609–625). New York: Jason Aronson.

Pittman, F. S. (1987). *Turning points. Treating families in transition and crisis*. New York: W.W. Norton.

Pollinger-Haas, A., & Hendin, H. (1983). Suicide among older people: Projections for the future. *Suicide and Life-Threatening Behavior*, *13*, 147–154.

Portwood, D. (1978). *Common sense suicide*. New York: Dodd-Mead.

Resnick, H. L. P., & Cantor, J. M. (1970). Suicide and aging. *Journal of the American Geriatrics Society*, *18*, 152–158.

Richman, J. (1975). *Precipitants and motives of attempted suicide in younger and older subjects*. Presented at the Fifth Annual Conference of the International Gerontological Association, Jerusalem, Israel.

Richman, J. (1981). Marital psychotherapy and terminal illness. In A. S. Gurman (Ed.), *Questions and answers in the practice of family therapy*. New York: Brunner/Mazel.

Richman, J. (1986). *Family therapy for suicidal people*. New York: Springer.

Sabbath, J. C. (1969). The expendable child. *Journal of the American Academy of Child Psychiatry*, *8*, 272–289.

Schuckman, T. (1975). *Aging is not for sissies*. Philadelphia: Westminster Press.

Shneidman, E. S. (1971). Perturbation and lethality as precursors of suicide in a gifted group. *Suicide and Life-Threatening Behavior*, *1*, 23–45.

Stanton, M., Todd, T. C., & Associates. (1982). *The family therapy of drug abuse and addiction*. New York: Guilford.

World Federation for Mental Health (1989, January). *The declaration of Luxor: Human rights for the mentally ill*. Adopted at the Annual Conference of the WFMH, Luxor, Egypt.

Ziegler, E., & Glick, M. (1988). Is paranoid schizophrenia really camouflaged depression? *American Psychologist*, *43*, 284–290.

IV

Correlates of Suicide

Suicide is probably best understood as a multidimensional malaise. It would seem most accurate to define suicide as an event with biological (including biochemical), neuropsychological, sociocultural, anthropological, interpersonal, psychological, and personal philosophical/existential aspects. These aspects—as already shown regarding psychological issues in Part III—may vary depending on the time-line. Part IV consists of three chapters: the biological correlates of suicide across the life span; social correlates of suicide by age (with special focus on media impact); and a cross-cultural perspective of suicide at different ages.

13

Biological Correlates of Suicide across the Life Span

Jerome A. Motto and Victor I. Reus

Much has been said about the psychological implications of the various stages of life as regards suicide. The life span is generally depicted as involving a dynamic, ever-changing interplay of both internal and external forces that largely determine the nature and stability of a person's emotional experience. A major focus has been on developmental tasks and goals that, if incompletely or tardily accomplished, become an obstacle to subsequent growth, and a source of psychic pain conducive to self-destructive activity.

Less evident has been the biological significance of the time of life, other than a keen awareness of hormonal changes during adolescence and in the menopause. The rapid development of interest in biological indicators of vulnerability to suicide prompts the question whether these ostensible "biological markers of suicide risk" are influenced by the time of life during which they are observed. Although the psychosocial correlates of suicide in different age groups is a time-honored approach, and a veritable flood of information has recently appeared regarding biological observations related to suicide, there has been relatively little consideration of the relationship of these biological indicators to the life span.

This discussion examines the significance of a person's stage of life in considering biologic observations that have been associated with suicide. In doing

JEROME A. MOTTO and VICTOR I. REUS • Department of Psychiatry and Langley Porter Psychiatric Institute, University of California, San Francisco, California 94143.

so, clinicians are challenged to become familiar with terms and concepts drawn from the languages of psychopharmacology, psychoimmunology, and neurochemistry, which might now be regarded as the mother tongue of biological psychiatry.

Suicide prevention and biological research are a relatively new combination, and there is still a wide chasm between workers in the two fields. One reason for this is what Carroll (1983) refers to in depression research as a "crisis of paradigm." That is, what are we trying to identify by examining biologic compounds? A past history of suicidal behavior? Future suicide or suicide attempts by means other than drug ingestion or a single wrist cut? A tendency toward violence, impulsiveness, or anxious distress? Until some clarity is developed as to the meaning of the observations made, the application of biologic research to clinical work is likely to be limited.

BIOLOGICAL CORRELATES OF SUICIDE

Urinary 17-hydroxycorticosteroids (17-OHCS)

A claim of primacy can be made for urinary 17-OHCS as the first biologic compound to be suggested as a possible indicator of suicide risk. Bunney and Fawcett (1965) proposed this idea when 3 of their 36 depressed research subjects committed suicide during or shortly after inpatient care, and these 3 patients were noted to have had some of the highest 17-OHCS levels in the entire sample. Even more striking was the observation that during their hospital stay, twice-daily clinical estimates of suicide risk had placed these 3 individuals below the mean for the entire patient group. The investigation postulated that urinary 17-OHCS levels reflected the intensity of psychic pain in certain depressed persons, especially in those with limited psychological defenses. They cautioned that the contrary finding of a low 17-OHCS level should offer no reassurance regarding suicide, as the implication of this compound for suicide risk might only apply to a certain type of depressed patient.

This caution was later underscored by Levy and Hansen (1969), who reported two suicides of patients with consistently low urinary 17-OHCS levels. They pointed out that the excretion of this metabolite is very dependent on body size, and that psychotherapeutic drugs could interfere with the laboratory test. Fink and Carpenter (1976) also reported two suicides in patients whose mean urinary 17-OHCS levels were well below those suggested by Bunney and Fawcett as cause for concern (9 mg/24 h by women and 14 mg/24 h for men). Meanwhile, Bunney, Fawcett, Davis, and Gifford (1969) had refined their view by recognizing "long-term" and "short-term" patterns of elevated urinary 17-OHCS levels, and emphasized that the significance of their findings remained to be determined.

Although little further has been reported of urinary 17-OHCS, current investigations focusing on free cortisol rather than 17-OHCS, the surface simplicity and logic of this ostensible measure of psychic pain retains some of its early appeal. Both Bunney (1984) and Fawcett (1988) continue to suggest that it may still have a useful role. A recent review of further studies in this area with subjects under varying kinds of stress reveals a wide range of individual responses to identical stressors and a weak correlation between 17-OHCS excretion rates and severity of psychopathological symptoms (Berger, Krieg, Bossert, Schreiber, & von Zerssen, 1988).

Although specific populations have been examined in stressful situations, we find no studies of urinary 17-OHCS and suicidal behavior over the life span. Normal values of urinary 17-OHCS increase with age, and reach adult values at ages 16 to 20 years in males (3.0–10 mg/24 h) and 12 to 16 years in females (2.8–6.8 mg/24 h). Because excretion is positively correlated with body weight, changes with age and body build are minimized by using a mean value of about 90 mg/kg/day after 9 years of age (Davis, Bishop, & Mass, 1989). It must also be kept in mind that 17-OHCS is an indirect indicator of the functional activity of the adrenal cortex, and many drugs that affect pituitary-adrenal activity will cause changes in urinary 17-OHCS excretion.

Cortisol in Plasma and Cerebrospinal Fluid (CSF)

The examination of cortisol excretion as a biological marker of suicide risk was a natural sequence to the interest in urinary 17-OHCS. Cortisol is the precursor of 17-OHCS, and measuring it in the blood is much simpler than gathering complete 24-hour urine samples. Krieger (1974) was unable to satisfactorily collect such samples from his psychiatric inpatients, and turned to determining blood cortisol levels as an easier and theoretically more accurate measure of a patient's emotional distress. He found that 13 patients who committed suicide within 2 years of the test had a significantly higher mean 8:30 a.m. serum cortisol level (21.08 μg/dL) than did 39 suicide-risk matched patients who did not suicide (16.5 μg/dL). On the basis of this finding, he recommended that if a patient who is recognized clinically to be at risk for suicide has a plasma cortisol level above 20 μg/dL, "in the absence of other causes for such a high level . . . [such a patient should] be recognized as having a high potential for suicide, be provided with more protective precautions, more frequent contact with his therapist, and prolonged after-care" (Krieger, 1975, p. 229). Krieger postulated a higher than normal basal level of cortisol in some individuals, which could make such persons more vulnerable to suicide in the presence of added stress in their lives. If, as recent studies suggest, the increased cortisol output is secondary to an augmented release of corticotropin-releasing hormone (CRH) from the hypothalamus, the altered "set point" in the hypothalamus might result either from genetic factors or from significant emotional stresses during critical periods in neuroendocrine development. He pointed out further that depressive and suicidal states are seen in various clinical situations involving steroids such as Cushing's disease, arthritis treatment with steroids, and certain contraceptive medications (Krieger, 1975). From a treatment perspective, the Sachar et al. (1980) report that small doses of intravenous dextroamphetamine sulfate reduced the elevated plasma cortisol levels in depressed patients to normal in 90 minutes seems pertinent to these observations.

Further data were provided by Agren (1983), who determined "suicide scores" for patients with a major depressive disorder, based on past and current suicidal ideation and behavior. He found high plasma cortisol levels in subjects with a history of serious suicide attempts "earlier in life," and a correlation of the "suicide score" with the ratio of the pre-post dexamethasone suppression test (DST) plasma cortisol levels. Though not a generally usable procedure, such research findings support the suggestions for clinical application made earlier by Krieger (1974).

Davis et al. (1989) point out that a plasma cortisol determination is preferable to any of the urine assays because it is both easier to perform and less subject to interference. He also notes that cortisol levels are increased with obesity or hyperthyroidism, and decreased with poor nutrition, liver disease, or hypothyroidism.

Recent studies of CSF in depression have examined CSF cortisol, which may or may not correlate with plasma levels. No clear relationship to suicidal behavior has been found. Both suicidal and nonsuicidal depressed patients show elevated values, while nondepressed suicide attempters have levels only slightly above normal controls (Traskman et al., 1980). More recent results (Banki, Arato, Papp, & Kurca, 1984) are even less encouraging, with no differences found in depressed "violent" suicide attempters, depressed "nonviolent" attempters (by drug ingestion or single wrist cut), or nonsuicidal subjects with varied diagnoses.

An effort to analyze the possible influence of age on the relationship of CSF cortisol to suicide, and to depression with and without suicide attempts, proved negative, in that no difference in cortisol levels at different ages could be found (Arato et al., 1989b). This reconfirmed the results of prior studies of this research group on suicide and CSF cortisol. CSF CRH, however, was subsequently found by these researchers to be elevated in completed suicides (Arato et al., 1989a). In contrast, both plasma and CSF cortisol levels clearly show significant though modest correlations with age (Kocsis et al., 1985). Another age-related study carried out on depressed prepubertal children (aged 6–12) likewise proved negative, in regard to suicide, in that plasma cortisol concentrations in suicidal subjects did not differ significantly from the nonsuicidal subjects (Puig-Antich et al., 1989).

The DST provides a special approach to the study of cortisol secretion. Similar to the rationale for 17-OHCS and plasma cortisol determinations, the DST is based on the observation of a hypersecretion of cortisol in persons with a major depressive disorder. Normally this hormone is regulated through interaction of the hypothalamus, pituitary, and adrenal glands. In nondepressed persons, the synthetic steroid dexamethasone will cause suppression of cortisol secretion for about

24 hours, while in about 50% of primary unipolar depressives, this suppression does not occur. This test is most specific for endogenous depression.

In a retrospective report of DST data, Coryell and Schlesser (1981) noted that four suicides among their primary depressed patients had all shown abnormal DSTs when previously seen as inpatients. One suicide also occurred in a patient with secondary depression whose DST had been normal. They postulated from this a type of primary depression with an associated hypothalamic-pituitary-adrenal dysfunction that is more likely to involve suicide than are other types of depression.

A profusion of reports followed, examining the association of the DST to suicidal behavior. No clear pattern emerged, and as the early enthusiasm for this procedure waned, it became apparent that if there is a relationship between the DST and suicide, or cortisol and suicide, it is not revealed by the methodology now being used. There are contrary views (Berger et al., 1988) but the only promising lead at present seems to be the elevated CSF CRH found in completed suicides. From the life-span perspective, one of the factors associated with a positive DST, that is, nonsuppression of cortisol secretion, is advanced age in depressed subjects. The effect of age on nonsuppression in normal subjects is less clear, though, and increased basal cortisol level is seen in older individuals. A possible explanation for this is the age-related reduction in activity and density of noradrenergic neurons in the central nervous system (Veith & Raskind, 1988). Davis et al. (1984) also pointed out that there is an increased plasma cortisol level with normal aging.

One explanation for this association is that the threshold of sensitivity of the hypothalamic-pituitary-adrenal system to negative feedback rises with increasing age. Thus, in later life there is progressively less response to the inhibitory effect of dexamethasone (Dilman, Ostrovmova, & Tsyrlina, 1979). At the other end of the spectrum, reports of the DST with suicidal adolescents show very mixed results. (Chabrol, Claverie, & Moron, 1983; Crumley, 1983; Robbins & Alessi, 1985), and in children aged 7 to 11 under stress, the highest cortisol excretion rates were in those who used intense denial to cope with the threatening event (Berger et al., 1988).

In summary, in the 1960s and 1970s cortisol was regarded as a measure of internal stress, and in the late 1970s and 1980s it was considered an indicator of endogenous depression and disturbed impulse control. Hormonal studies in suicidal behavior have focused predominantly on cortisol secretion, but the data are so far unconvincing. Information about different stages of life is very sparse. The 1990s will probably see the further exploration of cortisol production in states of outward directed aggression and in anxious distress.

Cerebrospinal Fluid 5-Hydroxyindoleacetic Acid

Of the numerous biologic compounds studied as possible indicators of suicide risk, the field has been clearly dominated by the interest in 5-hydroxyindoleacetic acid (5-HIAA), a metabolite of the neurotransmitter serotonin. This interest stemmed from the work of Asberg and her group in Stockholm, who observed that the distribution of CSF levels of this compound in 68 depressed patients was bimodal, and possibly reflective of two separate biochemical subgroups of depression. Reminiscent of Bunney and Fawcett's earlier experience, Asberg's group noted that the 2 patients in their sample who subsequently suicided were both in the lower-level mode, and they decided to compare the high- and low-level patients for various kinds of suicidal behavior (Asberg, Traskman, & Thoren, 1976). When they found a significantly greater proportion and severity of suicidal behavior in the low-level group, they reported that, in their sample, a low level of 5-HIAA in the CSF was a "predictor of suicidal acts" (p. 1194). The actual numbers were eight suicidal acts (two of them lethal) among 20 low-level subjects, and seven (nonlethal) among 48 high-level subjects.

The subsequent report by this group (Traskman, Asberg, Bertilsson, & Sjostrand, 1981) generated much interest in the world press and gave considerable impetus to the idea of CSF 5-HIAA as a biologic marker for suicide. The key finding was that in a complex sample of 119 subjects, six of the seven suicides were included in a group of 30 subjects who had made a suicide attempt before admission, and who also had CSF 5-HIAA levels below the median for the entire sample (92.5 nmol/L).

Many reports followed, relating low CSF 5-HIAA levels to a variety of impulsive or disinhibited behavioral patterns. For example, aggressiveness in borderline patients with a past history of suicide attempts (Brown et al., 1982), "violent" suicide attempts as distinguished from "nonviolent" attempts (Banki, Vojnik, Papp, Balla, & Arato, 1985), and suicidal schizophrenic patients in contrast to nonsuicidal schizophrenic patients (Ninan et al., 1984; van Praag, 1983). These findings of low 5-HIAA associated with pathologic behavior were quite consistent and cut across a number of diagnostic groups.

At the same time, research reports continued to involve small samples, and sometimes showed considerable overlap of values or ambiguity in the different risk groups. For example, Agren (1983) found, in considering current and past suicidal thinking and behavior, that present or recent suicidal ideation in depressed patients was associated with both low and high CSF 5-HIAA levels, while all past suicidal manifestations and current suicidal behavior (not ideation) were correlated with low levels. Other reports apparently contradicted earlier findings. Thus, Roy et al. (1985) postulated a low CSF 5-HIAA level in schizophrenic patients who had a history of suicide attempts, but their data showed no significant differences among those with no attempts, nonviolent attempts, and violent attempts. In a subsequent study of the brain tissue of deceased chronic schizophrenic patients, nonschizophrenic suicides, and normal controls, 5-HIAA was significantly elevated in the occipital cortex of the chronic schizophrenic patients, and nonschizophrenic suicides. This was considered possibly due to antipsychotic or antidepressant treatment (Korpi et al., 1986).

The examination of CSF to obtain direct evidence of central nervous system serotonin activity gradually gave way to analyzing receptor function in postmortem brain samples, focusing on measures of the maximum number of binding sites (B max) and the degree of affinity for the serotonin molecule (Kd). Though not a new technique, its increased use was apparently stimulated by the growing interest in exploring the biological aspects of suicide. Arora and Meltzer (1989), comparing findings from the frontal cortex of 32 suicides and age/sex matched controls, reported greater serotonin binding in the brains of violent suicides as compared with controls. They speculated that the increase in serotonin binding sites was a way of compensating for the diminished serotonin activity found in depression. Though the effects of age on receptor density and affinity were not significant, they noted a trend toward a negative correlation of age and receptor density in women.

The relationship of the life span to serotonin and CSF 5-HIAA activity has not been clearly defined. Banki, Arato, and Klitz (1986) found no significant relationship of age to CSF 5-HIAA, while Simpkins (1983) stated that although serotonin concentrations decrease, CSF 5-HIAA levels are elevated with age. Veith and Raskind (1988) also observed that postmortem studies of suicides and nonsuicides have found no consistent pattern of age-related changes in serotonin or 5-HIAA concentrations in various brain regions, in contrast to normal subjects, in whom CSF 5-HIAA has been shown to correlate positively, although modestly, with aging.

The most recent examination of this issue (Stanley & Stanley, 1989) reports that an analysis of 50 cases with an age range of 16 to 79 years) revealed no significant relationship of age and serotonin or 5-HIAA. Further, when serotonin-related dysfunction was found in persons who suicided, it was unrelated to diagnosis and was consistent across the age span. While agreeing that no clear relationship with age has been established with either serotonin or 5-HIAA, these investigators point out that studies targeting specific age groups at opposite ends of the spectrum, the young and the elderly, have yet to be carried out.

Tritiated Imipramine Binding

Consistent findings of reduced 5-HIAA in depression focused attention on measuring the level of serotonin metabolism in the brain. Since the receptor sites of blood platelets and of brain tissue possess virtually identical binding characteristics, and since there is evidence that tritiated imipramine binding is associated with the neuronal uptake mechanism for serotonin, it was predictable that the platelets of some depressed persons would show decreased binding sites for this compound. Stanley, Virgilio, and Gershon (1982) demonstrated that the brain tissue of persons who had committed suicide showed reduced binding as compared with brains of persons who died of other causes. Prior efforts to measure absolute serotonin levels in brain tissue of suicides had produced mixed results (Shaw, Camps, & Eccleston,

1967; Cochran, Robins, & Grote, 1976). The implied marker of suicidal risk, then, would be a determination of tritiated imipramine binding in platelets as an indicator of the level of serotonin activity in the brain, a lower level of activity implying a higher suicide risk. Follow-up postmortem studies of imipramine binding in brain tissue of suicide victims, however, have shown inconsistent results, with increased, decreased, and normal levels being reported (van Praag, 1986). Studies of platelet tritiated imipramine binding have had more agreement, with most finding a reduction of binding sites in drug-free depressed patients (Nemeroff, 1988).

From a life-span perspective, imipramine receptor density appears to be inversely related to aging in both normal and depressed individuals (Meltzer & Arora, 1986). Veith and Raskind (1988) have hypothesized that such a reduction may be secondary to the age-related increase in circulating cortisol.

Clarification of the inconsistent reports of imipramine binding in brain may be found in the work of Gross-Isseroff, Israeli, and Biegnon (1989), who examined 42 specific brain regions of suicides and matched controls. They found that imipramine binding was positively correlated with age over the 21- to 72-year range of their sample, the effect of age being most pronounced in portions of the basal and temporal cortex. There were 11 brain regions that showed an age-related positive correlation with imipramine binding, the head of the caudate nucleus showing an especially clear relationship. Region-specific differences in imipramine binding were found between the suicides and controls, with some regions in the suicide group showing increased binding, some decreased, and some no difference. The suggestion is made that more extensive mapping, with possible discovery of differences in pattern, may lead to an entirely different set of hypotheses regarding suicide, and the influence of age on serotonin activity.

3-Methoxy-4-Hydroxyphenylglycol and Homovanillic Acid

Although serotonin and 5-HIAA have been the primary focus of interest in biologic studies of suicide and depression, two other neurotransmitters deserve mention as being of interest in this context. Norepinephrine and dopamine as well as their respective metabolites, 3-methoxy-4-hydroxyphenylglycol (MHPG) and homovanillic acid (HVA), have also been examined to determine their possible role as indicators of suicide risk.

With the exception of the urinary norepinephrine:epinephrine ratio discussed below, the numerous efforts to define the relationship of these two compounds and their metabolites to suicidal thinking or behavior have thus far shown no specific association (Agren, 1983; Banki & Arato, 1983b; Banki et al., 1985; Roy et al., 1985; Traskman et al., 1981, van Praag, 1986). Roy, Pickar, DeJong, Karoum, and Linnoila (1989), aware that positive correlations between indices of noradrenergic function and age had been reported, included a consideration of age in their analysis, but found no significant relationship. Consistent with earlier findings, they indicated that the norepinephrine system is probably not a major determinant of suicidal behavior in depressed patients (p. 348). The same conclusion had previously been reached with schizophrenic patients as well (Roy et al., 1985; Pickar et al., 1986).

The data on HVA are similarly mixed, with a few reports of low cerebrospinal HVA in various suicidal behaviors (Agren, 1983; Roy et al., 1986) but others finding no correlation of HVA with either depression or suicidal acts (Oreland et al., 1981; Brown et al., 1982; Banki & Arato, 1983; Lidberg, Tuck, Asberg, & Scalia-Tomba, & Bertilsson, 1985).

As for age and life-span relationships, this issue is not specifically addressed in available reports. Banki et al. (1986) included age in a study of CSF metabolites in 141 female patients aged 21 to 71, including 52 who had made a recent suicide attempt but found no significant age effect on CSF HVA.

Urinary Norepinephrine:Epinephrine Ratio

Another logical extension of the examination of urinary 17-OHCS is exploration of the hypothesis that a high ratio of norepinephrine to epinephrine in the urine is related to a tendency to express anger outwardly onto the environment, and a low ratio to directing anger inward onto the self. That is, norepinephrine is related to externalized and epinephrine to internalized aggression. Thus, a high ratio would be associated with a risk of assault or other violent behavior, while a low ratio would be conducive to depression and suicidal acts. This idea was first presented by Funkenstein, King, and Drolette (1954), who tested it in a laboratory setting using college students subjected to a contrived stress, and examining subjective responses by interview. Woodman (1979) demonstrated its applicability to assaultiveness in prison inmates, and Ostroff et al. (1982) found support for its relationship to suicide in a small sample of 22 male subjects with two suicides and one serious attempt.

From the age and life-span perspective, Jenner, Harrison, Prior, Leonetti, and Fujimoto (1987) found that noradrenaline (norepinephrine) excretion tended to be positively related to age and to body weight, while adrenaline (epinephrine) excretion showed little or no relationship with either age or body weight. This suggests that the urinary norepinephrine:epinephrine ratio would gradually increase in the course of normal aging. The relationship of norepinephrine and epinephrine to age and weight varied considerably in the five diverse population samples studied, with the creatinine level a possible confounding factor. A universal decrease in creatinine excretion with age was noted, making interpretation of norepinephrine and epinephrine excretion a more complex task than initially believed.

To further confuse the issue, while several studies report a significant age-related reduction of norepinephrine in brain tissue (McGeer, 1978), Veith and Raskind (1988) demonstrated that CSF norepinephrine is increased in normal older as compared with younger men. This suggests an age-related increase in brain norepinephrine activity or turnover, assuming that CSF levels provide an index of brain activity, and that clearance of norepinephrine from the CSF may not be reduced in the elderly. Furthermore, normal aging in humans is associated with an elevation in blood pressure and plasma norepinephrine (Veith & Raskind, 1988). The age-related elevation of plasma norepinephrine is due principally to an increase in plasma norepinephrine release and a reduction in clearance. The mechanism of the reduced clearance is not known. The conclusion from these observations is, finally, that an understanding of the overall effect of aging on central nervous system norepinephrine function must await further studies.

Thyroid-Stimulating Hormone Response to Thyrotropin-Releasing Hormone

The hypothalamic-pituitary-thyroid axis became a center of interest in biological psychiatry in the same way as the hypothalamic-pituitary-adrenal axis, that is, by postulating dysregulation of that system as a marker for depression. Specifically, there is evidence of a suppressed response of thyroid-stimulating hormone (TSH) from the anterior pituitary to thyrotropin-releasing hormone (TRH) from the hypothalamus in depressive disorders. There are contradictory data as to whether this blunted response may be due to elevated serum cortisol, which would tie it in with the "stress" paradigm (Kierkegaard & Carroll, 1980; Loosen, Prange, & Wilson, 1978).

The relationship of this system to suicide was also introduced by a retrospective examination of data obtained from persons previously studied for depression. In a sample of 51 female depressed inpatients, Linkowski, van Wettere, Kerkhofs, Brauman, and Mendlewicz (1983) found four subsequent suicides after a mean follow-up of 5 years. All four had shown an absence of TSH response (less than 1 μU/mL) when first seen. One unexplained death had shown a blunted response (maximum change in TSH of 1.0 μU/mL), and three natural deaths had all shown responses greater than the suicides. The pattern was interpreted to suggest that a blunted TSH response to TRH might serve as a biological indicator of high suicide risk in depressed patients.

A subsequent report (Linkowski, van Wettere, Kerkhofs, Gregoire, & Brauman, 1984) added nine depressed female subjects and 42 normal female controls, and extended the follow-up to a mean of 8 years. Five of the seven suicides had very low TSH responses compared to the nonsuicide deaths and the controls. Subjects with a history of "violent" suicide attempts showed a significantly lower response than those with no history of suicidal behavior. The suggested use of this test as a marker of risk was limited to females, in view of an observed decrease in TSH response in normal males older than age 40.

Banki et al. (1984) found an opposite outcome with 141 female inpatient subjects, including 52 suicide attempts. The "violent" attempters showed a significantly higher mean TSH response than nonsuicidal subjects, and there was a marked overlap among the patient categories. Banki (1985) later refers to unpublished data indicating that the TSH response to TRH was more likely to be normal in "violent" suicide attempters. Another failure to support this approach was reported by Chabrol et al. (1983), who found blunted TSH response in only 2 of 20 adolescent suicide attempters, who, however, were not clinically depressed.

Age-related changes in this biological function are not clear. Simpkins (1983) states that TRH neurons maintain normal secretory capacity into late life, despite the decline in activity of norepinephrine, a neurotransmitter that clearly exerts a stimulating influence on TSH secretion. Snyder and Utiger (1972a) report diminished TSH response to TRH in elderly males, but this has not been confirmed (Hershman, 1978). No age-related fall in TSH has been found in women (Hershman, 1978). Davis et al. (1989) state that while TSH increases slightly with age, the response to a TRH stimulation test is suppressed in older men but not in older women, possibly because of the difference in normal levels of circulating thyroid hormone in men and women.

The significance of the TSH response to TRH as an indicator of suicide risk is still quite murky. When combined with the uncertainties of changes over the life span, it is not yet possible to assess the potential role of this procedure at any age.

OTHER BIOLOGICAL APPROACHES TO SUICIDE

Although the biological measures discussed above have received the most attention, a number of other observations deserve comment.

CSF magnesium levels were found by Banki et al. (1985) to be even more highly correlated with suicide attempts than CSF 5-HIAA. Subsequently, Banki et al. (1986) found that CSF magnesium showed a significant positive correlation with CSF 5-HIAA, but that it did not correlate significantly with age.

The neurotransmitter acetylcholine has been measured in brain samples of suicide victims, but no difference from controls was found. There was also no evidence of a change in cholinergic activity with normal aging (Veith & Raskind, 1988).

Electroencephalographic studies have found an association of paroxysmal dysrhythmia with suicidal ideation and attempts (Struve, 1979), though the relationship is not very strong. The base rate of paroxysmal electroencephalographic findings is increased in young patients, which makes interpretation more difficult (Struve, Sarof, Hrko, Klein, & Becka, 1977).

Finally, we note studies of the relationship of suicide to CSF corticotropin-releasing factor (Arato et al., 1989), gamma-aminobutyric acid (Cross, Cheetham, Crompton, Katona, & Horton, 1988), benzodiazepine receptors (Manchon et al., 1987), and growth hormone secretion in suicidal adolescents (Ash, Clark, Sandberg, Hunter, & Woodward, 1983). This list is far from complete, and we can probably look forward to a never-ending pursuit of new biologic aspects of suicide.

CONCLUSIONS

It seems clear that the concept of biological correlates of suicide across the life span is somewhat premature, in that the entire field is still in its nascent period. Although we now have a massive body of scientific literature, it does not have much cohesiveness, and so interpreting the available information is a formidable challenge.

It is pertinent to review the comments made some years ago by a distinguished researcher in biological psychiatry regarding the status of our knowledge about affective disorders:

> In reviewing the clinical metabolic studies in this field, one is forced to conclude that it is a tribute to the persuasiveness and attractiveness of current pharmacological theories concerning the biogenic amines that they have persisted in spite of conflicting and inconsistent clinical findings. Even the most cautious conclusions based on the clinical literature are hard to propose without fear of contradiction . . . Regardless of whether the currently available metabolic findings suggest interesting generalizations about groups of patients, it is not yet possible to base clinical decisions or predictions about a major affective illness on any known measure of amine metabolism. Another unhappy realization is that the amine hypotheses have not yet led to the prediction and rational development of a therapy which is better or safer than those known two decades ago. (Baldessarini, 1975, pp. 79–81)

These comments could be repeated at this stage of development of the topic at hand. Not only are we just getting acquainted with some biologic aspects of suicide, but relatively little knowledge regarding the neurobiology of aging in humans is currently available.

There is still ample reason for optimism. Despite our present limitations, we can remain confident that the remarkable rate at which new biological information about suicide is being reported will continue to bring us closer to the understanding that we seek.

REFERENCES

Arato, M., Banki, C., Bissette, G., & Nemeroff, C. (1989a). Elevated CSF CRF in suicide victims. *Biological Psychiatry*, *25*, 355–359.

Arato, M., Banki, C., Tothfulusi, L., Bissette, G., Nemeroff, C., & Akil, H. (1989b, May). *CSF neuropeptide changes in depression and suicide*. Presented at the American Psychiatric Association Annual Meeting, San Francisco, CA.

Agren, H. (1983). Life at risk: Markers of suicidality in depression. *Psychiatric Developments*, *1*, 87–103.

Arora, R., & Meltzer, H. (1989). Serotonergic measures in the brains of suicide victims: $5HT_2$ binding sites in the frontal cortex of suicide victims and control subjects. *American Journal of Psychiatry*, *146*, 730–736.

Asberg, M., Traskman, L., & Thoren, P. (1976). 5-HIAA in the cerebrospinal fluid: A biochemical suicide predictor? *Archives of General Psychiatry*, *33*, 1193—1197.

Ash, K., Clark, S., Sandberg, L., Hunter, E., & Woodward, S. (1983). The influences of sample distribution and age on reference intervals for adult males. *American Journal of Clinical Pathology*, *79*, 574–581.

Baldessarini, R. (1975). An overview of the basis for amine hypothesis in affective illness. In J. Mendels (Ed.), *The psychobiology of depression*. New York: Spectrum.

Banki, C. (1985). Biochemical markers for suicidal behavior. *American Journal of Psychiatry*, *142*, 147–148.

Banki, C., & Arato, M. (1983a). Amine metabolites and neuroendocrine responses related to depression and suicide. *Journal of Affective Disorders*, *5*, 223–232.

Banki, C., & Arato, M. (1983b). Amine metabolites, neuroendocrine findings, and personality dimensions as correlates of suicidal behavior. *Psychiatry Research*, *10*, 253–261.

Banki, C., Arato, M., & Kiltz, C. (1986). Aminergic studies and cerebrospinal fluid cations in suicide. In J. Mann, & M. Stanley (Eds.), *Psychobiology of suicidal behavior*. New York: New York Academy of Sciences.

Banki, C., Arato, M., Papp, Z., & Kurca, M. (1984). Biochemical markers in suicidal patients. *Journal of Affective Disorder*, *6*, 341–350.

Banki, C., Vojnik, M., Papp, Z., Balla, K. Z., & Arato, M. (1985). Cerebrospinal fluid magnesium and calcium related to amine metabolites, diagnosis, and suicide attempts. *Biological Psychiatry*, *20*, 163–171.

Berger, M., Krieg, C., Bossert, S., Schreiber, W., & von Zerssen D. (1988). Past and present strategies of research on the HPA-axis in psychiatry. *Acta Psychiatrica Scandinavica*, *341*, 112–125.

Brown, G., Ebert, M., Goyer, P., Jimerson, D. C., Klein, W. J., Bunney, W. E., & Goodwin, F. K. (1982). Aggression, suicide, and serotonin: Relationships to CSF amine metabolites. *American Journal of Psychiatry*, *139*, 741–746.

Bunney, W. (1984, October). *The future of biologic psychiatry*. Paper presented at the San Diego Psychiatric Symposium. San Diego, CA.

Bunney, W., & Fawcett, J. (1965). Possibility of a biochemical test for suicide potential. *Archives of General Psychiatry*, *13*, 232–239.

Bunney, W., Fawcett, J., Davis, J., & Gifford, S. (1969). Further evaluation of urinary 17-hydroxycorticosteroids in suicidal patients. *Archives of General Psychiatry*, *21*, 138–150.

Carroll, B. (1983). Neurobiologic dimensions of depression and mania. In J. Angst (Ed.), *The origins of depression: Current concepts and approaches* (Dahlem Conference). New York: Springer.

Chabrol, H., Claverie, J., & Moron, P. (1983). DST, TRH test, and adolescent suicide attempts. *American Journal of Psychiatry*, *140*, 265.

Cochran, E., Robins, E., & Grote, S. (1976). Regional serotonin levels in brain: A comparison of depressive suicides and alcoholic suicides with controls. *Biological Psychiatry*, *11*, 283–294.

Coryell, W., & Schlesser, M. (1981). Suicide and the DST in unipolar depression. *American Journal of Psychiatry*, *138*, 1120–1121.

Cross, J., Cheetham, S., Crompton, M., Katona, C., & Horton, R. (1988). Brain GABA B binding sites in depressed suicide victims. *Psychiatry Research*, *26*, 119–129.

Crumley, F. (1983). *The dexamethasone suppression test and adolescent suicide attempts*. Paper presented at the 16th Annual Meeting of the American Association of Suicidology, Dallas, TX.
Davis, B., Bishop, M., & Mass, D. (1989). *Clinical laboratory science: Strategies for practice*. Philadelphia: Lippincott.
Davis, K., Davis, B., Mathe, A., Mohs, R., Rothpearl, M., Levy, M., Gorman, L., & Berger, P. (1984). Age and the dexamethasone suppression test. *American Journal of Psychiatry*, *141*, 872–874.
Dilman, V., Ostrovmova, M., & Tsyrlina, E. (1979). Hypothalamic mechanisms of aging and of specific age pathology II. On the sensitivity threshold of the hypothalamic-pituitary complex to homeostatic stimuli in adaptive homeostasis. *Experimental Gerontology*, *14*, 175–181.
Fawcett, J. (1988). Predictors of early suicide: Identification and appropriate intervention. *Journal of Clinical Psychiatry*, *49*, 7–8.
Fink, E., & Carpenter, W. (1976). Further examination of a biochemical test for suicide potential. *Diseases of the Nervous System*, *37*, 341–343.
Funkenstein, D., King, S., & Drolette, M. (1954). The direction of anger during a laboratory stress-inducing situation. *Psychosomatic Medicine*, *16*, 404–413.
Gross-Isseroff, R., Israeli, M., & Biegon, A. (1989). Autoradiographic analysis of tritiated imipramine binding in the human brain post mortem: Effects of suicide. *Archives of General Psychiatry*, *46*, 237–241.
Hershman, J. (1978). Use of thyrotropin-release hormone in clinical medicine. *Medical Clinics of North America*, *62*, 313–325.
Jenner, D., Harrison, G., Prior, I., Leonetti, D., & Fujimoto, W. (1987). Twenty-four-hour catecholamine excretion: Relationships with age and weight. *Clinica Chimica Acta*, *164*, 17–25.
Kierkegaard, C., & Carroll, B. (1980). Disturbances of TSH and adrenocortical disturbances in endogenous depression. *Psychiatry Research*, *3*, 253–264.
Kocsis, J., Davis, J., Katz, M., Koslow, S., Stokes, P., Casper, R., & Redmond, D. (1985). Depressive behavior and hyperactive adrenocortical function. *American Journal of Psychiatry*, *142*, 1291–1298.
Korpi, E., Kleinman, J., Goodman, S., Phillips, I., Delisi, L., Linnoila, M., & Wyatt, R. (1986). Serotonin and 5-hydroxyindoleacetic acid in brains of suicide victims: Comparison in chronic schizophrenic patients with suicide as cause of death. *Archives of General Psychiatry*, *43*, 594–600.
Krieger, G. (1974). The plasma level of cortisol as a predictor of suicide. *Diseases of the Nervous System*, *35*, 237–240.
Krieger, G. (1975). Is there a biochemical predictor of suicide? *Suicide and Life-Threatening Behavior*, *5*, 228–231.
Levy, B., & Hansen, E. (1969). Failure of the urinary test for suicide. *Archives of General Psychiatry*, *20*, 415–418.
Lidberg, L., Tuck, J., Asberg, M., Scalia-Tomba, G., & Bertilsson, L. (1985). Homicide, suicide and CSF 5-HIAA. *Acta Psychiatrica Scandinavica*, *71*, 230–236.
Linkowski, P., van Wettere, J., Kerkhofs, M., Brauman, H., & Mendlewicz, J. (1983). Thyrotrophin response to thyreostimulin in affectively ill women: Relationship to suicidal behavior. *British Journal of Psychiatry*, *143*, 401–405.
Linkowski, P., van Wettere, J., Kerkhofs, M., Gregoire, F., & Brauman, H. (1984). Violent suicidal behavior and the thrytropin releasing hormone-thyroid stimulating hormone test: A clinical outcome study. *Neuropsychobiology*, *12*, 19–22.
Loosen, P., Prange, A., & Wilson, I. (1978). Influence of cortisol on TRH-induced TSH response in depression. *American Journal of Psychiatry*, *135*, 244–246.
Manchon, M., Kopp, N., Rovzioux, J., Lecestre, D., Deluermoz, S., & Miachon, S. (1987). Benzodiazepine receptor and neurotransmitter studies in the brain of suicides. *Life Sciences*, 24, 2623–2630.

McGeer, E. (1978). Aging and neurotransmitter metabolism in the human brain. In R. Katzman, R. Terry, & K. Bick (Eds.), *Alzheimer's disease: Senile dementia and related disorders*. New York: Raven Press.

Meltzer, H., & Arora, R. (1986). Platelet markers of suicidality. In J. Mann & M. Stanley (Eds.), *Psychobiology of suicidal behavior*. New York: New York Academy of Sciences.

Nemeroff, C. (1988). The neurobiology of aging and the neurobiology of depression: Is there a relationship? *Neurobiology of Aging*, *9*, 122–124.

Ninan, P., van Kammen, D., Scheinen, M., Linnoila, M., Bunney, W. E., & Goodwin, F. K. (1984). CSF 5-hydroxyindoleacetic acid levels in suicidal schizophrenia patients. *American Journal of Psychiatry*, *141*, 566–569.

Oreland, L., Widberg, A., Asberg, M., Traskman, L., Sjostrand, L., Thoren, P., Bertilsson, L., & Tybring, G. (1981). Platelet MAO activity and monoamine metabolites in CSF in depressed and suicidal patients and in healthy controls. *Psychiatry Research*, *4*, 21–29.

Ostroff, R., Giller, E., Bonese, K., Ebersole, E., Harkness, L., & Mason, J. (1982). Neuroendocrine risk factors of suicidal behavior. *American Journal of Psychiatry*, *139*, 1323–1325.

Pickar, D., Roy, A., Breier, A., Doran, A., Wolkowitz, O., Colison, J., & Agren, H. (1986). Suicide and aggression in schizophrenia. Neurobiologic correlates. *Annual of New York Academy of Science*, *487*, 189–196.

Puig-Antich, J., Duhl, R., Ryan, N. Novacenko, H., Goetz, D., Goetz, R., Twomey, J., & Klepper, T. (1989). Cortisol secretion in prepubertal children with major depressive disorders. *Archives of General Psychiatry*, *46*, 801–809.

Robbins, D., & Alessi, N. (1985). Suicide and the dexamethasone suppression test in adolescence. *Biological Psychiatry*, *20*, 107–110.

Roy, A., Agren, H., Pickar, D., Linnoila, M., Doran, A., Cutler, N., & Paul S. (1986). Reduced CSF concentrations of homovanillic acid and HVA to 5-HIAA ratios in depressed patients: Relationship to suicidal behavior and dexamethasone nonsuppression. *American Journal of Psychiatry*, *143*, 1539–1545.

Roy, A., Ninan, P., Mazonson, A., Pickar, D., van Kammen, D., Linnoila, M., & Paul, S. (1985). CSF monoamine metabolites in chronic schizophrenic patients who attempt suicide. *Psychological Medicine*, *15*, 335–340.

Roy, A., Pickar, D., DeJong, J., Karoum, F., & Linnoila, M. (1989). Suicidal behavior in depression: Relation to noradrenergic function. *Biological Psychiatry*, *25*, 341–350.

Sachar, E., Asnis, G., Nathan, S., Halbreich, U., Tabrizi, A., & Halpern, F. (1980). Dextroamphetamine and cortisol in depression. *Archives of General Psychiatry*, *37*, 755–757.

Shaw, D., Camps, F., & Eccleston, E. (1967). 5-Hydroxytryptamine in the hindbrain of depressed suicides. *British Journal of Psychiatry*, *113*, 1407–1411.

Simpkins, J. (1983). Changes in hypothalamic hypophysiotropic hormones and neurotransmitters during aging. In J. Meites (Ed.), *Neuroendocrinology of aging*. New York: Plenum Press.

Snyder, P., & Utiger, R. (1972a). Response to thyrotropin releasing hormone (TRH) in normal men. *Journal of Clinical Endocrinology & Metabolism*, *34*, 380–385.

Snyder, P., & Utiger, R. (1972b). Thyrotropin response to thyrotropin releasing hormone in normal females over forty. *Journal of Clinical Endocrinology & Metabolism*, *34*, 1096–1098.

Stanley, M., & Stanley, B. (1989). Biochemical studies in suicide victims: Current findings and future implications. *Suicide and Life-Threatening Behavior*, *19*, 30–42.

Stanley, M., Virgilio, J., & Gershon, S. (1982). Tritiated imipramine binding sites are decreased in the frontal cortex of suicides. *Science*, *216*, 1337–1339.

Struve, F. (1979). Clinical encephalography. In L. Hankoff & B. Einsidler (Eds.), *Suicide: Theory and clinical aspects*. Littleton, MA: PSG.

Struve, F., Saraf, K., Arko, R., Klein, D., & Becka D. (1977). Relationship between paroxysmal electroencephalographic dysrhythmia and suicide ideation and attempts in psychiatric patients. In

C. Shogass, S. Gershon, & A. Friedhof (Eds.), *Psychopathology and brain dysfunction*. New York: Raven Press.

Traskman, L., Asberg, M. Bertilsson, L., & Sjostrand, L. (1981). Monoamine metabolites in CSF and suicidal behavior. *Archives of General Psychiatry*, *38*, 631–636.

Traskman, L., Tybring, G., Asberg, M., Bertilsson, L., Lantto, O., & Schalling, G. (1980). Cortisol in the CSF of depressed and suicidal patients. *Archives of General Psychiatry*, *37*, 761–767.

van Praag, H. (1983). CSF 5-HIAA and suicide in nondepressed schizophrenics. *Lancet*, *2*, 1256.

van Praag, H. (1986). Biological suicide research: Outcome and limitations. *Biological Psychiatry*, *21*, 1305–1323.

Veith, R., & Raskind, M. (1988). The neurobiology of aging: Does it predispose to depression? *Neurobiology of Aging*, *9*, 101–117.

Woodman, D. (1979). Evidence of a permanent imbalance in catecholamine secretions in violent social deviants. *Journal of Psychosomatic Research*, *23*, 155–157.

14

Social Correlates of Suicide by Age
Media Impacts

Steven Stack

Sociological work on suicide has often neglected age-specific analysis. Although there has been a good deal of work on teenage suicide and some work on suicide among the elderly, people in midlife have been especially neglected (Stack, 1982, 1987b). The present study first discusses social correlates of suicide by broad age groups: young, middle-aged, and old. The shared-life circumstances of each group are used to predict age-group propensities to imitate suicide. A statistical model is then tested linking publicized suicide stories with age-specific suicide rates.

The literature on imitative suicide has neglected the role of life-cycle status in mediating any copycat effect (Phillips, 1974, 1977, 1979, 1982; Bollen & Phillips, 1981, 1982; Altheide, 1981; Wasserman, 1984a; Stack, 1983a, 1987a,b; Baron & Reiss, 1985a,b; Kessler & Stipp, 1984; Phillips & Bollen, 1985; see Phillips, 1986, and Stack, 1987b, for reviews). Generally, all suicide stories are lumped together, the stories involving midlife suicide are grouped along with those about teenagers as well as other age cohorts. The neglect of the age-specific analysis of copycat suicide is a sign of poor theoretical development.

The mood and receptivity of the audience needs to be taken into account in assessing media impacts on suicide. In particular, the receptivity of the audience might vary according to broad age groups. To the extent that different age groups experience different suicidogenic conditions, or different degrees of such, then

STEVEN STACK • Department of Sociology, Wayne State University, Detroit, Michigan 48202.

their receptivity to suicide stories should vary accordingly. The present study incorporates Blumer's (1969) concept of audience receptivity in its age-specific analysis of media impacts. That is, there is no automatic connection between news stories on suicide and suicidal behavior. People in different age groups experience different strains on the stage of society. Hence, the present study argues that people in a given age group will tend to identify the most with the stories about suicide victims of the same general age. These age-matched victims are the ones most apt to be marked by the same social correlates of suicide as in the audience. A matching of suicidogenic conditions common to both the audience and the victim in the story should increase the propensity toward copycat suicide.

SOCIAL CORRELATES OF SUICIDE BY AGE

The correlates of suicidal behavior that vary by age include the position of the age group in society's institutional structure: the economy, religion, and family, An age group's position in the institutional structure includes certain suicidogenic conditions common to many members of that group.

First, the young (teenagers through young adults) of the post 1960s have experienced a host of social changes that have increased their suicide rate and suicide potential. Family life has become more chaotic. The divorce rate, for example, rose from 9.5 to 21.9 per thousand married women between 1954 and 1978 (Stack, 1986). Teenagers often blame themselves for parental problems, a process that contributes to suicidal behavior. The financial pressures associated with divorce can also be an extra burden carried by teenagers. Routine contacts with one parent are greatly reduced, thereby decreasing the amount of social support. Families with teenage suicide victims are more likely than other families to be marked by recurrent yelling, less affection, a pattern of hostility, nagging parents, a symbiotic relationship between parent and child that permits little autonomy, depressed or dominant mothers, geographic mobility that breaks up social networks, and neglect of children for a career (Stack, 1986).

Given that the rate of divorce has increased more than 100%, the proportion of teenagers that carry the burden of a chaotic family life, and who bring the psychological baggage with them into young adulthood, has also increased. Such a burden was associated with an increase in the suicide rate by more than 200% in the space of one generation (Stack, 1985).

For young adults in their 20s, the divorce rate is the highest. Most marriages end within the first 7 years, and persons in the period under study generally were married for the first time by their early 20s (Stack, 1985). The increase in marital problems affects young couples directly as parties in divorce. Divorce, in turn, brings out psychological states, such as depression, which contribute to suicide potential (Gerstel, Riessman, & Rosenfield, 1985). That increases in divorce contribute to suicide is a well-documented generalization that applies to samples in the United States as well as foreign countries (Stack, 1985, 1989; see Stack, 1982, for a review).

With respect to the economic institution, young people have been faced with a negativistic life situation relative to middle-aged age cohorts. For example, the youth (16–24) unemployment rate rose from 10.6% in 1954 to 18.0% in 1982. A more widespread economic problem has been underemployment, or working below the level for which a person is trained, for example, a secretary with a master's degree in sociology. Demographers such as Easterlin (1980) have measured the phenomenon of underemployment with an index of relative cohort size (RCS). A large generation, such as the baby boomers, are faced with poor economic prospects since their numbers simply result in a glutted labor market. RCS, the proportion of young (15–29) to middle-aged (30–64) population increased from 0.49 in 1954 to 0.72 in 1978. RCS is one of the strongest predictors of youth as well as middle-aged suicide (Ahlburg & Shapiro, 1984). As RCS increases, youth suicide increases, but middle-aged suicide decreases.

Religious factors have also been linked to the incidence of suicide (Stack, 1980, 1983b, 1983c, 1985). One indicator of religiosity, church attendance, fell by nearly half for young people between 1954 and 1973. In contrast, for other cohorts, it remained relatively stable. This factor was more closely associated with the variance in youth suicide than other more commonly used predictors such as unemployment (Stack, 1983b). Religiosity is thought to be important to suicide prevention in a number of ways. These include teachings that suicide is morally wrong and that one should persevere in order to obtain eternal salvation (Stack, 1983c). If all else is equal, the religious person is thought to be better able to cope with underemployment, negativistic relations with parents, divorce, and other stressful life events, as compared with the nonreligious person. Given that religiosity declined substantially for the young, we would expect their suicide rate to increase.

Turning to the middle-aged, the complex of suicidogenic versus life-saving conditions is more complex than that of the young. First, divorce rates decrease considerably in midlife. Marital strain has subsided for most in their middle years.

The "midlife crisis" could possibly be a suicidogenic condition found among members of the middle-aged cohort. There is, however, considerable disagreement over whether or not this crisis is a pattern found only in the middle-ager. Levinson (1978) in a study of 44 men at midlife gave special attention to the anxiety and depression that may emerge as men re-evaluate their careers at midlife. Other authors such as Pearlin (1975) contend, however, that the experiences reported by people in "midlife crises" may be just as common among those in their 20s or 60s. A national study found no evidence of a piling up in the middle years of anxiety or depression or even of unique transitions and crises (Pearlin, 1975). With respect to women, research by Baruch (1984) indicates that the mental health of women at midlife is largely determined by their labor force participation, its presence or absence, and its quality. The "empty-nest crisis" may be largely a myth or mainly restricted to women who have invested themselves disproportionately in motherhood. Nevertheless, the suicide rate for females still peaks in the middle years, at around age 50.

With respect to religion, the much higher level of people at midlife compared to the young should protect the middle ager from suicidal impulses. Other indicators would predict low suicidogenic conditions for this age group. The RCS factor, for example, favors them in the prediction of labor market success.

The social correlates of midlife do not put the middle-aged group at as high risk for copycat suicide as the young. Still, it would seem reasonable to expect that of the thousands of people who do suicide at midlife, some would be copycat suicides emanating from publicized stories about midlife suicides.

The elderly encounter many stressful life events that are either absent or relatively uncommon to other age groups in society. They are relatively more socially isolated, physically ill, and likely to experience life's chief crisis: death of a spouse. In addition, financial hardship is widespread. Certain life changes, such as retirement, are also unique to the aged population. As Miller (1979, pp. 62–68) points out, however, most elderly persons who suicide do so because of multiple reasons. Although the discussion treats the meanings of various life stress factors individually, these normally must occur in simultaneous sets in order to drive aged people to self-destruction.

One key suicidogenic condition facing the elderly is serious physical illness. Strokes, heart attacks, bouts with cancer, and eventual death characterize the elderly cohort. Miller's (1979, p. 26) study of 301 consecutive aged, white male suicides found that more than 60% of the sample had extreme health problems. In intensive interviews with surviving spouses, the wives understood their husbands' suicides in relation to a quest for relief from intolerable physical conditions. In one study of suicide completers, 85% were ill and in 69% the illness contributed to their suicides (Dorpat, Anderson, & Ripley, 1968).

As Lyons (1984, p. 380) points out, the meaning of severe physical illness intermeshes with other suicidogenic conditions facing the elderly. For example, loss of mobility as a result of stroke contributes to social isolation, which in turn contributes to suicide. Some physical disorders, such as pancreatic cancer, can produce depression, a key suicidogenic psychological state, directly through biologic mechanisms. Self-esteem can be lost through disfigurement and increased isolation. Knop and Fischer (1981) contend that physical illness contributes to aged suicide indirectly through its association with alcoholism. Clearly, the link between physical illness and suicide is complex; nonetheless, it appears to be a suicidogenic condition that distinguishes the elderly from other age groups.

Social isolation among the elderly is generally greater than that for other age cohorts. Retirement, death of spouse, deaths of life-long friends, physical limitations to mobility, and fear of crime all contribute to greater isolation in later life.

An endemic condition facing the elderly is retirement. Retirement can contribute to suicide potential in a number of ways such as a substantial cut in income, loss of ties to co-workers, the loss of the routines associated with work, and the loss of status and self-esteem based on work (Miller 1978, 1979; Lyons, 1984, pp. 380–381; Osgood & McIntosh, 1986, pp. 10–11). As one retiree said, "I regret giving up work more than any decision I ever made. Now that I am retired I'm not worth anything. I'm just a vegetable" (Miller, 1979, p. 49). When combined with the death of a spouse, the cumulative role loss, representing two major social institutions, drives some elderly to suicidal behavior (Blau, 1956).

The increased social isolation of the aged from the economy, family, voluntary associations, and so on has been also interpreted from the standpoint of Durkheim's (1966) social integration perspective (Rosow, 1967). Such isolation contributes to egoistic suicides. Empirical work on aged suicides has confirmed a link between social isolation and propensity toward suicide among the elderly (Bock, 1972; see Osgood & McIntosh, 1986 for a review).

A key aspect of social isolation facing the elderly is loss of one's spouse through death. This is generally regarded as the most traumatic of stressful life events. Loss of a spouse has also been interpreted as contributing to suicide through the promotion of anomie (Durkheim, 1966). Such a loss leaves the individual relatively deregulated. Research indicates that the likelihood of suicide among widows and widowers is highest the first 2 years after loss of a spouse (Osgood & McIntosh, 1986, p. 10; Lyons, 1984).

Finally, financial pressures are endemic to the life circumstances of the elderly. Some elderly complete suicide because they perceive themselves to be financial burdens (Lyons, 1984, p. 380). Research indicates that suicide is more common among the elderly who are especially financially hard pressed (Breed & Huffine 1979, p. 294). Marshall (1978) contends that the decline in elderly suicide through 1972 was mainly attributed to the improved financial position of the elderly.

Given the high incidence of physical illness, social isolation, and financial hardship in the aged group, it is contended that their suicidal mood is higher than that of other age groups. In turn, their receptivity to suicide stories will be higher than other groups.

REVIEW OF THEORY AND RESEARCH ON COPYCAT SUICIDE

The recent sociological work on the effect of suicide stories on the suicide rate of a population can be divided into two broad categories: the simple suggestion model and the differential identification (DI) model.[1] These two models are probably best conceived of as related; the latter is, essentially, an extension or elaboration of the former. Briefly, the simple suggestion model is characterized by the lack of differentiation of the audience watching the suicide stories. In addition, it lacks differentiation of the suicide stories in terms of the social characteristics of the victims. Sometimes this lack of differentiation may be due to the lack of enough stories in the sample. Typically, a wide variety of stories are lumped together in an index. This aggregated index then becomes the key independent variable. In contrast, the DI model assumes that different social types of suicide victims in news stories will produce differential degrees of identification between the victim and the audience. For example, Wasserman (1984a) argues that the American audience will identify only with celebrities. Therefore, suicide stories on celebrities can be expected to trigger imitative suicides, but stories on noncelebrities are alleged to have no such impact.

Although the roots of the simple suggestion model can be found in the classic writings of Tarde (1903), modern authors have buttressed the classic formulations with explanatory mechanisms drawn from recent, mostly social psychological theories. Phillips (1979, pp. 1168–1171) outlines how behavior decision theory, reference group theory, and anomie theory can be used to explain the link between the appearance of a story and imitative suicides. In all cases, however, Phillips lumps all suicide stories together. For example, any suicide story can set an agenda for the suicidal population; any story is viewed as offering a solution for the anomie of the anomic population.

Much empirical support has been found for the simple suggestion model. This includes work on completed suicides (e.g., Phillips, 1974; Bollen & Phillips, 1982) and disguised suicides such as motor vehicle fatalities (Phillips, 1977, 1979; Bollen & Phillips, 1981; see Phillips, 1986 for a review). Throughout this research there was essentially no test for differential identification between the public and the suicide victim either in terms of celebrity status or in terms of social characteristics such as gender or age.[2]

[1] The present study's use of the concept of DI is restricted to other than face-to-face encounters with role models. It is assumed that few, if any, members of the audience have interacted on a face-to-face basis with the suicide victims in the news stories. The theory of DI, however, is flexible enough to take into account vicarious identification (Traub & Little, 1980, pp. 189–194).

[2] It would have been impossible for Phillips (1974) to test a theory of DI based on gender given that for the period he studied (1948–1967); no published data were available on age or sex-specific suicide rates. Such data are available only from 1969 on. Some of the past work incorporates aspects of a DI perspective but does so only in passing. For example, Phillips (1980, p. 1003) uses identification considerations to omit cases of foreign pilots involved in fatal airplane crashes from his study. He contends that American pilots would be more apt to identify with pilots of their own nationality. In a second study a significant correlation coefficient is presented, in passing, illustrating a link between the age of the victim in a suicide story and the age of the victims in real-life, single-car, automobile fatalities. This is noted as evidence of identification by age (Phillips, 1979, p. 1163).

In particular, the previous work on the impact of the electronic media on suicide is marked by some flaws. The study of Bollen and Phillips (1982) excluded at least one relevant two- or three-network story for the 1972 to 1976 period. In addition, it includes one story on a Soviet crew member that should have been excluded given the authors' rule that stories occurring 0 to 4 days after a holiday should be omitted. There are also some problems with a more recent study that adds the years 1977 to 1979 to the analysis (Phillips & Bollen, 1985).[3] These problems leave the question of the effect of television news stories on real-life suicides somewhat open. Furthermore, the effect of such stories was assumed implicitly to affect all social groups. That is, there was no test of DI. Finally, these studies did not provide a test of the hypothesis relating the amount of coverage given the suicide story to the suicide rate.

The second model, the DI perspective, has not been used explicitly in the suicide and suggestion literature, but the work often uses its assumptions.[4] The basic DI theory used herein has its roots in the criminology and deviance literature where it was developed in response to some of the shortcomings of Sutherland's classic theory of differential association (Matthews, 1968; Glaser, 1956; Thio, 1983,

[3] The excluded story in Bollen and Phillips (1982) is David Huffstedttler (2/73). They also exclude stories on Harvey McLeod (5/72), Sgt. Abel Kavanaugh (6/73), Tony Boyle (9/73), Gary Gilmore and Nicole Barrett (11/76), a later attempt by Gilmore (12/76), Avraham Ofer (1/77), Rudolph Hess (2/77), and Charles Boyer (8/78). Phillips and Bollen state clearly that Charles Boyer was omitted since his death occurred close to the Labor Day holiday. Reasons for the other omissions are not as clear. However, they probably excluded many of these persons for the following reasons. Harvey McLeod's suicide was close to the Memorial Day holiday; since they used daily data, the holiday may have been responsible for any immediate change in suicide. This may be the same reason for the exclusion of the 6/27/73 story on Sgt. Kavanaugh, although it appears that the story is far enough away from the Fourth of July holiday, which came 8 days later. In like manner this may have been the rationale for omitting the suicide of T.O. Gravitt (CBS: November 25, 1974 and NBC: November 27, 1974). The Phillips and Bollen (1985) study omits Avraham Ofer, whose suicide occurred a few days after New Year's Day. The present study includes these five cases since it employs monthly data. This has been the custom in work using the month as opposed to the day as the unit of analysis (e.g. Phillips, 1974; Wasserman, 1984a). Also, there is evidence that many holidays do not affect the suicide rate, including Fourth of July and New Year's Day (Bollen & Phillips, 1982, p. 805). If some holidays do not influence suicide, it does not seem appropriate to exclude suicides that occur around them. The stories on Boyle, Gilmore-Barrett, Gilmore, and Hess were probably omitted because they were suicide attempts as opposed to completions. However, the present study includes these suicide attempts for the following reasons. First, the reports on Barrett and Boyle indicated that they would probably die from their serious attempts. Although they eventually did recover, many persons in the audience probably believed that they would die. In addition, there are suicide victims who did not die the day of their story, but who were listed in critical condition and who are included in the past research (e.g., Freddie Prinze). In the case of Gilmore, the media made it clear that he was a man who genuinely wanted to die; as such, the story may have a triggering effect on suicide even though he survived his drug overdoses.

[4] An exception would be the study of fictional, soap opera suicides by Kessler and Stipp (1984). The present study, however, is limited to real suicide stories, not fictional accounts since it assumes that the former should have more of an impact on imitative suicides.

pp. 40–41; Sutherland & Cressey, 1980, pp. 92–93; Traub & Little, 1980, pp. 189–199). Unlike the differential association theory, which stresses the learning of positive definitions of deviance from real people, the adherents of the DI theory are more open to the learning of positive definitions of deviance from vicarious role models such as those in the mass media with whom members of the audience identify. Such identification can even entail "imaginary" persons in the DI theory (Traub & Little, 1980, p. 190).

The central hypothesis of the DI theory of suicide is the greater the identification of the audience with the suicide victim in the news story, the greater the effect on the probability of suicide among members of that audience. But, a key issue is what kinds of social characteristics are relevant to the measurement of the potential level of identification.

Two different views on the identification process have been put forth in the limited literature on suicide. Both were noted in Phillips' (1974, p. 352) call for future research, but little work has appeared on them. The present study will term these perspectives vertical and horizontal identification. In vertical identification people tend to identify with the famous, rich, powerful, or other nonordinary groups. For example, there is the view of Wasserman (1984a) that people tend to identify with others who are well known—celebrities. Suicides of celebrities will trigger suicides, but stories dealing with everyday people will not do so. Second, in the horizontal DI view, people tend to identify with people who are socially similar to themselves; in most cases this would mean ordinary people, not celebrities or elites. This view is often derived from the research on laboratory studies of imitation. In these studies, it is often found that the greater the social similarities between the character in a story and the audience watching the story, the greater imitative behavior of that audience (e.g., see reviews in Comstock, 1977; NIMH, 1982; Roberts & Maccoby, 1985). Vertical and horizontal identification are not necessarily mutually exclusive categories. They can be combined into a thesis that celebrity stories involving celebrities with social characteristics X,Y, and Z will provoke suicides among members of the audience with social characteristics X,Y, and Z. This synthetic version of the two perspectives will be tested in the present study by using age/gender-specific celebrity terms in its age/gender-specific equations.

Research on vertical identification and suicide is sparse. Wasserman (1984a) finds a significant association between the presence of a celebrity suicide story in the *New York Times* and the monthly rate of suicide (all ages and sexes combined together). In contrast, the presence or absence of a suicide story per se (celebrities and noncelebrities combined) had no effect on the national, overall suicide rate.

However, the Wasserman (1984a) study is marked by several flaws and as such the effect of celebrity stories on suicides remains an open question (Stack, 1987a). Most important, there are a total of 17 stories from the 1968 to 1977 period that were missed in the previous work (Wasserman, 1984a). This is 17 of 24 or 71% of the stories that made page 1 of the *New York Times* and that appeared in *Facts on File*. In addition, it included 6 stories that should not have been listed. Finally, it also misclassified a number of celebrities as noncelebrities.[5]

To date, there has been almost no work on the horizontal DI theory of suicide and the mass media. One study finds an association between the female suicide rate and the suicidal behavior on television's soap operas (Phillips, 1982). Phillips contends that given the high degree of devotion of millions of people (mostly female) to the watching of soap operas, there is probably a high degree of audience identification with the soap opera characters. However, Kessler and Stipp's (1984) reanalysis of the Phillips study finds that this relationship vanishes once errors are corrected. However, there was no control introduced for the age of the victims, leaving the possibility of age identification still open. Nevertheless, given that these suicides were fictional, the identification process may be significantly reduced, even for an age-matched audience.

In sum, the past work on imitative suicide has been based on a simple suggestion model. It typically has used a single, nondifferentiated measure of stories. In contrast, the present study extends the simple suggestion model by combining it with DI theory. This extension of the suggestion perspective provides a new conceptual framework that allows for analyzing disaggregated suicide rates.

METHODOLOGY

The time frame of the present study is the period from August 1968 through 1980. This period is chosen because it represents the only years for which age and sex-specific, monthly suicide rates were available at the time of data collection (June, 1985). August was the starting point of the time series since this is the first month for which data were collected on television news stories (Joint University Libraries, 1968–1982). Suicide rates were calculated for 11 groups classified on the basis of age and gender: the total population older than 15, males older than 15, females older than 15, population between 15 and 34, population between 35 and 64, population older than 65, males aged 15 to 34, males aged 35 to 64, males older than 65, females 15 to 34, and females 35 to 64. Females 65 and older are excluded as a separate group since there were no suicide stories on women in this group. The cutoff point between the young cohort (15–34) and the middle-aged (35–64) cohort is arbitrary. In all cases, the suicide rates refer to the number of suicides per 100,000 population at risk. In the case of the total suicide rate, the total male and

[5] These 17 stories that were missed include ones on U.S. Representative William Mills, Board Chairman Eli Black, and Jan Palach. Persons who should not be in the list include Gregg Sanders and Bernard Ploscowe. Misclassified celebrities include Yukio Mishima, Mark Rothko, and Abraham Feller. The inclusion of local suicide stories, such as the Van Dusens, Gregg Sanders, and Bernard Ploscowe, would certainly reduce the effect of noncelebrity suicides on triggering additional suicides (write the author for details).

total female rate, the population at risk is defined as the population 15 and older given that there are only a few hundred suicides per year for the population 0 to 14 years of age. Data on the size of the monthly population for each of the 11 population groups were taken from U.S. Bureau of Labor Statistics (1982, pp. 2–49). These monthly estimates are viewed as an improvement over the past study, which used linear interpolations of annual population data to estimate the monthly population of the United States (Wasserman, 1984a, 1984b). The present study does not, then, assume a constant rate of change in population from month to month within any given year.

The numerator of each suicide rate was derived from the annual mortality tapes of the National Center for Health Statistics. These were provided by the Inter-University Consortium for Political and Social Research at the University of Michigan. The mortality tapes are essentially files of computerized death certificates. All deaths corresponding to the death codes for suicide for each year were extracted from each tape. In all, there were more than 275,000 records of suicides for the 13-year period. Monthly frequency counts were generated for the 11 population groups using the array procedure in the Statistical Analysis System program.

The data on suicide stories are from the Vanderbilt Television News Archive (Joint University Libraries, 1968–1982). For the period 1968 to 1970, the staff at the Archives graciously provided the author with unpublished data on the amount of seconds of coverage devoted to each suicide story.

The present study follows a set of rules similar to those in the past study in constructing the set of suicide stories. For example, it includes only stories on specific individuals, and only those stories that aired on two or more networks (ABC, CBS, or NBC).[6]

Another issue involves the coding of suicides that occur at or near the end of the month. The present study departs slightly from Phillips' (1974, p. 342) arbitrary assumption that the effect of a suicide story would last 2 weeks. Phillips

[6] Stories on the general subject of suicide are omitted. The one story about a suicide that occurred in the distant past, Frank Olson, was omitted. All other stories were published either immediately following the suicide or, in a few cases, a few weeks later. As already noted in footnote 3, the study does include some stories that were excluded in past investigations. There has been some debate over the inclusion of Salvador Allende Gossen's death as a suicide (Wasserman, 1984, p. 428; Bollen & Phillips, 1982). Wasserman deletes it given the assumption that many people in the United States probably regarded it as a homicide. News stories on Allende's death were reviewed in light of the findings of Bollen and Phillips (1982) that imitative suicides peak on the day of the story, and the 6th and 7th day after the story. If news stories labeling the death as a possible murder fell within 7 days after Allende's death, it would seem desirable to omit the story from the study. However, news reports, including those of Mrs. Allende who was in exile in Mexico, from September 11th to 19th, labeled the death as a suicide. Only on September 20th was there a report that labeled the death a possible murder. Since 9 days passed before the mention of possible homicide in the news, it was decided that the critical period for imitative suicides had already passed and the Allende should remain in the sample.

classified all stories occurring after the 23rd of the month, in the month after the story. However, since the publication of this pioneering piece, there is evidence that the effect of a suicide story lasts 8 days with peaks on the day of the story and 6 and 7 days after the story (e.g., Bollen & Phillips, 1982; see Phillips, 1986, for a review). Given these three peaks, it was decided to code stories accordingly—ones appearing with less than 6 days left in the month are coded as affecting the following month's suicide since the 6th and 7th day peaks are in the following month. Given a variation in the length of months in days, 28 through 31, different days are used for different months for this cutoff. Only a minority of stories were matched with the month after the story using these criteria. Alternative schemes for recoding these stories make little difference since most of the stories were aired between the 28th and 31st of the month. Using this scheme instead of Phillips' scheme affected the coding of only two stories.[7]

An advantage of using network news stories on suicide is that one can assume that they reached a national audience (Bollen & Phillips, 1982). Stories on page 1 of the *New York Times*, an alternative measure of (potential) national stories, may be invalid in some cases (Bollen & Phillips, 1982, p. 803). For example, a previous study, using page 1 *New York Times* stories as its index, included a number of stories that failed to make either television news or page 1 in other major newspapers. For example, the story on Gregg Sanders, a youth who suicided after murdering his parents in New York, while making page 1 of the *New York Times*, failed to make the news in any other major newspapers that were checked (*Los Angeles Times, Washington Post, Chicago Tribune*) and was not listed in *Facts on File*. Mr. and Mrs. Van Dusen's suicide, while making page 1 of the *New York Times*, did not make television news, did not make page 1 of the other major papers, and did not make *Facts on File*. The inclusion of stories such as these in the previous research (Wasserman, 1984a) may lead to a bias in the results. Since they probably did not reach a national audience, the suggestion effect for noncelebrity stories will not be found in these cases. As Bollen and Phillips (1982, p. 803) point out, suicide stories on the front page of the *New York Times* may not be representative of suicide stories carried in the national media such as the six o'clock news.

The present study measures celebrity status the same way as in the previous

[7] A number of stories ran more than a single day. For example, Jan Palach, a Czechoslovakian student who burned himself to death in protest of the Soviet occupation of his country, was the subject of 10 stories during January 1969. Eight of these stories were carried on three days—2 three-network stories and 1 two-network story. Two stories were carried by one network so they are not counted in the present study. In calculating the seconds of TV time devoted to the 8 two- and three-network stories, the present study simply adds together the number of seconds of coverage from each network. For example, three stories on Palach aired on January 20, 1969. Each network devoted 20 seconds of coverage to his death. The sum of seconds of coverage for that day would be 60 seconds. This would be added to the sums of seconds of coverage from the other days of two- or three-network stories to obtain a total amount of coverage.

research (Wasserman, 1984a, p. 431). For a person to be regarded as a celebrity, his or her name must appear in the *New York Times* Index for at least 2 of the 5 years previous to his or her suicide. This index assumes a 5-year collective memory for the American population and that people will tend to recognize the names of such celebrities. Two cumulative name indexes to the *New York Times* were used to facilitate the completion of this task (Falk & Falk, 1977; 1984).[8]

The present study employs a series of 11 indicators of suicide stories. They correspond to the 11 suicide rates (e.g., stories on males only, stories on young males, and so on). Whenever possible, all equations contain both a celebrity and a noncelebrity term.[9] This will allow for inspecting the relative importance of each type of story in explaining suicide. All equations will test the two counter-hypotheses drawn from vertical and horizontal theory:

H1. Only celebrity stories will trigger imitative suicides.

H2. Only noncelebrity stories will trigger imitative suicides.

Third, each equation will focus on an age/gender-specific group of stories for an age/gender-specific suicide rate. This strategy will test horizontal DI theory as it applies to social similarities in age and gender.[10]

H3. Age/gender-specific indices of suicide stories should be associated with the corresponding age/gender suicide rates.

This strategy for analysis simplifies the presentation of a large amount of data.

[8] There were 13 persons who met the criterion for celebrity status in the news stories: Tony Boyle, Romain Gary, William Mills, Andreas Baader, Charles Boyer, Rudolph Hess, George Sanders, Salvador Allende Gossens, Avraham Ofer, Freddie Prinze, Jan Karl Raspe, Gudrun Ensslin, and Eli Black. All except three (Baader, Jan Karle Raspe, and Gudrun Ensslin) appeared as separate news stories. There were 11 separate television suicide news stories on celebrities.

The noncelebrity stories were on Jan Palach, Thomas Walton, Captain Charles Reid, Mr. Boehm—a defense clerk, Mr. Zajic—a Czechoslovakian student, a married East German couple, Jack Twinning, Clark Wiley, Nguyen Minh Pang, Harvey McLeod, David Huffstedttler, Captain James "Ed" Brudno, Abel Kavanaugh, Christine Chubbuck, T.O. Gravitt, Jason Howe, a Soviet plane crew member, David McRae, Gary Gilmore and Nicole Barrett, Gary Gilmore (a second attempt), Fred Cowan, George DeMohrenschildt, Jane Young, Thomas Hannan, Leonina Shevchenko, Rachel David and her six children, John Paisley, Thomas Hufnagel, Michael Prokes, Y. Vlasenko, Jean Seberg, and Wayne Culliname. The new 1980 stories are on James Hoskins, Babrak Karmal, and Paul Snider.

[9] To generate reliable estimates of the effect of age/gender-specific story indexes, it is assumed that there should be three or more cases per age/gender category. Fortunately, there were at least three persons in most age/gender categories even when we introduced the endemic celebrity versus noncelebrity dimension. The only exceptions are elderly females for which, surprisingly, there were no stories at all; all-female celebrity categories since there were no stories on female celebrities; and young male celebrities since there were only two stories in that group.

[10] Data on the age and gender of the suicide victims were taken from either the abstracts of the news stories (Joint University Libraries, 1968–1982) or from the stories in the *New York Times*. In a few cases in which the exact age was not available in either of these sources, it was obtained from the *Los Angeles Times*.

Twenty-two equations will be presented in two tables. The first table will measure the impact of the presence or absence of a story. The second will assess the impact of the amount of coverage given to the stories on the incidence of suicide.

The preliminary inspection of descriptive statistics on the amount of coverage in seconds of television time found high levels of skewness (e.g., 7.85 for total seconds per month). The skewness indicators ranged from 3 to 10. Hence, to normalize the distributions of these variables, they were treated with a logarithmic transformation.

The present study includes a series of control variables: season, the state of the economy, the vitality of family life, and war. One purpose for including these control variables is to weight their importance against that of the suggestion factor.

Given that suicide rates vary according to season and month, the suicide data need to be detrended. Seasonal effects on suicide are controlled out by introducing 11 dummy variables into the analysis for the months January through November. This is the same technique as employed in previous studies based on analyses of monthly data (Wasserman, 1984a;1984b).

As Wasserman (1984a) points out, it is important to control for the state of the national economy in assessing the influence of suicide stories on the suicide rate. That is, in a period of increasing unemployment, such as 1975, a suicide story is likely to be associated with an increase in suicide as a result of the worsening economy. Numerous explanations have been advanced for the linkage between unemployment and suicide (see Platt, 1984, for a review). The present study uses the percentage of the labor force that is employed as its measure of the state of the national economy. The data on the number of unemployed persons and the size of the labor force are from the U.S. Bureau of Labor statistics (1982).

The vitality of the family is another variable often included in sociological work on suicide (Wasserman, 1984b; Danigelis & Pope, 1979; Sholders, 1981). Much of this work connecting divorce and suicide is interpreted from the standpoint of Durkheim's (1966) theory of marital integration (Danigelis & Pope, 1979). The current study will include a measure of the vitality of the family, the divorce rate, in its analysis. The present study follows the lead by a previous work that assumes a 6-month delay between the filing for a divorce and the actual granting of the divorce (Wasserman, 1984b, p. 854). Therefore, divorce was treated as having a retroactive effect. For example, the divorce rate in July affects the suicide rate in January, 6 months earlier when the couples filed for divorce. This entailed gathering data for an additional 6 months (through June of 1981). The previous study on the subject has a flaw: its source of data on divorce (Wasserman, 1984b, p. 854). These data refer to the month of marriage for the persons getting divorced each month (U.S. Public Health Service, 1964–1978). These data resemble a marriage rate more than a divorce rate. Hence, the present study uses a different data source giving the number of divorces per se per month (U.S. National Center for Health Statistics, 1968–1982). These data are age adjusted by dividing by the population at risk, those older than 15 years old.

The final variable in the model is a dummy variable for the Korean and Vietnam wars; war has been thought to lower suicide through such mechanisms as increasing social integration and improving economic conditions (Durkheim, 1966; Marshall, 1981).

One methodological problem in the current study is that of autocorrelation, a situation where the error term and its own lag are significantly correlated. When autocorrelation is present, a fundamental assumption of regression analysis has been violated and the results are not reliable (Johnston, 1984). The present study found that ordinary least squares estimates of its suicide equations were almost all marked by the problem of autocorrelation as indicated by the standard Durbin Watson d statistic test. It therefore employed a commonly used technique designed to help purge series of autocorrelation, the Cochrane-Orcutt (C.O.) iterative first difference technique (Wasserman, 1984a, 1984b; Marshall, 1981; for a discussion see Ostrom, 1978, pp. 39–40). However, most of the equations were still not purged of autocorrelation through use of the C.O. technique. The equations were next estimated using their autoregressive form, that is, with a lagged dependent variable as an independent variable. These equations required a new test for autocorrelation since it can be shown that a lagged dependent variable combined with positive autocorrelation will bias the Durbin Watson statistic upward (Johnston, 1984, p. 316). To handle this problem the present study measures autocorrelation using a test developed by Durbin (1970), the Durbin's h statistic. If h is in the interval -1.64 to 1.64 one can conclude that autocorrelation is absent. However, in some equations Durbin's h statistic could not be calculated since the calculations involved taking the square root of a negative number. Durbin (1970) provides an alternative test for handling this problem. This alternative test is used herein when the h statistic is not calculable. It involves taking the residuals from the C.O. autoregressive equation and regressing them on the lag of these residuals together with the independent variables from the C.O. equation. If the coefficient of the lag of the residual term in this equation is significantly different from zero, then one accepts the presence of autocorrelation.

THE ANALYSIS

Table 1, panel A, provides the results of the C.O. analysis for the equations employing story variables measuring the presence or absence of a story.

Table 1, column 1, provides data to test vertical identification theory in the absence of any controls for horizontal DI based on age/gender. Overall, stories on noncelebrities are significantly associated with increases in the monthly suicide rate net of the independent variables. However, there is not a significant increase in suicide during months with stories on celebrities. Overall, vertical DI theory is not confirmed. However, the coefficient for the celebrity term just misses the point of statistical significance ($p = .06$). Hence, it is possible that vertical DI theory will be confirmed for some subgroups of the population.

To answer this question, which regards the validity of hypothesis 1 versus hypothesis 2, one can count the number of times each hypothesis is confirmed in the 11 equations. The noncelebrity dummy variable is significant in 6 of the 11 equations. The celebrity story variable was significantly related to suicide in 3 of the 6 equations with celebrity terms. Therefore, controlling for seasonal variation and the other independent variables, we can say that both celebrity and noncelebrity stories are often associated with increases in suicide rates. This is true for approximately half of the equations in each case.

With respect to horizontal DI on the basis of gender, columns 2 and 3 provide some relevant results. Controlling for the other independent variables, stories on male suicides (both celebrities and noncelebrities alike) are associated with increases in the male suicide rate. The results in column 3 indicate that the appearance of stories on female noncelebrities are significantly related to increases in the female suicide rate. These findings suggest that there is no clear differential impact of stories by gender. The level of statistical significance is, however, higher for the male story term than the female story term.

The data in columns 4 to 6 allow for a test of horizontal DI on the basis of age alone. Stories on young persons (15–34) are associated with increases in suicide independent of the other variables. Months with stories on young suicides have higher suicide rates than months lacking such stories. These stories refer to only noncelebrity stories. Column 5 gives the results for middle-aged (35–64) persons. For this group, controlling for the other variables, neither the noncelebrity nor the celebrity variables are significantly related to suicide. Whether or not stories on the suicides of celebrities or noncelebrities appear has essentially no impact on the suicidal behavior of this group. Finally, for the elderly (65 and older) age group, column 6 indicates support for DI in the case of celebrity stories only. Controlling for the other factors, months with stories on aged suicides tend to have higher aged suicide rates than months lacking such stories. In the case of the elderly, the stories concerning noncelebrities had no impact on aged suicide. Here horizontal DI theory must be combined with vertical DI theory to fit the data.

Columns 7 to 11 lay out the findings for the five age/gender-specific groups for which stories were available. Here the data can be used to test horizontal DI theory based on a combination of age and gender roles. For young males and young females, this perspective is supported (see columns 7 and 10). Months with noncelebrity stories have significantly higher suicide rates than months lacking such stories. Hence, the age-specific effect found in column 4 remains significant after we control for DI based on gender.

The equations run on middle-aged males and females (columns 8 and 11) indicate no support for DI theory. Neither celebrity nor noncelebrity stories are significantly associated with increases in suicide for these groups. Hence, control-

Table 1. A. The Effect of Television News Stories on Suicide; B. Heteroscedasticity Test; C. Two Bogus Models, 1968 to 1980

	Regression coefficients					
	(1) Total suicide rate	(2) Male rate	(3) Female rate	(4) Persons 15–34 rate	(5) Persons 35–64 rate	(6) Persons 65+ rate
A. Effects of Television News Stories						
Lag of suicide rate	.76[a]	.66[a]	.85[a]	.76[a]	.80[a]	.37[a]
Noncelebrity story	.37[a]	.33[a]	.23[a]	.41[a]	.34	.19
Celebrity story	.20	.45	—	—	−.04	1.61[a]
Unemployment	.10[a]	.16[a]	.05[a]	.07	.11[a]	.11
Divorce rate	−.002[a]	−.002	−.002[a]	.003	−.006[a]	−.007[a]
War	−.15	−.41[a]	−.06	−.20	−.28[a]	.26
Constant	4.88[a]	9.23[a]	2.11	1.34	7.06[a]	15.00[a]
R^2	.75	.74	.78	.86	.80	.72
Autocorrelation coefficient	−.021	.008	−.070	−.048	−.021	−.006
Durbin's h statistic	−.36	.20	−1.02	−.82	−.33	(a)
B. Glejser Test for Heteroscedasticity						
Story coefficients						
Noncelebrity story	.03	−.03	−.10	.17	.06	−.07
Celebrity story	.10	.27	—	—	−.12	.59
f statistic for equation	.71	.95	1.49	.72	.98	1.07
C. Bogus Models						
(1) Year-behind coefficients						
Noncelebrity story	.02	−.02	.04	−.23	−.18	.05
Celebrity story	−.24	−.37	—	—	−.20	−1.04
(2) Year-ahead coefficients						
Noncelebrity story	−.21	−.37	−.10	−.16	.05	−.62
Celebrity story	−.15	.20	—	—	−.31	—

Table 1. (Continued)

	Regression coefficients				
	(7) Males 15–34 rate	(8) Males 35–64 rate	(9) Males 65+	(10) Females 15–34	(11) Females 35–64
				(b)	
A. Effects of Television News Stories					
Lag of suicide rate	.75[a]	.67[a]	−.06	.67[a]	.81[a]
Noncelebrity story	.76[a]	.01	.34	.36[a]	.41
Celebrity story	—	.01	40.41[a]	—	—
Unemployment	.10	.27	−.09	.06[a]	.08
Divorce rate	.006[a]	−.01[a]	−.01[a]	−.0002	−.004[a]
War	−.46	−.52	.11	.09	−.15[a]
Constant	1.48	15.34[a]	4.49	−1.57[a]	−1.18[a]
R^2	.88	.74	.81	.41	.74
Autocorrelation coefficient	−.040	−.008	−.006	−.069	−.075
Durbin's h statistic	−.72	−.16	−.11	−1.50	−1.18
B. Glejser Test for Heteroscedasticity					
Story coefficients					
Noncelebrity story	.22	.10	−.53	.05	−.25
Celebrity story	—	−.45	.75	—	—
f statistic for equation	.96	1.15	.70	1.01	1.56
C. Bogus Models					
(1) Year-behind coefficients					
Noncelebrity story	−.29	−.27	.20	.16	−.50
Celebrity story	—	−1.21	−2.32	—	—
(2) Year-ahead coefficients					
Noncelebrity story	−.34	.02	—	−.06	−.40
Celebrity story	—	−.69	−.04	—	—

[a]Statistically significant at the .05 level.

Eleven monthly dummy variables that were introduced to deseasonalized the date series are not shown for the purposes of brevity and clarity. (a) Durbin's h statistic not calculable due to square root of negative number; an alternative test (Durbin, 1970) indicates no autocorrelation (residuals regressed on the lag of the error term and the independent variables). In the regression on the elderly suicide rate the coefficient of the lag of the residual was −.08; its standard error was .26. This yielded a t ratio of −.31, considerably less than what was needed to demonstrate significant autocorrelation. (b) Series purged of heteroscedasticity through the use of weighted least squares. A nondirectional t-test was used for the bogus models.

ling for gender, a relationship between stories and suicide fails to emerge for this group. There is no evidence of a suppressor effect. The results from column 5 where males and females were lumped together are replicated for age/gender-specific equations.

Finally, column 9 provides results for the equation on elderly male suicide. For this group, stories on noncelebrity, aged males have no imitative impact. However, stories on aged, male celebrities are significantly associated with increases in aged male suicide. Here horizontal DI theory works only when combined with vertical DI theory. This is consistent with the findings of column 6 where all elderly people were lumped together in one equation.

Table 2 shifts the analysis to the impact of the amount of coverage of suicide stories on suicide rates. The data in column 1 indicate that overall, the greater the amount of coverage of stories on noncelebrities, the greater the increase in suicide. The amount of coverage given to celebrity stories, however, is unrelated to suicide. However, given that celebrity stories did affect the suicide rates in Table 1, it is likely that the celebrity term will be significant, again, in the age/gender-specific runs.

As in Table 1, if we look at all 11 columns of results, stories on noncelebrities and celebrities tend to be about equally likely to affect suicide rates. One third (4 of 11) of the terms involving noncelebrity stories are significant. One third (2 of 6) terms involving celebrity stories are significant predictors of suicide. Overall, then, it seems that both vertical and horizontal DI theories are supported.

The amount of coverage given to noncelebrity male stories has a significant relationship to suicide (column 2). This is not true, however, for female suicide stories (column 3). In addition, the amount of coverage given male celebrity stories is not significantly related to suicide, although the term just misses the significance level ($p = .06$). These latter two findings do not supplement the significant relationships for the story dummy variables in Table 1 columns 2 and 3. While the appearance of these latter two categories of stories affects imitative suicide, the amount of seconds of coverage does not.

Columns 4 to 6 of Table 2 find the same patterns between stories and suicide as found in Table 1. The greater the amount of coverage of stories on young suicides, the greater the suicide rate. Neither the amount of coverage given to the suicides of middle-aged noncelebrities nor middle-aged celebrities affects the suicide rate of the middle ager. Even stories that receive the greatest amount of coverage, then, are apparently not related to the suicide rate. Finally, controlling for the other variables in the equation, the greater the amount of coverage of stories about elderly celebrities, the greater the suicide rate of the elderly.

The equations on age/gender specific suicide rates support the patterns of Table 1 for males, but not fully for females (columns 7–11). For young males, the greater the coverage of noncelebrity suicides, the greater the suicide rate. For elderly males, the greater the coverage of celebrity suicides, the greater the suicide rate. For both middle-aged males and females, all story variables are unrelated to suicide. For elderly males, the greater the coverage of celebrity suicides, the greater the increase in the suicide rate. For young females, however, the amount of coverage, unlike coverage per se, was unrelated to suicide. In no case did a new, significant relationship emerge once the amount of coverage was allowed to vary.

One consistent pattern found in both tables is that the suicide rates of the middle-ager are essentially unresponsive to suicide stories about the middle-ager.

In Table 2, since the suggestion factor is measured on a continuous variable, as opposed to a categorical dummy variable, beta coefficients can be interpreted. The absolute values of these will allow for ranking the variables' importance in explaining the variability in suicide. One way of putting the importance of the suggestion model into perspective is to count how many times it provides the most important variable in the 11 equations, and do the same for the other continuous variables. Only variables that are significant and have the right sign will be counted. The results are as follows:

Variable	*Times most important*
Noncelebrity seconds	1
Celebrity seconds	1
Unemployment rate	6
Divorce rate	2

One equation (column 11) did not have any qualified coefficients and was not counted. It is clear that the rate of unemployment tends to be the most important variable, having the largest beta coefficient in 6 of the 11 equations. While the suggestion factor is significant and important in many equations, its relation to suicide rates is usually secondary. Past research, by omitting control variables such as unemployment, has been unable to put the suggestion factor in its greater sociological perspective.[11]

DISCUSSION: A TEST OF AN ALTERNATIVE INTERPRETATION

The results in panel A of Tables 1 and 2 might be criticized from the standpoint of "artifact" theory (Baron and Reiss, 1985a, 1985b). That is, these relationships could be the product of such statistical conditions as heteroscedasticity and the timing of publicized stories. To address the artifact thesis, the present study

[11] One issue emerging from the analysis is the fairly consistent negative sign of the divorce term. These findings may, however, be a function of an inappropriate lag structure that taps into the divorce cycle at the wrong point. That is, the current study uncritically followed the previous research (Wasserman, 1984b) in constructing a retroactive divorce variable. In an analysis not reported here because of space limitations, it was determined that the signs became positive through the use of a different lag structure (write author for details).

Table 2. A. The Effect of the Amount of Coverage Given to Television Suicide News Stories on Suicide Rates; B. Heteroscedasticity Test; C. Two Bogus Models, 1968 to 1980

	Regression coefficients					
	(1) Total suicide rate	(2) Male rate	(3) Female rate	(4) Persons 15–34 rate	(5) Persons 35–64 suicide rate	(6) Persons 65+ suicide rate
A. Effect of Television News Stories						
Lag of suicide rate	.75[a] (.75)	.66[a] (.66)	.84[a] (.83)	.76[a] (.77)	.80[a] (.79)	.34[a] (.34)
Noncelebrity story	.07[a] (.152)	.05[a] (.07)	.03 (.05)	.11[a] (.10)	.06 (.05)	.05 (.02)
Celebrity story	.02 (.04)	.07 (.07)	—	—	.02 (.007)	.27[a] (.11)
Unemployment	.10[a] (.145)	.16[a] (.15)	.05[a] (.07)	−.08[a] (.06)	.12[a] (.10)	.12 (.07)
Divorce rate	−.002[a](−.19)	−.002 (−.11)	−.002[a](−.19)	.002[a](−.12)	−.006[a](−.29)	−.007[a](−.23)
War	−.15 (−.07)	−.41 (−.13)	−.07 (−.04)	−.17 (−.05)	−.27 (−.08)	.33[a] (.07)
Constant	4.93	9.22[a]	2.12[a]	1.26	7.05[a]	15.62[a]
R^2	.75	.73	.77	.87	.80	.72
Autocorrelation coefficient	−.016	.008	−.072	−.052	−.023	−.004
Durbin's h statistic	−.28	.21	−1.05	−.88	−.36	(a)
B. Glejser Test for Heteroscedasticity						
Story coefficients						
Noncelebrity story	.006	.004	−.02	.02	.009	−.02
Celebrity story	.007	.04	—	—	−.03	.10
f statistic for equation	.76	.98	1.48	.73	1.03	.99
C. Bogus Models						
(1) Year-behind coefficients						
Noncelebrity story	−.003	−.0002	−.003	−.06	−.04	−.02
Celebrity story	−.04	−.06	—	—	−.04	−.21
(2) Year-ahead coefficients						
Noncelebrity story	−.04	−.07[a]	−.02	−.02	−.21	—
Celebrity story	.03	.05	—	—	−.15	−.11

Table 2. (Continued)

	Regression coefficients				
	(7) Males 15–34 suicide rate	(8) Males 35–64 suicide rate	(9) Males 65+ suicide rate	(10) Females 15–34 suicide rate	(11) Females 35–64 suicide rate
A. Effects of Television News Stories					
Lag of suicide rate	.75[a] (.76)	.67[a] (.66)	.23 (.23)	.67[a] (.67)	.80[a] (.79)
Noncelebrity story	.17[a] (.08)	.03	.008 (.001)	.05 (.08)	.06 (.0007)
Celebrity story	— (—)	.03 (.01)	.37[a] (.09)	—	—
Unemployment	.10 (.04)	.27[a] (.18)	.03 (.01)	.06[a] (.14)	.07 (.04)
Divorce rate	.006[a](.14)	−.01[a] (−.42)	−.008 (−.15)	−.0003 (−.004)	−.004[a](−.24)
War	−.45 (−.06)	−.50[a] (−.11)	.43 (.05)	.09 (.06)	.15 (−.005)
Constant	1.38	15.21[a]	31.08[a]	1.58[a]	4.04[a]
R^2	.89	.74	.67	.41	.74
Autocorrelation coefficient	−.042	−.008	.0005	−.070	−.075
Durbin's h statistic	−.73	−.15	(a)	−1.55	−1.18
B. Glejser Test for Heteroscedasticity					
Story coefficients					
Noncelebrity story	.06	.02	−.12	−.0003	−.07
Celebrity story	—	−.10	.25	—	—
f statistic for equation	1.05	1.15	.88	1.04	1.69
C. Bogus Models					
(1) Year-behind coefficients					
Noncelebrity story	−.08	−.06	−.02	.02	−.11
Celebrity story	—	.24	−.52[a]	—	—
(2) Year-ahead coefficients					
Noncelebrity story	−.34	−.02	—	−.002	−.10
Celebrity story	—	−.12	−.02	—	—

Note:Numbers in parentheses are standardized regression coefficients.
[a]Statistically significant at the .05 level.
Eleven monthly dummy variables that were introduced to deseasonalize the date series are not shown for purposes of brevity and clarity. (a) Durbin's h statistic not calculable due to square root of negative number; an alternative test (Durbin, 1970) indicates no autocorrelation (residuals regressed on the lag of the error term and the independent variables). For the equation on elderly males the *t* ratio for the lag of the error term was .032, far below the valued needed for significant autocorrelation. This *t* ratio was −.240 for the equation for the elderly as a whole, again much less than what would be needed for a significant level of autocorrelation.

employs the same tests as Phillips and Bollen (1985). These tests are the Glejser (1969) test for heteroscedasticity (see Johnston, 1984, pp. 301–302, for a discussion), and both year ahead and year behind bogus models (see Phillips & Bollen, 1985, for a discussion).

Heteroscedasticity, or unequal variance in the error term across values of the independent variable, tends to bias regression coefficients upwards. Hence, if present, *t* ratios will be relatively high and a variable is apt to be artificially significant (Johnston, 1984).

A standard test for heteroscedasticity was developed by Glejser (1969). The residuals from the regression equation are regressed on the predictor variables. If any of the terms are significant, they are marked by heteroscedasticity.

Panel B of Tables 1 and 2 present the results of the Glejser test for each of the 22 equations. In all cases but one, the C.O.-generated equations were free of heteroscedasticity. The one exception was equation 9 in Table 2. That equation was re-estimated using a standard procedure, weighted least squares (Pindyck & Rubinfeld, 1981, pp. 145–146). That procedure successfully removed the heteroscedasticity, and the results are reported in the table. None of the story variables' coefficients was significant in the 22 equations. The coefficients of the story variables from the Glejser equations are given in the tables.

As a further check for heteroscedastic disturbance terms, the present analysis also inspected the f statistic for the entire equation. It is possible, for example, that all the variables taken together may create a situation of heteroscedasticity. The f statistic for the entire Glejser equation is also provided in panel B of the two tables. These f statistics proved to be rather small and insignificant. Many are, in fact, less than 1.

It is concluded that there is no support for the artifact hypothesis based on heteroscedasticity.

As a further test of the artifact thesis, Tables 1 and 2 present the results of bogus models in panel C. For the purpose of brevity only the coefficients of the story variables are given in the tables.[12] Two bogus models were run on each of the 22 suicide rate equations. In the first, the year-behind model, the effect of the suicide story is measured as occurring a year before the story even appeared. For example, a suicide story airing in January 1977 is matched with the January 1976 suicide rate. In the second bogus model, the year-ahead model, the effect of a suicide story is lagged a year into the future. For example, a story airing in June 1975 is matched with the suicide rate for June 1976.

Of the 32 story coefficients from the bogus panel C in Table 1, only one is significant (column 9, year-behind model). This is about what we would expect by chance.

[12] For the year-ahead bogus regressions, the number of elderly noncelebrities fell below the required number of three cases. Babrak Karmal's 1980 story was no longer in the sample. Hence, the bogus regressions were estimated without the noncelebrity terms.

Of the 32 bogus model coefficients presented in Table 2, panel C, only two are significant. Again, this is about what we would anticipate by chance.

It is concluded that since only 3 of the 64 bogus model story coefficients are significant, there is essentially no evidence in support of the artifact hypothesis. Given that approximately 1 in 20 coefficients would be significant by chance, 3 of 64 coefficients indicate chance fluctuations.

CONCLUSION

The present study tested several specifications of the suggestion/imitation theory of suicide. The simple suggestion model was extended to take into account the process of DI. DI, in turn, was conceptualized in terms of two subprocesses: horizontal and vertical identification. This conceptual framework differs substantially from the past work, which has been almost entirely based on a simple suggestion model.

The findings on vertical DI are significantly different from those in the past work (Wasserman, 1984a). While celebrity suicides certainly did trigger suicides in some population groups, noncelebrity suicide stories were just as related to real-life suicides. The present study contends that for the electronic news story, it does not always matter whether or not a suicide victim is a celebrity, what matters is whether or not the story is aired nationwide and reaches a truly national audience. The apparent contradiction between the findings of Wasserman (1984a) and the present study may also be due to the former's flaws in sampling procedures, which included missing 71% of the relevant suicide stories. The findings that celebrity as well as noncelebrity stories trigger suicide support the stream of research findings based on a simple suggestion model (Phillips, 1979, 1980, 1982; Bollen & Phillips, 1981, 1982).

The findings on vertical identification suggest that the identification process is marked by a duality. That is, people identify both upwards and laterally. This duality in the process of identification has been noted for many years in the field of advertising (Mandell, 1984, pp. 252–253). Sometimes advertisers select high-status persons, other times ordinary people, for their ads. The public seems to identify well with either group as evidenced by data on consumer purchases.

The present study also extended DI theory to the neglected gender and age dimensions of identification. These are taken as key dimensions of social life upon which people build a sense of identity. The regressions based on age and sex found strong support for this version of the theory for the relatively young, and the elderly. The horizontal DI theory also worked for both males and females. Further work is needed to explain the relative lack of an association between news stories on the middle-ager and the suicide rates of that group. The suicide rates of the middle-ager stood out as being consistently unrelated to imitative suicide.

For the moment, it is speculated that the failure of the suggestion perspective to work for the data on the middle-ager may be due to the relatively low level of suicidogenic life conditions for that age group. For example, unlike the elderly group, the middle-aged group is in comparatively good health and is financially well off. Compared to the young, they are more settled into society's institutional framework, including marriage, the family, work, and politics. The middle-aged group tends to hold a disproportional amount of the power positions in society. Further, the middle-aged group was the chief beneficiaries of a phenomenon termed RCS for the period under study. As social demographers such as Easterlin (1980) have noted, a high ratio of young to middle age usually has a considerable negative impact on the quality of life of the young and a substantial positive impact on the lives of the middle-ager. Ahlburg and Shapiro (1984) develop this argument in explaining annual suicide trends in the United States. RCS may be taken as a contextual factor that acts as a buffer against suicide for the middle-ager; the labor market and other benefits derived from being in a relatively small-sized generation may protect an age cohort from suicidal behavior. Finally, if these speculations are correct, as the baby-boom generation becomes middle-aged, the relationship between age and suicide should reverse. Research on this issue will have to wait, however, since the large-sized baby-boom cohort is just beginning to enter their 40s. Caution should be exercised in generalizing the findings of the present study on age and imitative suicides; 20 or so years from now the middle-aged cohort, suffering from a large generation effect, may have the highest propensity for imitative suicide.

Finally, while support was found for both the horizontal and vertical versions of DI theory, the analysis indicated that the state of the national economy was generally more important to the explanation of suicide. However, there are a number of age/gender groups that are in need of further work. In particular, future work should inspect the relationship between female celebrity suicide stories and female suicide. For the 1968 to 1980 period there were no female celebrity suicides at all. Data for the 1980s may uncover some cases for analysis of this important category. In addition, there were absolutely no suicide stories on elderly females. For these reasons, some caution needs to be exercised in accepting the hegemony of the economic model.

ACKNOWLEDGMENT. This study was supported by grants MH38209 and MH41510 from the National Institutes of Mental Health, Bethesda, MD. The author is indebted to the staff of the Vanderbilt Television News Archive for making unpublished data available. Tapes containing suicide records were provided by the Inter-University Consortium for Political and Social Research at the University of Michigan.

REFERENCES

Ahlburg, D., & Shapiro, M. (1984). Socio-economic ramifications of relative cohort size. *Demography*, *21*, 97–108.

Altheide, D. (1981). Airplane accidents, murder, and the mass media: Comment on Phillips. *Social Forces*, *60*, 593–596.

Baron, J., & Reiss, P. (1985a). Same time next year: Aggregate analysis of the mass media and violent behavior. *American Sociological Review*, *50*, 347–363.

Baron, J., & Reiss, P. (1985b). Reply to Phillips and Bollen. *American Sociological Review*, *50*, 372–376.

Baruch, G. (1984). The psychological well being of women in the middle years. In G. Baruch & J. Brooks-Gunn (Eds.), *Women in midlife* (pp. 161–180). New York: Plenum.

Blau, Z. N. (1956). Changes in status and age identification. *American Sociological Review*, *21*, 198–203.

Blumer, H. (1969). Suggestions for the study of mass media effects. (pp. 183–194). In Herbert Blumer (Ed.), *Symbolic interactionism*, Englewood Cliffs, NJ: Prentice Hall.

Bock, E. W. (1972). Aging and suicide: the significance of marital, kinship, and alternative relations. *Family Coordinator*, *21*, 71–79.

Bollen, K., & Phillips, D. (1981). Suicidal motor vehicle fatalities in Detroit: A replication. *American Journal of Sociology*, *87*, 404–412.

Bollen, K., & Phillips, D. (1982). Imitative suicides: A national study of the effects of television news stories. *American Sociological Review*, *47*, 802–809.

Breed, W., & Huffine, C. L. (1979). Sex differences in suicide among older white Americans: A role and developmental approach. In O. J. Kaplan (Ed.), *Psychopathology of aging* (pp. 289–309). New York: Academic Press.

Comstock, G. (1977). Types of portrayal and aggressive behavior. *Journal of Communication*, *26*, 189–198.

Danigelis, N., & Pope, W. (1979). Durkheim's theory of suicide as applied to the family. *Social Forces*, *57*, 1081–1106.

Dorpat, T. L., Anderson, W. F., & Ripley, N. S. (1968). The relationship of physical illness to suicide. In H. L. P. Resnik (Ed.), *Suicidal behaviors: Diagnosis and management*. Boston: Little, Brown.

Durbin, J. M. (1970). Testing for serial correlation in least squares when some of the regressions are lagged dependent variables. *Econometrica*, *38*, 410–421.

Durkheim, E. (1966). *Suicide*. New York: Free Press.

Easterlin, R. (1980). *Birth and Fortune*. New York: Basic Books.

Falk, B., & Falk, V. (1977). Personal name index to the *New York Times*. Succasunna, NJ: Roxbury Data Interface.

Falk, B., & Falk, V. (1984). Personal name index to the *New York Times* Index, 1974-1979 Supplement. Verdi, NV: Roxbury Data Interface.

Gerstel, N., Riessman, C. K., & Rosenfield, S. (1985). Explaining the symptomatology of separated and divorced women and men: The role of material conditions and social networks. *Social Forces*, *64*, 84–101.

Glaser, D. (1956). Criminality theories and behavioral images. *American Journal of Sociology*, *61*, 433–444.

Glejser, H. (1969). A new test for heteroscedasticity. *Journal of the American Statistical Association*, *64*, 316–323.

Johnston, J. (1984). *Econometric methods* (3rd ed.). New York: McGraw Hill.

Joint University Libraries. (1968-1982). Vanderbilt Television News Archives. Nashville: Vanderbilt University.

Kessler, R., & Stipp, H. (1984). The impact of fictional television suicide stories on U.S. fatalities. A replication. *American Journal of Sociology*, *90*, 151–167.

Knop, J., & Fischer, A. (1981). Duodenal ulcer, suicide, psychopathology, and alcoholism. *Acta Psychiatrica Scandinavia, 63*, 346–355.

Lester, D. (1983). *Why people kill themselves* (2nd ed.). Springfield, IL: Charles C Thomas.

Levinson, D. C., Darrow, N., Klein, E. B., Levinson, M. H., & McKee, B. (1978). *The seasons of a man's life*. New York: Ballantine.

Lyons, M. J. (1984). Suicide in later life: Some putative causes with implications for prevention. *Journal of Community Psychology, 12*, 379–388.

Mandell, M. I. (1984). *Advertising*. Englewood Cliffs, NJ: Prentice Hall.

Marshall, J. (1978). Changes in white male suicide: 1948–1972. *Journal of Gerontology, 33*, 763–768.

Marshall, J. (1981). Political integration and the effect of war on suicide in the United States, 1933–76. *Social Forces, 59*, 771–785.

Matthews, V. (1968). Differential identification: An empirical note. *Social Problems, 15*, 376–383.

Miller, M. (1978). Geriatric suicide: The Arizona study. *The Gerontologist, 18*, 488–495.

Miller, M. (1979). *Suicide after sixty: The final alternative*. New York: Springer.

National Institute of Mental Health. (1982). *Television and behavior: Ten years of scientific progress and implications for the eighties*. Washington, DC: U.S. Government Printing Office.

Osgood, N. J., & McIntosh, J. (1986). *Suicide among the elderly: An annotated bibliography*. New York: Greenwood Press.

Ostrom, C. (1978). *Time series analysis*. Beverly Hills, CA: Sage.

Pearlin, L. (1975). Sex roles and depression. In N. Datan & L. H. Ginsberg (Eds.), *Life span developmental psychology: Normative life crises*. New York: Academic Press.

Phillips, D. (1974). The influence of suggestion on suicide. *American Sociological Review, 39*, 340–354.

Phillips, D. (1977). Motor vehicle fatalities increase just after publicized suicide stories. *Science, 196*, 1464–1465.

Phillips, D. (1979). Suicide, motor vehicle fatalities, and the mass media: Evidence toward a theory of suggestion. *American Journal of Sociology, 84*, 1150–1174.

Phillips, D. (1980). Airplane accidents, murder, and the mass media: Towards a theory of imitation and suggestion. *Social Forces, 58*, 1001–1024.

Phillips, D. (1982). The impact of fictional television stories on U.S. adult fatalities. *American Journal of Sociology, 87*, 1340–1359.

Phillips, D. (1983). The impact of mass media violence on US homicides. *American Sociological Review, 48*, 560–568.

Phillips, D. (1986). The found experiments: A new technique for assessing the impact of mass media violence on real-world aggression. In *Public Communication and Behavior* (Vol. 1; pp. 259–307). New York: Academic Press.

Phillips, D., & Bollen, K. (1985). Same time last year: Selective data dredging for negative findings. *American Sociological Review, 50*, 364–371.

Pindyck, R. S., & Rubinfeld, D. (1981). *Econometric models and economic forecasts* (2nd ed.). New York: McGraw Hill.

Platt, S. (1984). Unemployment and suicidal behavior: A review of the literature. *Social Science and Medicine, 19*, 93–115.

Roberts, D. F., & Maccoby, N. (1985). Effects of mass communication. In G. Lindzey & E. Aronson (Eds.), *The handbook of social psychology, volume 2: Special fields and applications* (pp. 539–598). New York: Random House.

Rosow, I. (1967). *Social integration of the aged*. New York: Free Press.

Sholders, M. A. (1981). *Suicide in Indianapolis*, 1976–1980. *Sociological Focus, 14*, 221–231.

Stack, S. (1980). Religion and suicide: A reanalysis. *Social Psychiatry, 15*, 65–70.

Stack, S. (1982). Suicide: A decade review of the sociological literature. *Deviant Behavior, 4*, 41–66.

Stack, S. (1983a). The effect of Jonestown on the suicide rate. *Journal of Social Psychology, 119*, 145–146.

Stack, S. (1983b). The effect of the decline in institutionalized religion on suicide, 1954–1978. *Journal for the Scientific Study of Religion*, *22*, 239–252.

Stack, S. (1983c). The effect of religious commitment on suicide: A cross national analysis. *Journal of Health and Social Behavior*, *24*, 362–374.

Stack, S. (1985). The effect of domestic/religious individualism on suicide, 1954–1978. *Journal of Marriage and the Family*, *47*, 431–447.

Stack, S. (1986, May 26). A leveling off in young suicides. *Wall Street Journal*, p. 34.

Stack, S. (1987a). Celebrities and suicide: A taxonomy and analysis, 1948-1983. *American Sociological Review*, *52*, 401–412.

Stack, S. (1987b). Sociological study of suicide: Methodological issues. *Suicide and Life-Threatening Behavior*, *17*, 133–150.

Stack, S. (1988). Suicide: Media impacts in war and peace. *Suicide and Life-Threatening Behavior*, *18*, 342–357.

Stack, S. (1989). The impact of divorce on suicide in Norway, 1951-1980. *Journal of Marriage and the Family*, *51*, 229–238.

Sutherland, E. H., & Cressey, D. (1980). Criminology (10th ed.). Philadelphia: J. B. Lippincott.

Tarde, G. (1903). *The laws of imitation*. New York: Holt.

Thio, A. (1983). Deviant behavior (2nd ed.). Boston: Houghton Mifflin.

Traub, S., & Little, C. B. (1980). *Theories of deviance* (2nd ed.). Itasca, IL: F.E. Peacock.

U.S. Bureau of Labor Statistics. (1982). Labor force statistics derived from the current population survey: A databook (Vol. 1). Washington, DC: U.S. Government Printing Office.

U.S. National Center for Health Statistics. (1968–1982). *Monthly vital statistics*. Washington, DC: U.S. Government Printing Office.

U.S. Public Health Service. (1964–1978). *Vital statistics of the U.S.* Washington, DC: U.S. Government Printing Office.

Wasserman, I. (1984a). Imitation and suicide: A reexamination of the Werther effect. *American Sociological Review*, *49*, 427–436.

Wasserman, I. (1984b). A longitudinal analysis of the linkage between suicide, unemployment, and marital dissolution. *Journal of Marriage and the Family*, *46*, 853–859.

15

Suicide in Different Ages from a Cross-Cultural Perspective

Dorothy Counts

The advantage of an anthropological approach to understanding suicides that occur at different times in the life cycle and in different cultures is that anthropology offers an analytical perspective that is concerned with understanding the cultural context in which suicides occur. Anthropology seeks to explain suicide as being a culturally constructed act that is performed in the context of a system of meaning. The system of meaning communicates, in a variety of ways as we shall see below, the rules of suicide for those who would kill themselves and a code of understanding for the survivors who must interpret the message that the suicide was attempting to convey. These rules are part of culturally shared understanding about the meaning of death: They identify those who may legitimately commit suicide as well as why and how it is to be done. The rules specify, in effect, that under some circumstances it is appropriate for certain types of persons to commit suicide. They also provide a script that the actor should follow if he intends for his death to communicate an appropriate message to his survivors. This script establishes what steps precede the deed and what method the suicide should use. If he follows the rules, the suicide can expect relatives and friends to respond to his death in predictable ways. The person who is contemplating suicide will refer to these publicly shared understandings in planning his act for, by so doing, he can

DOROTHY COUNTS • Department of Anthropology, University of Waterloo, Waterloo, Ontario, Canada N2L 3G1.

legitimize and give meaning to his death, both for himself and for others. He may also be able to control the consequences of his suicide and establish an agenda for his friends and kin to follow in response to his death.

In other societies, under certain circumstances, suicide may be made known as an acceptable option in a variety of ways. It may be so central to the culture that it is a theme in children's play as it was in Arawe on the south coast of West New Britain, Papua New Guinea. In this society, when school children were asked by researchers to draw a picture of a shamed person they drew the figure of an individual with a noose around his neck, and when they played they dramatized suicide by knotting a rope around their throats and dropping limply to the ground (Hoskin, Friedman, & Cawte, 1969, p.206). Or suicide may be a theme in oral literature as is true among the Kwara'ae and the Kwaio of Malaita in the Solomon Islands where most of the myths portray only females as suicide victims (Akin, 1985; Gegeo & Watson-Gegeo 1985). Suicide is also an integral part of the culture in Kaliai, West New Britain, Papua New Guinea where myths, legends, and folk tales recount the conditions under which people may legitimately kill themselves, describe the methods to be used, and depict the procedures that a suicide should follow in order that the deed will communicate a powerful message (Counts, 1980).

As we will see, the cultural patterning and stereotyping of suicide may result in a particularly dramatic case becoming a model to be followed by people who are in a similar unhappy plight and who share an interpretation of the act. In this circumstance, people may perceive suicide to be an appropriate or effective strategy in a given situation and, consequently, suicide may reach epidemic proportions. This has happened since the mid-1970s in Micronesia among adolescent and young adult males.

Suicide is a strategy that is also used by women of reproductive age in some Melanesian communities, and early in this century, it was common in some New Guinean societies for the widows of powerful men to demand that their relatives kill them following their husbands' deaths. I will, in this chapter, discuss suicides among these three age groups—young unmarried Micronesian men, married or marriageable Melanesian women, and elderly New Guinean widows—to illustrate the importance of cultural context in understanding the meaning of suicide in a particular society.

SUICIDE AMONG YOUNG MICRONESIAN MEN

Micronesia is a vast area in the western South Pacific that includes a vast number of small islands, some of the best known being Guam, Pohnpei, Truk, Palau, Yap, and Bikini. Although there is a population of only about 125,000 people in Micronesia, there are a dozen different languages and cultural groups. Social and economic change has been rapid and profound in these islands, especially since World War II. The indigenous economy, which was based on fishing and gardening, has been largely replaced by a cash economy based on government jobs and on the construction, educational, and health service projects that have been subsidized by the American government, which administers the area.

The leading cause of death for Micronesian males between the ages of 15 and 30 is suicide (Marshall, 1979, p.78). Rubinstein (1986, p.4) reports that between the mid-1960s and the 1970s the suicide rate for young males doubled every 4 years. By 1983 the annual suicide rate for the Micronesian population had increased from 8 per 100,000 to 48 per 100,000 (Rubinstein, 1985, pp.89, 91), with the highest rates being among men between the ages of 15 and 24 years. The median age of suicide for Micronesian males is slightly under 20 years (Rubinstein, 1986, p.4). By 1986 the annual suicide rate among young Micronesian men was 150 per 100,000, while in Truk it had reached 200 per 100,000, more than 10 times the suicide rate for American men of the same age (Rubinstein, 1986, p.5). In other words, 1 of every 50 Trukese men die by suicide between the ages of 15 and 24. The suicide rates for adolescent females followed a similar pattern but were only 10% of the male rate (Rubinstein, 1985, pp.89-90).

The young men who commit suicide share a number of personal and situational characteristics. The typical suicide victim is a single male who lives at home with his parents in a rural village a few miles from town. He either is a student or is employed as a manual or semiskilled laborer. The suicide occurs after an emotional argument with a close friend or relative, and it takes place near or inside the victim's home, usually at night. About one third of the suicides had been either drinking alcoholic beverages or using marijuana before their death (Rubinstein, 1986, p.5), and many had a history of moderately heavy drinking. The method of suicide is usually (85% of the time) by hanging (Hezel, 1976; Rubinstein, 1985), but often the body is not suspended off the ground. Instead the victim places his head in the noose, leans forward from a sitting or standing position, and dies from anoxia after losing consciousness (Rubinstein, 1986, p.5).

The typical pattern of events is for a young man to withdraw in anger and hang himself after being scolded by a parent or older sibling for violating family rules or following the refusal of some minor request. These deaths appear to be impulsive, and the family is frequently taken by surprise, for the incident that triggers the suicide is often trivial and out of proportion to the violent response. For instance, Rubinstein recounts one case of a young man who tried to hang himself after his father refused to give him $5 (Rubinstein, 1985, pp.94–96), and another of a 17-year-old who hanged himself following an angry scolding from his father because he was late to help his parents in their garden (Rubinstein, 1986, p.6). Hezel reports that within a month in Truk an 18-year-old who had been drifting from one relative's house to another hanged himself over a perceived insult from an older kinsman; a 9-year-old boy hanged himself after watching television in a friend's house because he was afraid his father would spank him for staying out so late; and a 24-year-old man took his life after he was denied credit in the family store (Hezel, 1987).

Anthropologists seeking to explain the high rate of suicide among young Micronesian men and the apparently trivial incidents that frequently trigger the deaths have focused on two interactive aspects of Micronesian life: (a) the rapid and pervasive change that has occurred in the organization of family life and the socialization of young men since the end of World War II, and (b) a unique emotional state that characterizes the feelings of a young person who feels anger toward his elders but who is prohibited by traditional values from directly expressing his frustration and rage.

Those aspects of social change that have created tensions between parents and their teenaged sons and that are especially relevant to adolescent male suicide are as follows (Rubinstein, 1986, pp.3–4):

1. The size and composition of the family unit has changed. The extended household and cooperative land-owning economic unit that was focused on sisters and their husbands has become a nuclear family, usually centered around a wage-earning father. In this new, smaller nuclear unit parents spend more time with and have more responsibility for their children, and there are fewer places where young people who are in conflict with their parents or older siblings can go to cool off.
2. The meeting houses where adolescent males traditionally lived, were socialized, and went for refuge have mostly disappeared. Today teenagers are more likely to live with, and be dependent on, their parents.
3. The introduction of American culture has widened the gap between an older generation of poorly educated parents who have little tolerance of things American and their children who are involved in consumer culture.

When these changes, which exacerbate the tensions between family members and lead to family conflict, are combined with an emotional state that is characteristically Micronesian, the result is an epidemic of adolescent male suicide. Pacific Islanders perceive, talk about, and experience emotion in culturally distinct ways (White, 1985). If we fail to understand their unique emotional experience we risk the error of applying Western psychological concepts to their behavior, thereby misunderstanding what suicide means to them.

As already noted, Trukese suicide usually occurs in the context of conflict between family members, a situation that gives rise to a complex of feelings termed *amwunumwun*. This term signifies the mixture of anger, frustration, and resentment that an individual feels toward higher status family members with whom he is in conflict. Hezel (1985) explains this complex emotion in the following way:

> When a Trukese is hurt and angered by someone he loves and respects, he commonly uses a strategy that is called *amwunumwun*. The refusal of a boy to eat when his parents have offended him is an example of *amwunumwun*. . . . [It] is a strategy of withdrawal or self-abasement used to show to those one must both love and obey that one is hurt by them. The act of *amwunumwun* is intended not principally to inflict revenge—although it would be naive to maintain that there is nothing of this in the act—but to dramatize one's anger, frustration, and sorrow in the hope that the present unhappy situation will soon be remedied. If the one who employs *amwunumwun* is trying to shame the one who has offended him it is always with the intention of showing the offending party the sad state into which their relationship has fallen so that he will take steps to restore it to what it once was or should have been. . . . Suicide, in the overwhelming majority of Trukese cases, must be understood as a kind of *amwunumwun*. Indeed, it is the extreme form of *amwunumwun* since it means inflicting the ultimate harm upon oneself in order to compel the parents or others to recognize the damage they have done and to repair it. (pp.115–116)

As White (1985) also points out, *amwunumwun* is part of a culturally recognized scenario that permits youths to appeal to higher ranking relatives indirectly, without expressing anger or resentment. Such expression would violate values of respect that are due to older family members. Micronesian culture favors resolving conflict by denial or withdrawal, methods that are nonconfrontational. Ideally, after an offended young person withdraws from further interaction with his elders, he is approached by a relative who attempts to soothe him and repair the breach. However, as a result of changes in the size and composition of the family unit, the demise of the meeting house, and the cultural gap between youths and their parents' generation this intervention often does not occur. There may be no appropriate person to repair the breach, or perhaps those who could step in to soothe the hurt and angry child do not recognize the seriousness of his despair. The consequence of the breakdown of the traditional method of conflict resolution is teenage suicide, a deed that Micronesians interpret as being the ultimate act of withdrawal (Rubinstein, 1986, pp.6–7).

Rubinstein (1986, p.7) is quick to point out that Micronesians do not approve of adolescent suicide, and that it does not affirm cultural values. However, local attitudes toward it are ambivalent and contextual and vary from one community to another. He also observes that the clustering of multiple adolescent suicides in one small community in a short time has become commonplace in Micronesia, and that this patterning may give suicide a specific local cultural meaning. It may be, for instance, locally understood as a boy's final appeal to his family for recognition and love. When suicide becomes stereotyped and imbued with meaning in this way, it may become acceptable and acquire legitimacy, especially for others in the high-risk category.

Suicide is also stereotyped, culturally patterned, and meaningful for Melanesian women of reproductive age. We will now investigate the pattern that suicide takes among these women and consider what meaning suicide has for them and for their survivors.

SUICIDE BY MELANESIAN WOMEN

Melanesia covers the southwestern South Pacific from the island of New Guinea to Fiji and includes the countries of Papua New Guinea, Vanuatu, New Caledonia, the Solomon Islands, and Fiji. It is difficult to make any general statement that would hold true of all of Melanesia for it contains a great variety of languages, cultures, and colonial experiences. It is accurate to say, however, that the area has undergone rapid political, economic, and social change since World War II, that there is an ethos of male domination of females throughout Melanesia, and that suicide is endemic in many Melanesian communities. A common pattern is for a young woman to commit suicide after a confrontation centering around marriage. If she is unmarried, she has probably been involved in a controversy with her relatives over whom she will marry. She may have been beaten by her kin and will either be compelled to marry against her wishes or forbidden to marry the husband of her choice. If she is married she is likely to have had a conflict with her husband in which she was shamed or beaten, and it is probable that her own relatives failed to support her or provide her with sanctuary. Whereas in Micronesia the element of revenge is apparently only a minor component of the suicide of adolescent males, Melanesian suicide is often revenge suicide. A Melanesian woman may decide to kill herself because she expects her death to shame her relatives or to force them to avenge her death, thus allowing her, vicariously, to take revenge on her tormentors.

The first anthropologist to identify revenge suicide in a non-Western culture was Jeffreys (1952) who discovered it in Africa and called it samsonic suicide after the Biblical figure who pulled a temple down around his own head in order to kill his enemies. Revenge suicide is, of course, not exactly the same everywhere it is found, but there are a number of cross-cultural similarities:

First, powerless people who lack an effective, more direct way of influencing the behavior of others are the most likely to commit revenge suicide. These powerless people are often women. Panoff (1977) reports, for example, that among the Maenge of East New Britain, Papua New Guinea, revenge suicide occurs chiefly among two categories of persons—orphans and women: ". . . precisely those [categories] whose members have the fewest opportunities to pour out their aggressiveness" (p.55). According to Panoff the Maenge do not consider suicide to be proper behavior for everyone; rather, it ". . . is a type of death appropriate only to 'rubbish men' and women" (p.50).

Second, the society must hold someone other than the victim culpable for the suicide, and it must have some culturally recognized way of identifying and punishing the guilty person(s).

Identification of the culpable party may be the responsibility of the victim and may be part of the ritual accompanying the suicide. Alternatively, the identification may occur as the result of a public moot during which the events leading up to the death and the relationship of people close to the victim are analyzed in detail, or at which someone offers to pay compensation to the victim's survivor, thereby acknowledging culpability. Or a religious ritual, such as a divination or an interview with the ghost of the deceased, may identify the guilty person(s) (for examples of such a ritual, see Counts & Counts, 1974; Counts, 1980; Mitchell, 1978, pp.153–155).

Punishment of the guilty may be accomplished by supernatural entities, because people may believe that the ghost of the suicide has the power to torment the person responsible for the death. The Lusi-Kaliai, for instance, consider the ghosts of suicides to be fearful spirits who are malevolent and dangerous. Their shame and anger prevents them from entering the world of the dead and condemns them to exist on the fringes between human and spirit society where they may be captured to become the familiars of sorcerers. The survivors of a suicide victim know that, if they do not revenge her death either by physical violence, sorcery, or by demanding heavy compensation payments from her tormentor, they will see her ghost wandering near the edge of the village at dusk, reminding them that they have not done their duty.

The punishment of those who cause someone to commit suicide may also take a mundane form. It is common in Melanesia for the indigenous political system to impose a penalty on the person who provoked the suicide or confirm the right of the survivors to exact compensation from or take revenge on the guilty party. For instance, Akin (1985, p.201) notes that in Malaita, Solomon Islands, before pacification a husband who was held responsible for his wife's suicide might have been executed by her relatives, while today he may be forced to pay them compensation for her death.

Culpability and revenge are important aspects of the cultural pattern of suicide in many Papua New Guinea societies. For example, a Huli man whose wife commits suicide because of his ill-treatment is held responsible for her murder (Frankel, 1986, p.135), while the Jale of the highlands of Irian Jaya (the western, Indonesian portion of the island of New Guinea) consider suicide to be a vengeful act that is intended to harm those who are responsible for the death. The guilty persons feel regret and self-reproach and are expected to pay compensation to the victim's relatives (Koch, 1974, pp.74–76). Similarly, a shamed Fore woman who has no other recourse may commit suicide in order to punish her tormentors because her death will "set in motion the machinery of revenge" (Berndt, 1962, p.204).

A Gainj woman who kills herself following physical abuse or shaming by her husband can inflict both supernatural harm and mundane disaster on him (Johnson, 1981). In her discussion of the Gainj rules for revenge suicide and the effects of the death on the provocateur, Johnson (1981) says

> Gainj women do not kill themselves discreetly. They do it at a time which will preclude their being rescued (usually just before dawn), in a way that leaves no question as to intent (hanging from a tree), and in locations that demand public acknowledgement (usually next to a well-travelled path). It is perhaps the only time in a woman's life when she creates a public event, one calculated, moreover, to thoroughly humiliate her husband. . . . Thus the husband of a suicide loses assets—his wife, the brideprice he paid for her and the compensation he now must pay, and status. He is a man who has been thoroughly and publicly bested by a woman. (p.332)

Among the Maring of Papua New Guinea only women commit suicide, and they usually do so following violent domestic conflict (Healey, 1979, p.95). Their deaths are vengeful acts that are especially potent when they also kill their young daughters, as happened in half the cases of suicide (three of six) that Healey analyzed. Healey (1979) says:

> Destruction of a child in suicide is particularly vengeful, for not only is the husband deprived of a wife, but also of children who can care for him in his old age, and who will forge new affinal alliances for him. Further, he must provide the customary death-payments for both wife and child to the woman's agnates, and face the anger and possible vengeance of his affines by physical attack or witchcraft. (p.96)

In Kaliai, West New Britain Province, Papua New Guinea, suicide has become increasingly common and, in recent years, has been restricted to women of reproductive age (Counts, 1988). Between 1975 and 1985 I recorded four completed suicides and two suicide attempts in one rural village of about 250 people (the population fluctuated during the 10-year period). All of the deaths and one of the attempts were by women, and three of the women were closely related—in fact, two were mother and daughter. Before 1975 the only suicides in this community had been committed by two related men in the early part of this century. All of the recent incidents occurred as a result of conflict over marriage, either by young women who were shamed because they were unable to marry the men of their choice or in the context of domestic violence in which the women were beaten. In one case it was unclear whether the death was a suicide or was the result of injuries suffered as a result of multiple severe beatings (Counts, 1987; Counts, 1988). The first death, that of a 17-year-old girl (which is discussed in detail in Counts, 1980), seems to have become a model for the other female suicides, and my informants cite her death as setting the precedent for the others.

The cultural pattern of suicide in Kaliai is similar to patterns of revenge suicide in other Papua New Guinea societies. In Kaliai, suicide is an alternative available to shamed, abused, and powerless women. People consider suicide to be an act of homicide for whom someone other than the victim is responsible. Mechanisms for ascertaining the identity of and punishing the guilty party are in place, and there are widely known rules of procedure that permit a person to commit a culturally meaningful (revenge) suicide. These procedures are communicated through oral tradition and by gossip around evening cooking fires. These rules are as follows:

1. The victim should not kill herself impulsively or in secret. Rather she should warn others of her intent. She can do this in a number of ways: by destroying the things she uses every day, things such as her cooking pots, her canoe, or personal items such as her shell arm bands; by leaving her footprints in ashes; or by leaving a written message, one that is inscribed on paper or that is carved on the husks of green coconuts, where it is sure to be found.
2. She should dress herself in her finest Western clothing or traditional costume, decorate herself, and anoint herself with sweet smelling oils.
3. She should kill herself in the presence of others or where others will be sure to find her body soon after her death. The dramatic message of a suicide is enhanced if there are witnesses who helplessly see the death and hear the victim's last words, words which identify those whom she holds responsible for her suicide.
4. She should use one of the following methods: drinking poison, traditionally a concoction made of *derris* root (a rotenone poison) but now extended to include drinking household bleach, taking an overdose of chloroquine phosphate tablets (readily available malaria suppressants), or a mixture of the poisons; hanging herself; or jumping from the top of a tall tree. People sometimes combine two or more of these methods.
5. Finally, it is essential that she reveal to others the identity of the culpable person. This message is so important to the successful implementation of a revenge suicide that survivors may report that the person responsible for the suicide has been identified by the suicide's ghost.

A Lusi-Kaliai woman who follows these rules commits a culturally patterned and meaningful suicide and is said to have been "killed with talk." Consequently, she can expect her survivors to consider her to have been murdered by slander or abuse and to retaliate in the same way that they do to other forms of homicide: by demanding compensation and, sometimes, by ensorceling the guilty parties as well (Counts, 1980, 1984, 1987). In all of the cases of suicide for which I have data, the people who were held responsible for the deaths paid compensation to the relatives of the victim, but in two cases the payment did not adequately avenge the deaths. Consequently, the survivors of the suicide victims reportedly employed sorcerers to kill either the culpable party or one of his close relatives by malevolent magic.

Clearly, then, revenge suicide is a culturally patterned act that has meaning for the community as well as for the victim and that enables the victim to take revenge, albeit vicariously, on those whom she holds responsible for the misery leading to her death. As with the suicide of Micronesian adolescents, suicide rates are not enough. We must know the cultural context surrounding the suicide in order to understand the message that the death gives to the community and the social consequences of the deed.

A variation on the theme of revenge suicide—and one that leads nicely into the discussion on assisted suicide by widows to follow—is found in precontact Malaita where a woman who had been sexually assaulted could, by forcing her own kin to kill her, also bring about the death of her assailant (Akin, 1985). In precontact times the sacred zone surrounding the men's house was tabooed to women, and a woman who entered this forbidden area was killed by her male kin. A woman who had been raped could use this prohibition to, in effect, commit suicide by forcing her kin to kill her. She did this by climbing onto the roof of the men's house and demanding death, at the same time explaining the reason why she wished to die and naming the man who had raped her. As a result, "the rapist himself was seen as the girl's actual murderer, and in every case he was hunted down and killed" (Akin, 1985, pp.200–201).

WIDOWS AND ASSISTED SUICIDE

The final type of suicide that I wish to discuss here is the ritual killing of a widow following the death of her husband. It is somewhat similar to the Indian practice of *suttee* in which a widow was burned on her husband's funeral pyre. Widow killing is reported to have existed in a number of Papua New Guinea societies before white contact when it was outlawed by German and Australian administrators. Although technically the killing of a widow at her request, even at her insistence, was judged by German and Australian authorities to be ritual homicide, scholars have considered it to be a form of suicide. It has been called altruistic suicide (Durkheim, 1951, p.219), religious suicide (Rao, 1975, p.232), or institutional suicide because the act was approved by members of the society and because the culture prescribed under what circumstances it was to occur and the form it should take (Farberow, 1975, pp.1–2).

Although most reports of widow killing come from West New Britain, it was a custom that was also practiced in the New Guinea Highlands as recently as the years following World War II. In a personal communication to Edgerton (1976, p.40), L. L. Langess reports that a widowed Bena Bena woman who did not wish to be inherited by another man might ask her brother to help her to kill herself instead. The procedure was that the widow's brother bent down a tree limb while she stood on his back and placed a noose around her neck. When she signaled, he walked away. Edgerton considers the death to be suicide because the woman's brother reportedly "sees the decision as hers to make without interference. . . . No rule is violated, and no trouble results."

Todd (1935–1936, p.423), who briefly did research in the early part of this century among the people of the Kandrian area on the southwest coast of New Britain, declared that it was customary for a widow of an important man to request her relatives to strangle her and bury her in the grave with her husband. Todd also says that if a widow's kin were reluctant to kill her she would shame them into doing it by taunting them that they wanted her to remain alive so that they could commit incest with her. Goodale and Chowning (1971, p.8) also report that before pacification, widows among the Kaulong and Sengseng of the Passismanua area of interior southwest New Britain could expect to be strangled within 24 hours after their husbands' deaths.

My Lusi-Kaliai consultants state that a widow was not shamed if she did not ask to be killed and that only the elderly widows of important leaders were strangled, and then only at their insistence and with the agreement of their relatives. If her kin unanimously agreed, the widow knelt on a pandanas mat and one of her close relatives—usually her oldest son—either garotted her or broke her neck at the base of her skull with a wooden sword that had been especially carved for the purpose. Sometimes both methods were used. One of my consultants who witnessed the death of his grandmother in this fashion said that her behavior following her husband's death indicated that she intended to ask to be killed. Instead of isolating herself in deep mourning, she was inappropriately cheerful and went about her business as usual. There were few expressions of grief following the woman's death, for she was buried with her husband, and her spirit was thought to join his in the land of the dead where they would continue the close and affectionate relationship that they had enjoyed during life.

I have argued elsewhere that our Western categories of homicide and suicide, derived from our own legal assumptions and cultural experience, are inappropriate to and distort the meaning of the assisted suicide of widows that the Lusi-Kaliai describe (Counts, 1980, pp.342–343). Although by European legal standards this type of death was homicide, by Lusi-Kaliai criteria it was not. My informants interpreted the widow's request to be slain as a rational one. They assumed that the elderly widow, who had enjoyed the prestige of being married to a leader, was unwilling to tolerate her new status, one that would make her dependent on her children who might resent having an unproductive mouth to feed, or even neglect her, when she became incapacitated with age. The ritual associated with her death avoided the social disruption and accusations of culpability that are usually associated with either homicide or suicide. Instead the widow had control over her death. She insisted on dying; her relatives, the persons who ordinarily revenged homicide or suicide, were all required to agree to it; and it had to be done by one of her closest kin. If she were killed with a wooden sword, it would become a treasured heirloom to be passed down to her descendants, together with the story of her death, and to be displayed in her memory on ceremonial occasions.

Obviously our legal categories, homicide and suicide, are inadequate for discussing this form of death. Neither term describes the act nor the social relationships in which it is imbedded. They do not instruct us about the attitude that people had toward the widow and the man who assisted her in her death, nor do they inform us as to the social consequences of it. This is an act for which we have no linguistic gloss and no relevant legal category. It is imbedded in a particular cultural context and has meaning for us only if we understand that context and the pattern of expectations and behavior that lead up to it and flow from it. Indeed, there is an ironic twist to this understanding: what the Lusi-Kaliai thought of as the *only* blameless form of suicide was regarded by colonial authorities as a form of homicide; what the authorities defined as *suicide* the Lusi-Kaliai almost invariably considered to be a form of homicide.

CONCLUSION

In this chapter I have described suicides that are characteristically committed by people who are at different stages in the life cycle: adolescent Micronesian males, Melanesian women of reproductive age, and elderly Papua New Guinean widows. These suicides each occur in a unique cultural context, they are patterned differently, and they have a distinctive meaning for the victims and for their survivors. The suicide by the adolescent Micronesian is interpreted as being an act of withdrawal from conflict that communicates a plea for love and recognition by his family. Both the adolescent Micronesians and the Melanesian women express their anger by their deaths, but the consequences of the acts are different in the two cultures. By following a widely known cultural script, a powerless Melanesian woman communicates her shame to her kin who are forced, by the suicide, to take revenge on those whom the victim identifies as being responsible for her misery and death, while the survivors of the Micronesian youths have no culpable others to hold responsible and, apparently, no aggressive outlet for their grief and guilt. In contrast, the type of suicide that is most similar to the Western legal category of homicide is the least socially disruptive. Elderly widows of powerful men insist that their kinsmen assist them to die, an act that is, strictly speaking, neither homicide nor suicide but one that brings honor to the woman and is remembered with pride by her descendants.

These three species of self-killing have demonstrated that suicide in other cultures is embedded in the society's cultural context. In all three types described above, people invest their actions with meaning that is based on stereotyped cultural models that are communicated to members of the society in ways that range from child's play to mythic tradition, models that are widely known and clearly understood. Contemporary societies view rising rates of suicide with alarm and often devise programs of intervention hoping to solve the social problems assumed to underly such socially disruptive action. Those who have as their goal the prevention of suicides must first understand the cultural patterning of self-destruction, and intervention must be appropriate to such patterns if it is to be successful.

ACKNOWLEDGMENTS. The field research on which major parts of this chapter are based was conducted in West New Britain, Papua New Guinea in 1966 to 1967, 1971, 1975 to 1976, 1981, and 1985. Support for the research was provided by Southern Illinois University, the National Science Foundation, the Canada Council, the Wenner-Gren Foundation, the University of Waterloo, and the Social Sciences and Humanities Research Council of Canada.

REFERENCES

Akin, D. (1985). Suicide and women in East Kwaio, Malaita. In F. X. Hezel, D. H. Rubinstein, & G. M. White (Eds.), *Culture, youth and suicide in the Pacific* (pp. 198–210). Papers from an East-West Center Conference, September 1984, Honolulu, Hawaii.

Berndt, R. M. (1962). *Excess and restraint: Social control among a New Guinea mountain people.* Chicago: University of Chicago Press.

Counts, D., & Counts, D. (1974). The Kaliai Lupunga: Disputing in the public forum. In A. L. Epstein (Ed.), *Contention and dispute: Aspects of conflict resolution in New Guinea* (pp. 113–151). Canberra: Australian National University Press.

Counts, D. A. (1980). Fighting back is not the way: Suicide and the women of Kaliai. *American Ethnologist, 7*, 332–351.

Counts, D. A. (1984). Revenge suicide by Lusi women: An expression of power. In D. O'Brien & S. Tiffany (Eds.), *Rethinking women's roles: Perspectives from the Pacific* (pp. 71–93). Berkeley: University of California Press.

Counts, D. A. (1987). Female suicide and wife abuse: A cross-cultural perspective. *Suicide & Life-Threatening Behavior, 17*, 194–204.

Counts, D. A. (1988). Ambiguity in the interpretation of suicide—female death in Papua New Guinea. In D. Lester (Ed.), *Why women kill themselves* (pp. 87–110). Springfield, IL: Charles C Thomas.

Durkheim, E. (1951). *Suicide: A study in sociology*. Glencoe, IL: The Free Press.

Edgerton, R. B. (1976). *Deviance: A cross-cultural perspective*. Menlo Park, CA: Cummings.

Farberow, N. L. (1975). Cultural history of suicide. In N. L. Farberow (Ed.), *Suicide in different cultures* (pp. 1–15). Baltimore: University Park Press.

Frankel, S. (1986). The Huli response to illness. Cambridge: Cambridge University Press.

Gegeo, D., & Watson-Gegeo, K. A. (1985). Patterns of suicide in West Kwara'ae, Malaita, Solomon Islands. In F. X. Hezel, D. H. Rubinstein, & G. M. White (Eds.), *Culture, youth and suicide in the Pacific* (pp. 182–197). Papers from an East-West Center Conference, September 1984, Honolulu, Hawaii.

Goodale, J., & Chowning, A. (1971). *The contaminating woman*. Paper read at 70th Annual Meeting, American Anthropological Association, New York City.

Healey, C. (1979). Women and suicide in New Guinea. *Social Analysis, 2*, 89–106.

Hezel, F. X. (1976). Tragic end for troubled youth. *Micronesian Reporter, 24*(4), 8–13.

Hezel, F. X. (1985). Trukese suicide. In F. X. Hezel, D. H. Rubinstein, & G. M. White (Eds.), *Culture, youth and suicide in the Pacific* (pp. 112–124). Papers from an East-West Center Conference, September 1984, Honolulu, Hawaii.

Hezel, F. X. (1987). Truk suicide epidemic and social change. *Human Organization, 46*, 283–291.

Hoskin, J. O., Friedman, M. I., & Cawte, J. E. (1969). A high incidence of suicide in a preliterate-primitive society. *Psychiatry*, *32*, 200–210.

Jeffreys, M. D. W. (1952). Samsonic suicide or suicide of revenge among Africans. *African Studies*, *11*, 118–122.

Johnson, P. L. (1981). When dying is better than living: Female suicide among the Gainj of Papua New Guinea. *Ethnology*, *20*, 325–334.

Koch, K. F. (1974). *War and peace in Jalemo: The management of conflict in Highland New Guinea*. Cambridge, MA: Harvard University Press.

Marshall, M. (1979). *Weekend warriors: Alcohol in a Micronesian culture*. Palo Alto, CA: Mayfield.

Mitchell, W. (1978). *The bamboo fire: An anthropologist in New Guinea*. New York: W. W. Norton.

Panoff, M. (1977). Suicide and social control in New Britain. *Bijdragen: Tot de Taal-land-en Volkenkunde*, *133*, 44–62.

Rao, A. (1975). Suicide in India. In N. L. Farberow (Ed.), *Suicide in different cultures* (pp. 231–238). Baltimore: University Park Press.

Rubinstein, D. H. (1985). Suicide in Micronesia. In F. X. Hezel, D. H. Rubinstein, & G. M. White (Eds.), *Culture, youth and suicide in the Pacific* (pp. 88–111). Papers from an East-West Center Conference, September 1984, Honolulu, Hawaii.

Rubinstein, D. M. (1986, April). *Local cultural patterning of youth suicide: An anthropological study in the Pacific islands*. Paper prepared for the 19th annual meeting of the American Association of Suicidology, Atlanta, GA.

Todd, J. A. (1935–1936). Redress of wrongs in south-west New Britain Territory of New Guinea. *Oceania*, *6*, 401–440.

White, G. M. (1985). Suicide and culture: Island views. In F. X. Hezel, D. H. Rubinstein, & G. M. White (Eds.), *Culture, youth and suicide in the Pacific* (pp. 1–14). Papers from an East-West Center Conference, September 1984, Honolulu, Hawaii.

V

Survivor Issues

Loss of a loved one due to suicide is a traumatic event. Reactions vary depending on one's time-line. Indeed, it is a myth that children and adolescents do not truly experience the pain associated with such a loss. A developmental perspective is essential in understanding any survivor. Part V presents two chapters: survivorship in children and adolescents and survivorship in adults.

16

Child and Adolescent Survivors of Suicide

Bonnie Frank Carter and Allan Brooks

Loss of loved ones due to death has been empirically ranked among the highest stresses possible, both for adults and adolescents (Holmes & Rahe, 1967; Rogan & Hussey, 1977). We must recognize, however, that the difficulties a suicide death poses for children and adolescents extend far beyond the short-term stress of the immediate confrontation with death. Death by suicide adds the exacerbating factors of inadequate or inaccurate information; stigmatization with its emotional distancing from relatives, friends, and other potentially supportive individuals, both young and old; and seemingly unacceptable feelings of guilt and anger that complicate the already painful experience of sudden and absolute loss. Grief is a normal process, necessary and predictable after loss, but its impact on children and adolescents has often been overlooked, and the further jolt ensuing from suicide survivorship can have physical and emotional consequences, even in children who otherwise seem normal. Although increasing in use, the term "suicide survivor" continues to present some confusion (as discussed by Dunne, McIntosh, & Dunne-Maxim, 1987). Any discussion of this subject must begin with the clarification that a survivor of suicide is someone left behind to deal with the psychological distress and daily turmoil in the aftermath of a completed suicide. This is distinct from a parasuicide, an individual who attempts suicide and survives. While certain

BONNIE FRANK CARTER and ALLAN BROOKS • Department of Psychiatry, Albert Einstein Medical Center, Philadelphia, Pennsylvania 19141.

aspects of the emotional pain may be similar, a survivor of suicide is typically *not* someone who has attempted suicide.

To elucidate the pain and needs of child and adolescent suicide survivors, we will first review "Normal" or Uncomplicated Bereavement, including the inherent developmental differences that affect youngsters at different ages. Next, we will present Bereavement Complications for Suicide Survivors, including a Case Presentation to illustrate the complexities. Posttraumatic Stress Disorder (PTSD) will be reviewed as it applies to children, because this psychiatric condition (Diagnosis 309.89 of the *DSM-III-R* Classification, American Psychiatric Association, 1987) delineates much of the distress posed by suicide survivorship, and provides a sizable literature from which we can learn (Leenaars, 1989). Extending our purview beyond the distress posed by suicide survivorship, we next discuss the situation where disturbances appear to be mitigated by factors of Resilience or Invulnerability. Our combined clinical activities have provided much experience with increased suicidality following exposure to suicide, and we address this issue next. That section, Suicidality and Suicide Survivorship, includes comments on contagion following a completed suicide. As our experience has also emphasized the role of good social supports in the mitigation of negative aftermath, this chapter continues with an overview of Postvention procedures, which is a structured means of enhancing both the supports available to suicide survivors and their possible positive outcomes. In the Conclusion, we again use the clinical approach of providing a Case Presentation, this time showing the role of professional intervention in redirecting suicide survivorship's thwarted grieving toward healthy bereavement.

The current increased concern about suicide survivorship is partially predicated on the growing numbers of people affected by the suicide death of a close friend or relative. McIntosh recently (1989) calculated the existence of approximately 3,100,000 suicide survivors living today in the United States. Of those, possibly 1 million became survivors during childhood years (Small & Small, 1984; Dunne-Maxim, Dunne, & Hauser, 1987).

NORMAL OR UNCOMPLICATED BEREAVEMENT

Freud's landmark study of war's effects on children (Freud & Burlingham, 1943) notes the fact that children's cognitive development and emotional development proceed at different paces, and that this often causes children to present a misleading constellation of statements, behaviors, and affects. When, for example, the child of 4, 5, or 6 accurately and dispassionately recounted events of air raid attacks, evacuations, or distant locations of a missing mother or a father away in the military (even though the child's real understanding was likely to be very different from the adult-perceived referrent), adults were misled into believing the child had adequately processed the underlying affects. Similarly, when a toddler of 1 or 2 exhibits grieving behaviors only briefly (e.g., seeming complete within 36 to 48 hours), adults may fail to recognize that the intensity is comparable to the grief work an older person would experience through a full year. The conclusion that children do not mourn with the same intensity as adults continues to be accepted by many investigators (e.g., van Eerdewegh, Bieri, Parilla, & Clayton, 1982), despite the fact that the difference in presented symptoms and duration belies similar psychological significance for the child.

In contrast to such earlier notions that children could not truly experience mourning because of their incomplete understanding of death, Bowlby (1960, 1961, 1980) fully elucidated the process of mourning in childhood. Through his earlier works on attachment and separation (Bowlby, 1969, 1973, 1982), he recognized children's full capability of forming a true bond to their parents and other significant caregiving figures in their lives. Consequently, he concluded that a child is capable of feeling true loss, and needs to process the loss through mourning in order to establish new attachments (see Chapter 8, in this volume).

While some grief manifestations in children are similar to those of adult mourners (such as anger, crying, diminished affect, sleeplessness, diminished appetite, and irritability), other expressions do not fit with the general saddened affect expected of adult mourners. Children are much more likely to externalize or act out their grief, often by reverting to regressed behaviors of younger ages. The expected reactions of shock, guilt, helplessness, fatigue, separation anxiety, and physical complaints are likely, but children must be asked about these as they are unlikely to volunteer such information. Symptoms are also likely at school, including socially withdrawing from peers or from the teacher, widespread daydreaming, inability to concentrate or other inefficiency in school work, behavioral regressions to behaviors characteristic of younger ages, profound sadness, fatigue, irritability, and conduct problems. Teachers are excellent resources for accessing this information. It must also be remembered that children cannot resolve their grief as readily as adults, as the child will review the earlier attachment and the death at each successive level of development. A further difference from adults is the typical absence of previous experience with death, so that the child has no internal basis for adapting to the loss.

Inaccuracies in factual knowledge and limitations in cognitive abilities of children must be accommodated in considering death's impact on children (Orbach, Gross, Glaubman, & Berman, 1985), although these should not be construed as a basis for dismissing the legitimacy of their bereavement. A child's concept of death is often vague and incomplete. Young children, up to the ages of 3 to 5, think death is reversible, that a person can live again after dying. The natural progression away from this inaccuracy is frequently delayed by exposure to the pervasive distortions of death and violence in television cartoons and dramas. Nevertheless, somewhere between 5 and 9, death is recognized as final, although still seen only as something that could happen to other people and in other families. It is not until the age of 9 or 10 that the child recognizes death as an absolute biological fact *and* as something that could happen in one's own family and even to oneself (Bowlby, 1960, 1961, 1980). Thereafter, the child continues the life-long endeavor of truly understanding death, not only as an irrefutable biological fact, but as an event with some individually accepted meaning and purpose.

It is common to try to protect children from the reality that life is finite and the omnipresent possibility of loss. When a close person dies, the child's pre-existing confusion is further increased if significant adults accept the mistaken view that the truth would be too upsetting, and instead present the child with some partial, euphemistic, or otherwise inaccurate version of the facts. These problems become compounded when children, frustrated in their attempt to develop a realistic and consistent understanding of death, "compare notes" with one another, and the already uncertain messages become further garbled.

Our exploration of death's impact on children must also acknowledge age differences in the central issues concerning youngsters. For example, not having a true understanding of the finality of death, a toddler might ask if the "death" will change where he lives, where he goes to school, his playmates, or other concrete daily issues. Far from being insensitive or self-centered, the child is simply translating the uncertainty being expressed by adults into his own terms; continuing access to the same playmates can be as crucial a source of stability and self-cohesiveness for a young child as is continued life with a marital partner for an adult. A further example of age-dependent differences is the varying effect of the lost person's gender, according to the developmental stage and sex of the child or adolescent (Weller & Weller, 1989; further described under the "Pessimist School").

Once death supervenes upon the family from any cause, a tremendous focus on death develops. Family members individually and as a group are full of concern about death and related topics. It seems as if nothing else, and no one else, gets any attention until intense bereavement ends. Consequently, children begin to identify themselves as belonging to a family where somebody died, as the brother of a dead sister or the daughter of a deceased father. This focus contrasts with the general lack of talk outside the family about any death, with the result that bereaved youngsters feel "different," and that everyone knows their changed status and will view it negatively.

Although not formally organized, the literature on childhood bereavement clusters into three schools of thought (as first conceptualized by and adapted from Weller & Weller, 1989). These approaches are differentiated by the adaptive course expected in a child's life following a psychologically significant loss. The Affective School focuses on the child's feelings (Bowlby, 1961, 1980; Rutter, 1983), particularly the likelihood of severe bereavement symptoms when the loss occurs before age 5. The young child is extremely focused on himself because of age-appropriate egocentrism, but this becomes exaggerated in response to the real and imagined threats inherent in an experience of death in the family. The child is likely to develop enormous concern about being deserted by family or friends, or an obsession with the impermanence of relationships in general. In addition, a feeling of helplessness is typical after the loss, and these feelings can remain very strong. Similar issues can affect youngsters at older ages, as well, as reported in recent work documenting increased depression in adolescent boys who experienced death during adolescence (Rutter, 1976; Wolfenstein, 1966, 1969).

The second approach, the Optimist School, embodies the simple faith that children always grow beyond adversity, and therefore can be expected to progress inevitably and naturally through bereavement. Some individuals who endured a childhood loss of a parent go so far as to credit that loss, and the subsequent necessity of surmounting it, as the source of certain of their capabilities in adulthood. Clearly, there are individual differences in the ability to adapt to loss as with all other aspects of personality and behavior, and these will be addressed later in terms of Resilience or Invulnerability. We would caution, however, that an emphasis on positive adaptation in the face of adversity can blind us to the obvious needs of youngsters struggling with loss (whether from suicide or other deaths), and similarly may detract from the validity of utilizing support potentially available from family, friends, social and religious institutions, and the mental health professions.

The third focus emphasizes only the most dire of outcomes and so is termed the Pessimist School. These outcomes include such psychiatric difficulties as schizophrenia or major depression and extreme behavioral consequences such as addictions, parasuicide, or suicide. Also included is the "long-range sleeper effect," where a child or adolescent does not show any drastic effect immediately after the death of a loved person but is expected to experience detrimental ramifications after a delay of some 5, 10, or 15 years.

The Pessimist School is based on evidence that very young children are likely to exhibit rebelliousness or other bad conduct, and that adolescents are likely to become depressed, sexualized, truant, and abusive of drugs or alcohol. A recent follow-up 4 years after the death of a parent (Elizur & Kaffman, 1982, 1983) found severe psychological problems in 70% of the children studied. This risk of dysfunction was increased two- or threefold when it was the psychologically significant parent who was lost, that is, the one upon whom the child was most dependent for nurturance or the one with whom the child experienced the most emotional conflict. Although the literature includes some contradictory data on the issue of suicidality for those with same-sex versus opposite-sex parental loss (Adam, Lohrenz, Harper, & Streiner, 1982), Weller and Weller (1989) categorize risk of negative outcome according to the sex of the deceased parent. Boys generally fare worse with the loss of the father, while girls may experience greater difficulty from loss of either sex parent, depending on the specific developmental issues being addressed at the time of the death. Additional risk factors include the sex and age of the bereaving child, the type of death, previous psychiatric disorders in the child or the family, and the presence and degree of family dysfunction.

The "best-case" (terminology from Bowlby, 1980) scenario for the nevertheless tragic situation of death would be a normal child at a relatively stable point in development in a healthy family with well-established and functional communication skills, who is honestly told the basic facts at the time the tragic event occurs. This child would also hear about the real finality of death from adults in a supportive environment where the emotional significance is similarly honestly shared. While immersed themselves in grief work, adult relatives and friends would provide a protective, buffering network available for help throughout the mourning period. Where more support is required or certain vulnerabilities appear, young mourners and their families would seek outside intervention while mastering the necessary adjustments entailed in the crisis of bereavement. With open communication and continuing self-help, these youngsters can be expected to work through their grief successfully over an appropriate period of time, become ready to proceed with their lives, and eventually accept substitute gratification including "replacements" for lost parents or peers.

BEREAVEMENT COMPLICATIONS FOR SUICIDE SURVIVORS

In contrast to the normal or "best-case" bereavement posed above, suicide survivorship poses several additional burdens on the grieving child or adolescent. Identifying the proximal and distal outcomes in the aftermath of suicide, as for any violent event, provides one way of understanding the overlapping symptoms constellations presented here. As shown in Figure 1 (adapted from Pynoos, 1988), a suicide survivor (and worse, a direct witness of suicide) experiences grief at the loss, worry about someone else committing suicide, reminders of previous loss experiences, overwhelming feelings of loss and hopelessness, and identification with the decreased, which lead, respectively, to PTSD, normal bereavement, incomplete bereavement, separation anxiety, exacerbation or renewal of pre-existing symptoms, loss of self-esteem, and depression and suicidal behavior. Rarely, however, are these occurrences evident in any pure or isolated form. Rather, suicide survivors are prone to many of these outcomes simultaneously, since grief, depression, PTSD, and suicide are behavioral categories that overlap in reality despite any theoretical separations.

Table 1 delineates the overlap in symptoms between normal bereavement and suicide survivorship by listing first the normal manifestations of bereavement identified in children (as described in the previous section), showing extensions of that normal grief in suicide survivorship due to the inherent loss and bereavement. (Additional overlap exists with the general realm of depression, but is not delin-

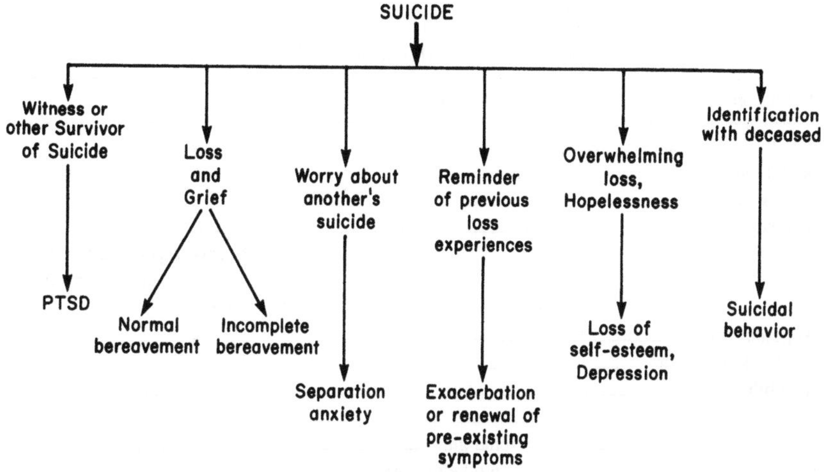

Figure 1. Outcomes of suicide survivorship (adapted from Pynoos, 1988).

eated here.) Affective and behavioral ramifications that accrue to suicide survivorship beyond normal grief are listed next. Finally, Table 1 lists the manifestations of PTSD (as documented in children by Terr, 1979, 1983a,b, and elaborated in the section below). The juxtaposition of symptoms from these three categorizations of grief and trauma reactions show that suicide survivorship includes all the components of normal bereavement, plus the added factors specific to the aftermath of suicide. Furthermore, as an exposure to a definite trauma, suicide survivorship would seem to constitute one type of PTSD, a logical conclusion that warrants further exploration in clinical investigations and empirical research. The overlapping of these categories is spatially represented in Figure 2.

Death by suicide presents a sudden loss for which the child could not have been prepared. Emotional as well as physical violence is typical. Many (although not all) pre-suicidal situations involve the family in emotional distress and dysfunctional communication. Regardless of the level of the family's communication competence prior to the suicide, problematic communication is likely as an aftermath because of continuing stigma and fear surrounding suicide. Surviving family members are at risk for contagion, in that they are in danger of copying the actions of the deceased, whether in the days and weeks immediate after the suicide or eventually years later. Interpersonal relationship difficulties diminish the availability of otherwise supportive resources, and psychological disturbances, depression, and other emotional stressors, including the circumstances of earlier attempts, exacerbate emotional distancing and feelings of blame. The essential sense of trust (developed by children in response to reliable caregiving; Erikson, 1968) is

Table 1. Symptom Comparison across Grief, Suicide Survivorship, and PTSD as Manifested in Children

Normal grief	Suicide survivorship	PTSD
Anger	—	
Agitation	—	
Crying	—	
Sleeplessness	—	—
		Dreams: repeat the trauma; include death, prophetic dreams
Appetite loss	—	
Regressed behaviors	—	
Irritability	—	—
Shock	—	—
Guilt —	Extreme guilt	—
Helplessness —	Extreme helplessness	—
		Extreme terror
		Panic attacks
		Extremely cautious
		Easily overwhelmed
Fatigue	—	
Separation fears	—	—
Anxiety	—	—
Physical complaints	—	—
		Perceptual distortions
		Visual distortions
Academic difficulties	—	
Social withdrawal	—	—
Daydreaming	—	Excessive daydreaming
	Denial or covering of the suicide —	Denial via "screen" memory or cover story
		Repetitive play
Search for meaning —	Exaggerated search	
		Search for omens
Inability to concentrate	—	
Repeated grieving at later developmental levels	—	
Abandonment fears	—	—
Distrust of relationship permanence	—	Relationships seen as fragile
Depression —	Chronic depression	
	Stigma	
	Contagion	
	Dysfunctional communication	
	Blame, of self and others	—
		Extreme shame
	Breach of trust —	Profound distrust
	Personality disorganization	
		Intrusive thoughts of the trauma

Table 1. (Continued)

Normal grief	Suicide survivorship	PTSD
Preoccupation with death ——	Preoccupation with suicide ——	Preoccupation with death
Fear of self dying ——	Obsession with suicide ——	Fear of self dying
Fear of others' dying ——	Fear of others' suicide	
	Suicidal behavior	
		Fear of further local disasters
		Futurelessness: foreshortened view; profound distrust
		Skewed sense of time
Interference with development ——	Greater interference with normal development	
Adversary reactions ——	Includes suicidality ——	Includes renewed posttraumatic repetitions

breached when a caregiving family member commits suicide and thereby renounces caring for the family and the child in particular.

The direct effects of suicide survivorship can be more readily comprehended by dividing them temporally into immediate, intermediate, and long-term effects. Within the first week following the loss, survivors experience the *immediate* effects of shock, denial, emotional paralysis, sadness, fatigue (with or without sleeplessness), suppressed appetite, agitation, irritability, extreme anger, any of a wide range of physical symptoms, helplessness, hopelessness, anguish, guilt, and feelings of blame directed at themselves and others. *Intermediate* effects occur after the first week and through as much as the first year (and longer, when necessary medical or mental health attention is neglected). These intermediate effects can include personality disorganization, acute PTSD, depression, morbid

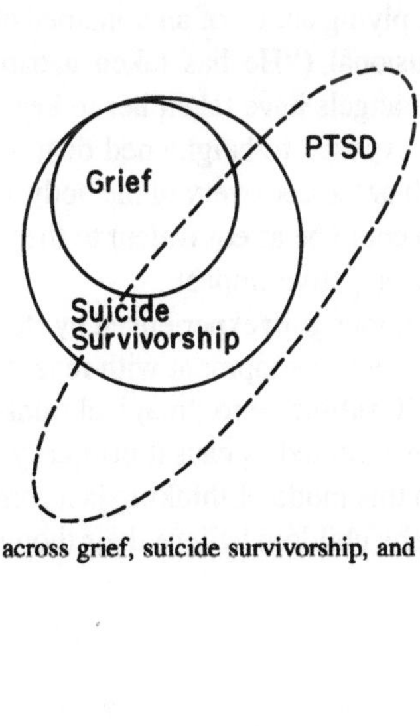

Figure 2. Symptom overlap across grief, suicide survivorship, and PTSD as manifested in children.

preoccupation with death, one's own suicidal ideation or activity, obsessive fears of others' suicidal behavior, and loss of trust in others including one's normal supports. The *long-range* effects of suicide survivorship in childhood or adolescence include unrelenting depression, chronic PTSD, suicidal behavior, interference with normal development (Nagera, 1970), distortions of identity due to the loss of role models (and inability to adopt new ones), use of unhealthy problem-solving strategies as role-modeled by the deceased relative or friend who took the proverbial "permanent solution to a temporary problem," and various other severe emotional disturbances, including a chronic mistrust of ordinarily dependable support systems. These long-range effects essentially constitute unresolved grief where the normal bereavement process has been interrupted or impaired. Yearning for the deceased continues unabated, and inevitably disorganizes the child or adolescent in his daily work, study, play, and social functions.

When death occurs in a family, children are often expected to take on the parenting role, for themselves, for other siblings, or even for the parents themselves who may be incapacitated by grief. This is due to the diminished behavioral competence and decreased emotional accessibility experienced by all survivors, which is particularly true following a parent's suicide. The remaining parent frequently becomes incapable of usual affective care for the children in the family. It is at such times that assistance from individuals beyond the immediate family becomes so crucial. The resources available from relatives, social and religious institutions, and the mental health professions will be discussed below under Postvention.

Distortions about death occur frequently around suicide. Denial of the death itself or of the circumstances, such as falsifying the cause of death, exacerbates the trauma for young survivors and increases their risk for negative outcomes. Talk about death in nonfinal terms is damaging, as this is contrary to the child's need for honest facts in order to internalize a realistic understanding of the true finality of death. Confusion can result whether the unrealistically nonfinal ideas are magical ("She is under a spell," implying action of an unnamed other who could similarly reverse the "spell"), delusional ("He has taken a trip," implying a someday return), or religious ("The angels have taken her to keep her safe"). Conversely, some young survivors are exposed to heightened distress through excruciatingly brutal detail about the death or the discovery of the body. It is possible that learning morbid details of the death could be as equivalent to the trauma of seeing the dead body itself in the extent of negative impact.

The prevalent and enormous guilt experienced by children when someone dies is based on immature cognitive development with regard to the laws of cause and effect. Children up to age 10 subscribe to "magical thinking," whereby logically impossible connections are accepted as causal primarily on the basis of temporal contiguity. Contributing to this mode of thinking is a continuing, age-appropriate sense of grandiosity, whereby children believe their thoughts are powerful enough to "cause" significant consequences. For example, if a family member dies at a time a child is harboring anger toward that individual, the child is wont to believe the anger "caused" the death. The same is likely with naughty or otherwise punishable behaviors, which the child views as the "cause" of the death. In the case of suicide, where all survivors experience self-recriminations as they evaluate any and all events preceding the death, young children can suffer as magical thinking combines with their self-evaluation. A healthy, growing sense of personal responsibility can be distorted into an extreme and punitive self-blame.

Contributing to the psychological damage experienced by young survivors of a close relative's suicide is the sense that they cannot talk about it, that no one really wants to hear it. People always seem willing to hear about other things that happen in the family, about illnesses, accidents, and other misfortunes, but not about suicide. Instead, people will come to the house and talk as little as possible, filling the time with trivia or gossip but not expressing the concern and fear they are most certainly feeling. The implicit message from society is "Don't talk about it." This reinforces the child's fear the suicide indicates something is very wrong with the family, that the family as a whole and all its members individually are "bad."

Siblings of children or adolescents who commit suicide are often the "forgotten mourners" (Morse, 1984). They are likely to require individual attention for their intense emotions but are often put in the background while center stage is occupied by the deceased sibling, stigmatization, or putative blame. The common "conspiracy of silence" (Cain & Fast, 1972), based on the mistaken notion that all knowledge about a suicide should be kept from youngsters, decreases their chances of processing emotions about the deceased sibling, emotions that will differ according to the actual relationship of the given children. Pre-existing sibling rivalry is both increased by anger at natural childhood experiences lost because of the suicide *and* is more fully thwarted since one "must not speak ill of the dead."

Further lack of support can accrue to the young suicide survivor by not being present at the funeral. This can happen because final rituals are denied to individuals who completed suicide, but access to the funeral may also be denied on the misguided grounds that such exposure would be damaging. Young survivors of suicide have already been exposed to death in a way that will remain with them throughout their lives. Allowing them to participate in a funeral or other memorial service provides a ritually designated place for mourning and does nothing to increase their despair, whereas denying them that access further separates them from needed social supports.

The stigma attached to suicide survivorship further burdens the youngster and impedes efforts to resolve the grief and move on with healthy sadness rather than destructive chronic mourning. This stigma tends to follow survivors throughout their lives, a veritable albatross around the neck or a seemingly visible ghost, ever-ready to emerge from the family "closet." Even more than other mourners, suicide survivors identify themselves as "the brother of the kid who committed suicide" or "the daughter of a mother who took an overdose of pills." Sometimes the lurking family "skeleton" feels like a birthright or an inheritance, as if time were just passing meaninglessly until it becomes "your turn to do it." In contrast, some suicide survivors create a healthy identity from the "surviving" aspect of their bereavement (Bolton, 1983; Dunne, McIntosh, & Dunne-Maxim, 1987; Wrobleski, 1989).

This negative scenario provides inadequate outlets for the unavoidable feelings of sadness, anger, helplessness, blame, and guilt that constitute grief. Where other deaths or significant losses generate support for those stricken, family and friends can become distant or even hostile after a suicide. It is more likely, therefore, that someone would suggest the survivor be "brave," or enjoin the child from displaying emotions openly for fear of appearing "weak." Advocating the stifling of these essential feelings or otherwise not allowing them worsens the impact of any death, especially a suicide. The underlying fear and hostility create a climate where minor fights are likely to occur in previously close relationships, such that emotional or even physical abandonment is possible if blame for the suicide is placed on the survivor.

Overall, suicide survivorship in children and adolescents can be expected to entail a progressive process initially involving shock, protest, yearning, enormous anger, irritability, and anxiety even to the point of panic, then moving through some behavioral disorganization with apathy and aimlessness, obsessive review of the deceased, the death, and the lost relationship, followed by renewed protest and despair, and finally, healthy detachment. Emergence from suicide survivorship grief is marked by reorganization, emotional and behavioral stability, social participation, renewed hopefulness about gratification, and re-established capacity for trust. Attainment of this stage brings with it an ability to cope with loss, and the willingness to use other people as resources to adapt to this crisis as well as other obstacles in life.

Case Presentation

The following composite (as well as the other two in this chapter) is constructed from several cases to protect the confidentiality of the actual patients. Highlighted in *italics* are the specific burdens of suicide survivorship, as illustrated in this case of children surviving a parent suicide.

Mr. R. died at the age of 40, after suffering from a degenerative disease and the attendant treatments for more than a year. The disease affected his personality and he argued frequently with his wife, whereupon she would quiet the children, telling them their father needed his rest. At times of anger, statements were made implying the children were to blame for relapses suffered by their father. Tommy was the noisy one at age 7 and more frequently held culpable, while 13-year-old Louise was the responsible one, serving as

Tommy's babysitter, companion, and disciplinarian. Louise also fulfilled a number of additional responsibilities around the house, including shopping, housecleaning, and some cooking, because of her mother's preoccupation with her father's health care.

One year before his death, the father attempted suicide by overdosing on analgesics and was rushed to the hospital. This parasuicide was initially *kept a secret* from both children, but Louise later learned of it. After a protracted siege of depressive, withdrawn behavior and one day before his completed suicide, Mr. R. had an argument with his wife and Tommy. Tommy was distinctly aware of *thinking to himself. "I wish you were dead."* The next morning, while the children were in school and Mrs. R. was at the market, Mr. R. took the final and fatal steps—swallowing a lethal amount of tranquilizers and lacerating one wrist. Mrs. R. returned home in the afternoon, much too late for any rescue, and Mr. R. died on the way to the hospital. Louise came home to the blood in the bedroom but was told by neighbors only that the ambulance had taken her father away. She arranged for Tommy to be met at school and kept with friends until the house was cleansed of their father's blood. When he did return home, *Tommy was told* his father was ill and in the hospital; this *falsehood was repeated* when his mother came back, weeping and openly distraught. The next day, Mrs. R. and Louise together told Tommy that his father had died but did not explain the circumstances. They *told him only* that Mr. R. had finally died from his illness.

The next day, a few of Mrs. R.'s friends came by ostensibly to offer their condolences, but the *death was never openly discussed.* Instead, all *visitors left* as *quickly* as decency permitted. At this time, all three survivors were in shock and *feeling abandoned.* The mother was in a constant state of hysteria, Tommy was in a dream-like stupor, and Louise was trying to hold them and herself together. Tommy asked to attend the *funeral* but this was *not permitted* for fear it would upset him too much. Louise did go, and the limited number of other attendees numbered mostly her friends and their parents.

Insufficient consolation was available to all three survivors throughout the mourning period. Tommy was *generally ignored* and had to fend for himself. He began having *upsetting dreams* of his father still being alive. Louise lost her usual poise, became *inhibited,* and experienced *terrifying nightmares* of her father lying in a pool of blood, as well as *daydreams* reliving that awful day when she returned to the house and found his blood all over the bedroom. The mother functioned only marginally for the next 6 months. Friends and relatives on both sides of the family avoided her, and she was left with feeling her husband's suicide was her fault.

A marked contrast existed in the social support systems for Tommy and Louise. Several close friends spent time listening to Louise's anguish. Although she never felt ready to discuss her father's suicide itself, she was able to accept the support of her friends. Tommy experienced *distancing from his close playmates and taunts from children of other ages.* In an unkind and unfortunately not atypical manner, children pointed at him, saying, "You're the kid whose father died." Later on these cruel remarks were replaced by more devastating *accusations*: "You're the kid whose father shot himself" and "Your dad killed himself." *Wholly unprepared* for this spectre of suicide, he ran to his mother and sister for comfort or verification, but they *perpetuated the myth* that his father's illness had caused his death. When Tommy finally did learn that his father had killed himself, he was suddenly aware of an *overpowering guilt.* He was convinced that his disputes with his father had caused him to take his life, particularly as reinforced by his awareness of wishing his father would die just the day before his death. Tommy became *preoccupied with fears* that his father would come back to *haunt* him and *accuse* him. He *obsessively daydreamed* of reliving the recent past and reviewed in his mind the multiple ways he could improve his behavior. Ultimately, Tommy *wanted to take his own life* in order to rejoin his father and make peace with him. In school, he *looked sad, spent much of his time daydreaming, and withdrew from peer friendships.* At home, his main activities were *daydreaming* in bed and watching television *alone.*

Eventually, the family sought professional assistance and Tommy was seen in individual therapy. He was *reluctant to reach out and accept help*, and it was difficult for him to begin the long road to his recovery. His entire base of *trust* in others had been *eroded.* His *grief* was pathologic and *incomplete*, as it had never been addressed directly, and the resulting drain of energy costly to his *emotional development.* Louise required treatment for symptoms of *PTSD* resulting from the complicated bereavement she experienced in the aftermath of her father's suicide. Her caring network of friends helped her achieve some measure of recovery fairly quickly. Mrs. R. required intensive therapy for the guilt and subsequent suicidal behavior she suffered following her husband's suicide.

PTSD

As indicated earlier (see Table 1), PTSD in children designates much of the symptom constellation experienced by young suicide survivors. The following is taken from the very complete description compiled by Terr (1979; 1983a) in her work with the Chowchilla, California bus kidnapping. After an experience of extreme violence or trauma, children initially feel overwhelming terror and helplessness. Rather than the sudden flashbacks that adults experience following trauma, children experience intrusive thoughts of the violent event and excessive daydreaming focused on the tragic events. Some children develop a cover or "screen" memory as a protection from more horrible specific reminiscences. They are usually very fearful of dying and of being separated from their parents, and view relationships as inevitably fragile. They become extremely cautious, easily overwhelmed, fearful even of fear itself. After an initial period when open discussion of the event is relatively easy, traumatized children become exceedingly reluctant to discuss their experiences. This can be understood on the basis of their intense feelings of shame, as they inaccurately believe they are to blame for the traumatic event, or somehow remiss in not averting or avoiding it. The sense of guilt is further expressed in pervasive worries about further disasters occurring locally.

Perceptual disturbances are likely for children suffering PTSD, including visual distortions and skewed time perception. Physical manifestations of their psychological pain can include muscle spasms, headaches, stomachaches, and dizziness. They frequently have a profound distrust or foreshortened sense of the future. Traumatized children search for omens that could have forewarned of the violent event. Dying occurs in their dreams at a rate inappropriate to their age.

Other repetitive phenomena in dreams and play activity present re-enactments of the original terrorizing event while secondary reparative attempts include overgeneralizations and prophetic dreams. These children have tremendous fears of any item related to the event, and experience panic attacks at the "anniversary" and other times. Post-traumatic play can depict the violent event by re-enacting it directly, by having it happen to others, or by somehow averting the event. This play becomes contagious to other children and is further replayed by them.

Attention to the congruence of PTSD and suicide survivorship sequelae is well warranted (Leenaars & Wenckstern, 1989). Child and adolescent suicide survivors displace their fears of suicide onto other people, just as survivors of other traumatic events. While Pynoos (1989) stipulates discovery of the body or knowledge of ghastly details as necessary precursors to the development of full PTSD following suicide or homicide, we have seen troublesome symptoms even in survivors who have been spared exposure to these more extreme stimuli.

RESILIENCE OR INVULNERABILITY

An individual's inherent ability to bounce back may provide some explanation for the wide range of outcomes after a loss such as a loved one's suicide. Sometimes people respond to crises with positive changes so significant they emerge seemingly transformed (see e.g., Erickson, 1968). External support systems (Caplan, 1964, 1974) are so clearly significant that approaches for enhancing previous resources and introducing additional ones have evolved into the strategy of postvention (described more fully later). In contrast to those individuals benefiting from postvention of some type, some people seem to accommodate to a crisis and achieve higher levels of functioning post-trauma *without* the benefit of professional intervention. So many unknowns enter the determination, however, that the final outcome may seem ascribable to random chance, or the "mazal factor" (Brooks, 1971). This resilience or invulnerability (Anthony, 1974; see, e.g., White, 1959, 1963; Kliman, 1968; Murphy & Moriarty, 1976; Cohler, 1987; for similar ideas with different terminology) has been described as exclusive of other survival factors such as support group or therapeutic intervention, and contrasted to vulnerability, or the likelihood of experiencing lasting damage following a trauma.

In contrast to the idea that some inherent unknown quality can provide a capacity for surviving a crisis with no great harm (basically a statement from the Optimist School described earlier), Terr (1979, 1983a,b) provides data indicating some degree of traumatic aftermath in *all* the youngsters she has assessed in the aftermath of many tragic events, regardless of varying proximity to the event (Pynoos, 1988) or source and form of the news (Bowlby, 1980). We would suggest a compromise position. Exposure to traumata such as suicide always has an impact on the survivors. Where positive outcomes seem to occur without benefit of professionally organized support, to simply call the individual "invulnerable" or in some other way "fortunate" is to do no more than acknowledge ignorance about the means of his or her survival. There are knowable factors that differentiate among more and less vulnerable youngsters. These factors include cognitive competence, peer acceptance, maternal acceptance, and physical competence (Earls, Beardslee, & Garrison, 1987). Major sources of support in the caregiving environment are further delineated such as being first-born, living with fewer siblings, or having a high activity level in infancy resulting in increased attention from caregivers, responsivity to people resulting in the availability of additional caretakers beyond the mother, adequate communication skills resulting in access to close peer friends, and so on (Werner & Smith, 1982), or a healthy identification with something larger than oneself (Anthony, 1984). Survivors of suicide and other tragedies would be well served by additional research to identify these variables, so that we might strengthen these factors where they already exist, and introduce them where they are absent. It is also important to differentiate truly healthy invulnerability from apparent invulnerability actually predicated on the dangerous "gift" of subordinating one's own needs in favor of the psychological requirements of parent figures (Miller, 1981; Anthony, 1987). In the case of suicide survivorship, this would be the need to believe the child is not significantly affected and to have the child available for assuaging the parent's own bereavement symptoms. These covert distinctions also warrant further clinical research.

SUICIDALITY AND SUICIDE SURVIVORSHIP

Child and adolescent survivors of the suicide of a significant loved one not only are at risk for a wide range of emotional difficulties, but are also a group at very high risk of suicidal behavior themselves (Cain & Fast, 1966, 1972). Suicidality in a parent or other family member rates risk scores of 9 and 6, respectively (on a 10-point scale) for completed suicides, and are ranked similarly for parasuicides, scoring 8 and 5, respectively (Victoroff, 1983). The literature provides data on the later risk of suicide or parasuicide following early parental loss from death separate from the increased burden posed when parental death occurs by suicide.

Early parental death has been associated with suicide attempts in adults (Birtchnell, 1970; Greer, 1966). Nonhospitalized suicide attemptors (Greer, Gunn, & Koller, 1966) and university students with suicidal ideation (Adam, Lohrenz, Harper, & Streiner, 1982) showed greater risk from loss of both parents in childhood. Other studies have associated suicidality with parental deprivation in general, recognizing the clinically significant fact that psychological damage from parental neglect (where the parent is alive but physically or emotionally unavailable due to abuse or abandonment) is comparable to that posed by parental absence due to death (Adam, Lohrenz, Harper, & Streiner, 1982; Walton, 1958). The completeness of the loss has also been associated with the degree of suicidality, with more death of parent(s) among completed suicides and more divorce of parents among parasuicides (Dorpat, Jackson, & Ripley, 1965). Where recent loss was found to be a precipitating factor in parasuicide, early parental loss has also been found (Lester & Beck, 1976). Overall, the empirical evidence more than adequately supports the clinical fact that parental loss is detrimental to healthy psychological development.

Clinical observations (Orbach & Glaubman, 1979), case study analysis (Orbach, Gross, & Glaubman, 1981), and research surveys (Pfeffer, Conte, Plutchik, & Jerrett, 1979; Pfeffer, Zuckerman, Plutchik, & Mizrucki, 1984) confirm an association between a parent's suicidal tendencies and the child's later suicide. One study (Teicher & Jacobs, 1966) identified parental suicide in one-fourth of the suicidal adolescents interviewed. In a staggering statistic, the parents of suicides evaluated through psychological autopsies were found to have committed suicide themselves at 88 times the expected rate (Farberow & Simon, 1969). While the loss of a parent to suicide poses a risk of suicidal behavior at any age, greater risk is attendant when the loss occurs during childhood (younger than 20) than in adulthood (Roy, 1983).

Family cases involving multiple suicides and parasuicides suggest a genetic inheritance of some suicidal tendency (Dabbagh, 1977; Zaw, 1981). Twin studies (Tsuang, 1977) have indicated greater congruence of suicidality between identical twins (who share all genes in common) than fraternal twins (who share one-quarter of their genes in common, as do all full siblings, but additionally are somewhat more likely than separately born siblings to share common experiences). The notion of suicide being "inherited" is further complicated by continuing controversy over whether suicidality is best understood as a communicative behavior (Stengel, 1969; Richman, 1986) with psychosocial bases only very distally heritable, or as a definitive symptom of psychiatric illness with a biologic basis (Mann & Stanley, 1986; Shaffer, 1986; Brent & Kolko, in press) with the possibility of more proximal heritability. It must be recognized that answering this question is as limited as any other issue in behavior genetics, where the appealing resolution of finding a single gene for a problematic human condition must be tempered by the reality of the multiple steps comprising the complex gene-to-behavior readout of encoded genetic information (Ginsburg, 1977, 1978), as well as the multiple paths whereby a single expressed characteristic (or phenotype) can arise from any of several underlying "genotypes" (Ginsburg & Laughlin, 1966, 1971).

Depression and suicidal behavior have been documented at increased rates among the first-degree relatives of suicidal children (Hersov, 1976) and among first- and second-degree relatives of suicidal adults (Roy, 1983), whether due to biological transmission or psychosocial learning. Children demonstrate their susceptibility to suicide contagion (and identification with the deceased) through a propensity for parasuicides and completed suicides enacted on an anniversary of the original suicide. Similarly, these survivors often choose the same means of self-destruction to which they were originally exposed (Cain & Fast, 1972). Not a biological phenomenon, suicide contagion (or the "Werther effect," so-named after the protagonist who died by ambiguous means in a novella by Goethe) embodies the idea that suicidal activity spreads through the psychosocial means of teaching by example or role modeling. In an effort to further understand and ultimately prevent suicide, especially teenage suicide and suicide clusters (Coleman, 1987), there has been wide discussion and research on the contagion notion (Gould & Shaffer, 1986; Gould, Shaffer, & Kleinman, 1988; Phillips & Carstenson, 1986; Terr, 1988). This theory states that suicide and parasuicide spread through knowledge about a complete suicide and that such spreading can be to individuals otherwise not at risk for suicidality. It is commendable that such concern has been heard by the media, and generated certain modifications, for example, in the way the print media reported the Philadelphia suicide of Edgar Rosenberg (Avery, 1987) and the Bergenfield cluster suicide (Grace, 1987). Additional attention to this matter is certainly critical, as evidenced by the publication of Proposed Media Guidelines by the American Association of Suicidology (1987). Nevertheless, we strongly caution it would be dangerous to generalize concern about contagion into perpetuation on the myth that talking about suicide encourages suicidal activity (Bonner, 1987; Carter & Brooks, September, 1986).

POSTVENTION

Suicide postvention is designed to prevent bereavement complications for individuals, families, and groups, by meeting immediate needs of distressed suicide survivors through interventions incorporating education and treatment (Schneidman, 1971, 1975; Webb, 1986). The immediate goal is to diffuse toxic affects and prevent further suicidal activity among the survivors, who are themselves at extreme risk of suicide (Smith & Crawford, 1986). Additional goals are the repair of damaged support systems and accessing previously unused internal, interpersonal, and professional resources. While the general goals and principles of postvention remain constant across difference target audiences, certain practices vary for family support versus school-based interventions. The following descriptions address the similar components first, then the approaches for family support, and finally the components for postvention at schools.

There are three approaches to suicide postvention therapy, all based on the original crisis intervention model (Lindemann, 1944). Short-term postvention (1–3 sessions) provides didactic and evaluative consultations that enable assessment of suicide aftermath symptoms in individuals identified as likely to be at risk, and provides referral for therapy beyond the postvention setting as needed (Leenaars,

1985; Leenaars & Wenckstern, 1986; Zinner, 1986; Bozigar, 1989). Intensive therapy (3 months to several years) is the long-term approach to postvention, where the full gamut of ramifications from the suicide are addressed for the individual. An intermediate protocol (10–12 weekly sessions) is called convergent postvention, as it "converges" between the two extremes (Baldwin, 1980; Yalom, cited in Farberow, 1976). Our own convergent postvention activities have been conducted on school grounds and in an outpatient clinic, assisting youngsters with the cognitive and emotional adjustments following suicide deaths and the similar psychological distresses after serious, and fortunately incomplete, parasuicides. An additional form of convergent postvention, specifically based on the tenets of Self-Psychology, is being investigated as a method of addressing the effects on families of other forms of violence (Carter, 1989).

Attention is warranted for the bystanders in all instances of suicidality. Orbach (1988) cites the example of "David" to confirm the comparably damaging impact of suicidal tendencies, even where a completed suicide, or even an overt suicide attempt, has not occurred. As a 10-year-old, David's suicidality could be traced directly to comparable ideation in his mother. Her suicidal tendencies were most significantly connected to this middle child by her plan to commit suicide by conceiving a medically contraindicated pregnancy (i.e., David) after bearing a disabled older sibling.

Postvention increases participants' social skills and awareness of their own competence, clarifies sources of family, peer, and community support, and generates constructive alternative expressions for feelings and conflicts that could create future suicidal ideation. Addressing the affect is particularly significant because sadness, fear, and anger inevitably are experienced after someone dies by suicide. This objective is accomplished by directly discussing current feelings of the survivors in the postvention setting. It is critical to provide an arena for expressing extreme emotions. Feelings of shock, denial, guilt, fear, and anger are all normal in the aftermath of suicide.

As the main source of support for children, the family warrants strenuous reinforcement when weakened in the aftermath of suicide. As noted earlier, suicide survivor families have far less support at the time of their grief than usually provided other mourners. They are also more heavily burdened as they search for meaning for the particularly senseless death. The adult survivors may suffer emotional numbing and behavioral disorganization or be unable to direct angry or guilty feelings constructively. In the chaotic, overwhelmed setting that ensues, children are often neglected.

The following recommended practices augment resources available to the family, and thereby increase the likelihood that children's needs will be met. Professionals visiting the family, whether mental health professionals, clergy, liaison school staff, or family physicians, should be prepared to address the suicide honestly and compassionately in order to counteract the silence and distortions likely from other sources. Attending the funeral is appropriate for these same people, as part of facilitating the family's search for an explanation of the suicidal death. Through a postvention that creates a forum for distressed feelings, the mental health professional or suicide expert offers assistance at a time the family very likely does not recognize their own needs. The family may need assistance gathering information about antecedents to the suicide and about positive aspects of the deceased previously unavailable to them. Access to such knowledge helps the family progress in their bereavement past denial and anger. The essential closure derived through knowing the strengths *and* the pains of the deceased is functionally equivalent to final burial rituals such as recovery of a body lost in an air disaster. The family should also be given information regarding the emotional and physical reactions of bereavement and the exacerbations that occur as a result of suicide, as a basis for recognizing long-range needs for help. While postvention can only be the initial step in the necessarily long-term recovery following a suicide, it can provide an invaluable introduction to more extensive individual or family therapies.

When responding to a school after the recent experience of a student suicide, a proactive or "pursuant" strategy is often required because school personnel and students usually recognize only a limited need for help. A previously established protocol defining the usual needs and services of postvention will facilitate such an offer to a school, but postventionists need to recognize that offered assistance may be accepted defensively or refused altogether because of general anxiety and fear of stigmatization. The general approach is to hold open discussions, again to prevent the factual and psychological distortions and evasions generated by other sources. Discussions should start with school personnel who are connected themselves with the student survivors or are identified as available resources for postvention support. Immediate consultation establishes facts about the student, the death, and the general school milieu.

The next step is identification of student survivors showing emotional and behavioral symptoms indicative of suicidality or other severe outcomes. Convergent postvention continues with a group session for selected students. Usually this is best limited to close friends and classmates of the suicide, but siblings may be included if they attend the same school. Participants are immediately told the purpose of providing a "safe place" for ventilating grief and other turbulent feelings. The setting can be at the school or may be moved to a mental health setting. As the therapeutic alliance develops (quickly for some participants and more gradually for others), that relationship can be used safely as a focus for anger and fear. Since interpersonal changes are inevitable among suicide survivors, participants' relationships require vigilant monitoring in order to provide needed support at times of "break-ups" and avert extreme reactions to situations perceivable as additional losses. Postvention discussions also address the warning signs of suicide, effective interventions, and alternatives other than suicidal activity for seeking assistance and resolving life crises.

Ending convergent postvention comes after 8 to 12 weeks, and is always prearranged. Termination renews issues of separation and loss, and anticipation of anniversary reactions is critical. Students are reassured about access to additional treatment resources, and the continuous process of evaluating for further treatment frequently is completed at this time. Elsewhere (Carter & Brooks, 1986; Brooks & Carter, 1987), we have provided further specific content of child and adolescent postventions. In addition, the School Program Committee of the American Association of Suicidology has prepared comprehensive guidelines for school postvention procedures, including a detailed recommended sequence of steps.

While direct evaluation research on school postvention continues to be minimal (Shaffer, Garland, Gould, Fisher, & Trautman, 1988), the effectiveness of suicide postvention is necessarily limited by the inherent vulnerability of the individual survivors. Most youngsters will continue to be at risk for the multiple potential negative outcomes detailed earlier, and therefore should be considered for more extensive therapy.

Countertransference impediments in postventionists are very likely due to the complexity, volatility, and inevitable anxiety connected to suicide. It is for this reason that we strongly recommend postvention be conducted by two co-therapists, to prevent unwise decisions motivated by countertransference feelings and safeguard against overload and burnout. Having another professional equally involved in the specific situation decreases the actual burden and enhances support available to each postventionist. Where this is absolutely impossible, we recommend review with another postventionist outside the situation, not so much for a critique of events and actions but for diffusing toxic affects (Carter & Brooks, 1986). After all "Who takes care of the caretaker when the caretaker is busy taking care?" (Weingarten & Magran, 1983). The necessity for co-therapy teams highlights an additional limitation of suicide postvention—the scarcity of experienced mental health professionals trained to provide this intervention. The statistics cited earlier clearly indicate the growing need for postvention, but the demand for trained professionals is additionally hampered by fears about suicidality, a stigma that continues to thrive within the mental health professions just as it does in the general public.

Case Presentation

This second composite clinical example delineates the typically difficult situation when suicide touches a school. As in the earlier case presentation, *italics* highlight issues specific to suicide survivorship as well as the aftermath concerns particular to a school-related suicide.

After a learning disability necessitated a transfer from his neighborhood junior high school, implicitly creating a *loss of status, friends, and familiar surroundings*, 14-year-old Karl died in a shooting incident of *uncertain intentionality*. Following that weekend death, school administrators found themselves facing more *open grief* among the boy's friends and the other students than could be addressed adequately by available counseling staff. A local community mental health agency met with counseling and teaching staff to structure the *emotional processing* and *screening for at-risk behavior* needed by the students, and to assuage the *inevitable guilt* among the staff.

Sensitive members of the administration soon recognized that a small group of Karl's *close friends and classmates needed more* than brief support. They *hesitated*, however, because the *family denied the possibility of suicide*, and the resulting confusion was increased by continuing *official uncertainty about the nature of the death*. After a few days, the decision was reached to bring in a therapist with *suicide postvention experience* and a meeting was scheduled for the *most seriously affected students*, many of whom had *experienced loss and feared abandonment* much like the suicide. In fact, several of Karl's friends had experienced *suicide or parasuicide survivorship before* his death.

The *first postvention group contact* further *assessed the emotional needs* of the suicide survivors and *provided immediate support*. Most important, that first session established realistic options for assessing *further therapeutic support*. Overall, the immediate need was to *prevent additional deaths* among these suicide survivors. *Crying* was *accepted* and even facilitated; a show was made of the availability of tissues. This stood in marked *contrast to* certain other messages the students were hearing, that is, *stop crying already*.

The first contact developed into a full *clinical postvention* with weekly meetings continuing for 3 months, plus three later follow-up contacts. *Anger* was a major theme for the group. Some expressed their anger directly at Karl, but most *directed their anger at authority figures*, blaming the required school transfer for Karl's death. The *family's denial* of the suicide (as it was eventually officially designated) was also a prominent topic, and these emotionally "gifted" (Miller, 1981) youngsters struggled to *balance* their own *need for honest information and emotional candor* with the family's experience of shock and *need for some initial denial*. Throughout the postvention, all *emotions* were *acknowledged as valid*, as this acceptance facilitates progressive changes and growth.

The supraordinate theme of the group was the inevitability of *losses*, and means of accepting or surviving this. The group explored the conflict of protecting oneself while still getting close enough for interpersonal commitment in the context of their own relationships. These friends had a well-established history before the start of the postvention group, and they experienced many *changes in* their *alliances during the postvention period*. At the time of Karl's death, Anita was an outcast from the group, in part due to a conflict with Beth over romantic involvements with Peter. Over time, Beth and Anita mended their friendship, and Anita regained her original status as a fully accepted group member. The focus on Anita as an outcast and then as a returning pilgrim initially appeared to be a distraction from needed focus on irretrievable losses, specifically Karl's death. Later it became evident that attention to retrievable losses functioned as means of working through the ultimate loss to death. Thus, as Anita returned to the group, Sam took on the outcast role. He channeled his energies into new friendships and school activities and became so separated from his former friends that he attended neither the last session, nor the 3-month follow-up "reunion" session.

The *clinical postvention* was provided by a *co-therapy team* composed of a senior level therapist and a psychiatry resident, with additional consultation on policy, countertransference, and medical issues. *Further school consultation* for staff and other students was offered, but *declined*. Despite this successful implementation of clinical postvention for the school-related aftershocks after a suicide, the *fear* that talking about suicide will increase the problem *remained* at this school as it does elsewhere.

CONCLUSION

We have seen that a suicidal death is a far more complicated loss to a child survivor than loss due to other deaths. Usual bereavement factors of shock, stigma, shame, anger, guilt, blame, and numbness are exaggerated. Customary societal acceptance of loss and support for the bereaved is frequently withdrawn or curtailed. Adult survivors are themselves entangled in grief and less likely to be sufficiently available for these youngsters. Even therapists and other professionals touched by the reverberations of a completed suicide can experience decreased capacity to access necessary resources for young survivors. These multileveled stresses weaken the support system available to the youngsters and diminish their prospects for healthy bereavement and recovery.

Rebuilding and augmenting essential support systems is vital for the recovery of child and adolescent suicide survivors. Some families may accept therapeutic interventions readily, others only with strong reluctance, and even others refuse the assistance entirely, exercising denial as a futile defense against the intrinsically shattering experience of suicide survivorship. Families sometimes allow postvention into their system but only for certain members of the family. An avenue of support for peers of a young suicide is through postvention at school, providing opportunities for shared feelings and pooled resources.

Case Presentation

We will close with a third composite clinical example, this time of a potentially worst case scenario reoriented to cautious but realistic optimism through open discussion and acceptance of therapeutic support. *Italics* highlight the issues specific to suicide survivorship (as in the earlier case presentations) and the components of bereavement resolution.

At 10 years old, Lenny M. was the younger of two children whose mother died 4 weeks before his contact with a child psychiatrist. His sister, 14, appeared to be experiencing "appropriate mourning" while Lenny concerned his overwhelmed father with *agitated and suicidal behavior*. Lenny's mother died of heart failure, the direct result of chronic malnourishment from severe anorexia nervosa of 10 years' duration. The anorexia was the pervasive condition of Mrs. M.'s repertoire of psychologically disturbed behaviors that included several more overt *suicide attempts* known to her husband and daughter but *kept secret* from Lenny. Mrs. M. also had a bizarre regimen of exaggerated exercise (several hours per day) and miniscule intake of food. All family members, including Lenny, had sought to dissuade Mrs. M. from her self-destructive anorexic behaviors and urged her to obtain professional assistance. Mr. M. was unsuccessful in his somewhat passive attempts to budge his single-minded wife who seemed "hell-bent on self-destruction." Her physical strength gradually failed, but never her iron will.

The immediate family perceived Mrs. M.'s death as a *long-term suicide completion*. Lenny was inconsolably hysterical when "Mommy killed herself," and he *tried to take his own life* by throwing himself into the street to await being hit by a car. He experienced various grief reactions of *moroseness, oppositional behavior, hyperactivity, and fearfulness*. He *angrily disparaged* his sister, his overwhelmed but attentive father, the therapist and *the entire world. Social isolation* from his schoolmates worsened, and eventually included complete truancy. In addition, he alternated between one-day hunger strikes and several-day eating binges. A complicated, difficult but nevertheless time-limited psychotherapy focused on Lenny's *feelings of anger, guilt, blame, and fear of the future*. Particular attention was needed concerning the feeling of isolation that arose from his *being "shielded" from knowledge of his mother's previous suicide attempts*, and from *fears about stigma* resulting from her peculiar death.

Psychotherapy for Lenny went hand-in-hand with brief individual counseling for his bereaved sister, intensive psychotherapy for his stricken father, and family therapy for all three of them. *Eventually* these treatment efforts enabled Lenny to *accept support systems* he had *previously spurned*. These included accepting a daily housekeeper, bringing friends to the home, joining usual as well as special school functions, participating in extracurricular activities, and allowing his sister to resume her previous position as a valued confidant. Lenny ceased his disturbed eating patterns, *regained behavioral stability*, and in essence, *allowed the beginning of his future*. Treatment ended after 3 months, when Lenny had learned enough about the turbulent *feelings of abandonment* that followed his mother's "crazy" suicide to attain the comfort of some *understanding and acceptance*.

REFERENCES

Adam, K. S., Lohrenz, M. D., Harper, D., & Streiner, D. (1982). Early parental loss and suicidal ideation in university students. *Canadian Journal of Psychiatry*, *27*, 275–281.

American Association of Suicidology. (1987). Proposed media guidelines. *Newslink*, *18*(2), 10.

American Psychiatric Association. (1987). *Diagnostic and statistical manual of mental disorders (3rd ed. revised)*. Washington, DC: Author.

Anthony, A. J. (1974). The syndrome of the psychologically invulnerable child. In E. J. Anthony & C. Koupernik (Eds.), *The child in his family: Children at psychiatric risk (International yearbook, Vol. 3)*. New York: Wiley.

Anthony, E. J. (1984). The St. Louis Risk Research Project. In N. F. Watt, E. J. Anthony, L. C. Wynne, & J. Roth (Eds.), *Children at risk for schizophrenia: A longitudinal perspective*. Cambridge, England: Cambridge University.

Anthony, E. J. (1987). Risk, vulnerability, and resilience: An overview. In E. J. Anthony & B. J. Cohler (Eds.), *The invulnerable child*. New York, London: Guilford.

Avery, R. (1987, August 15). River's Edgar takes life: Depressed by illness, Rosenberg downs valium overdose. *Philadelphia Daily News*, p. 3.

Baldwin, B. A. (1980). Styles of crisis intervention: Toward a convergent model. *Professional Psychology*, *11*(1), 113–120.

Birtchnell, J. (1970). The relationship between attempted suicide, depression and parent death. *British Journal of Psychiatry*, *116*, 303–313.

Bolton, I. (1983). *My son . . . my son . . .: A guide to healing after death, loss or suicide*. Atlanta, GA: Bolton.

Bonner, R. L. (1987). Everyone knows asking people about thoughts of suicide won't put the idea in their heads—Don't they? *Newslink*, *13*(2), 8,12.

Bowlby, J. (1960). Grief and mourning in infancy and early childhood. *Psychoanalytic Study of the Child*, *15*, 9–52.

Bowlby, J. (1961). Childhood mourning and its implications for psychiatry. *American Journal of Psychiatry*, *118*(6), 481–498.

Bowlby, J. (1969, 1982). *Attachment (Attachment and loss: Vol. 1 [2nd Ed.])*. New York: Basic Books.

Bowlby, J. (1973). *Separation, anxiety and anger (Attachment and loss: Vol. 2)*. New York: Basic Books.

Bowlby, J. (1980). *Loss: Sadness and depression (Attachment and loss: Vol. 3)*. New York: Basic Books.

Bozigar, J. A. (1989). Postvention: A standards manual. In D. Lester (Ed.), *Proceedings, Twenty-Second Annual Meeting, American Association of Suicidology* (pp. 140–141). Denver: AAS.

Brent, D. A., & D. J. Kolko. (1990). Suicide and suicidal behavior in children and adolescents. In B. D. Garfinkel, G. Carlson, & E. Weller (Eds.), *The medical basis of child and adolescent psychiatry* (pp. 372–391). Philadelphia: Saunders.

Brooks, A. (1971). *Lectures on child resilience: The "major" factor*. Unpublished manuscript, Creative Arts Therapy Program, Hahnemann University, Philadelphia.

Brooks, A., & Carter, B. F. (1987). Suicide postvention using convergent intervention strategies. In R. I. Yufit (Ed.), *Combined Proceedings, Twentieth Annual Meeting, American Association of Suicidology and Nineteenth International Congress, International Association for Suicide Prevention* (pp. 243–245). Denver: AAS.

Cain, A. C., & Fast, I. (1966). Children's disturbed reactions to parent suicide. *American Journal of Orthopsychiatry*, *36*(5), 873–880.

Cain, A. C., & Fast, I. (1972). The legacy of suicide: Observations on the pathogenic impact of suicide upon marital partners. In A. C. Cain (Ed.), *Survivors of suicide* (pp. 145–154). Springfield, IL: Charles C Thomas.

Caplan, G. (1964). *Principles of preventive psychiatry*. New York: Basic Books.

Caplan, G. (1974). *Support systems and community psychiatry*. New York: Behavioral Publications.

Carter, B. F. (1989). Applications of self psychology for postvention. In D. Lester (Ed.), *Proceedings, Twenty-Second Annual Meeting, American Association of Suicidology* (pp. 210–212). Denver: AAS.

Carter, B. F., & Brooks, A. (1986). An exploration of group postvention techniques. In R. Cohen-Sandler (Ed.), *Proceedings, Nineteenth Annual Meeting, American Association of Suicidology* (pp. 242–243). Denver: AAS.

Carter, B. F., & Brooks, A. (September, 1986). Stopping suicide [Letter to the editor]. *Philadelphia Inquirer*, p.A8.

Cohler, B. J. (1987). Adversity, resilience, and the study of lives. In E. J. Anthony & B. J. Cohler (Eds.), *The invulnerable child*. New York: Guilford.

Coleman, L. (1987). *Suicide clusters*. Winchester, MA: Faber & Faber.

Dabbagh, F. (1977). Family suicide. *British Journal of Psychiatry*, *130*, 159–161.

Dorpat, T. L., Jackson, J. K., & Ripley, H. S. (1965). Broken homes and attempted and completed suicide. *Archives of General Psychiatry, 12*, 213–216.

Dunne, E., McIntosh, J. L., & Dunne-Maxim, K. (Eds.). (1987). *Suicide and its aftermath*. New York: W. W. Norton.

Dunne-Maxim, K., Dunne, E. J., & Hauser, M. J. (1987). When children are suicide survivors. In E. Dunne, J. L. McIntosh, & K. Dunne-Maxim (Eds.), *Suicide and its aftermath*. New York: W. W. Norton.

Earls, F., Beardslee, W., & Garrison, W. (1987). Correlates and predictors of competence in young children. In E. J. Anthony, & B. J. Cohler (Eds.), *The invulnerable child*. New York: Guilford.

Elizur, E., & Kaffman, M. (1982). Children's bereavement reactions following death of the father: II. *Journal of American Academy of Child Psychiatry, 21*(5), 474–480.

Elizur, E., & Kaffman, M. (1983). Factors influencing the severity of childhood bereavement reactions. *American Journal of Orthopsychiatry, 53*(4), 668–676.

Erikson, E. H. (1968). *Identity: Youth and crisis*. New York: W. W. Norton.

Farberow, N. L. (1976). Group psychotherapy for self-destructive persons. In H. J. Parad, H. L. P. Resnik, L. G. Parad, & M. D. Bowie (Eds.), *Emergency and disaster management: A mental health source book* (pp. 169–185). Bowie, MD: Charles.

Farberow, N. L., & Simon, M. D. (1969). Suicides in Los Angeles & Vienna: An intercultural study of two cities. *Public Health Reports, 84*, 389–403.

Freud, A., & Burlingham, D. T. (1943). *War and children*. New York: International University Press, Foster Parents' Plan for War Children.

Ginsburg, B. E. (1977). Genetic models of behavior disorders. In I. Hanin & E. Usdin (Eds.), *Animal models in psychiatry and neurology* (pp. 307–314). New York: Pergamon.

Ginsburg, B. E. (1978). The genetics of social behavior. In P. P. G. Bateson & P. H. Klopfer (Eds.), *Perspectives in Ethology, Vol. 3* (pp. 1–15). New York: Plenum.

Ginsberg, B. E., & Laughlin, W. S. (1966). The multiple bases of human adaptability and achievement: A species point of view. *Eugenics Quarterly, 13(3)*, 240–257.

Ginsberg, B. E., & Laughlin, W. S. (1971). Race and intelligence: What do we really know? In R. Cancro (Ed.), *Intelligence: Genetic and environmental influences* (pp. 77–87). New York: Grune & Stratton.

Gould, M. S., & Shaffer, D. A. (1986). The impact of suicide in television movies: Evidence of imitation. *New England Journal of Medicine, 315*, 690–693.

Gould, M. S., Shaffer, D. A., & Kleinman, M. (1988). The impact of suicide in television movies: Replication and commentary. *Suicide and Life-Threatening Behavior, 18*(1), 90–99.

Grace, J. (1987, March 12). Mental health experts alert for a local fall-out. *Philadelphia Daily News*, p. 5.

Greer, S. (1966). Parental loss and attempted suicide: A further report. *British Journal of Psychiatry, 112*, 465–470.

Greer, S., Gunn, J. C., & Koller, K. M. (1966). Aetiological factors in attempted suicide. *British Medical Journal, 2*, 1352–1355.

Hersov, L. (1976). Emotional disorders. In M. Rutter & L. Hersov (Eds.), *Child psychiatry: Modern approaches* (pp. 428–454). Oxford: Blackwell.

Holmes, T. H., & Rahe, R. H. (1967). The Social Readjustment Rating Scale. *Journal of Psychosomatic Research, 2*, 213.

Kliman, G. (1968). *Psychological emergencies of childhood*. New York: Grune & Stratton.

Leenaars, A. A. (1985). Suicide postvention in a school system. *Canada's Mental Health, 33*(4).

Leenaars, A. A., & Wenckstern, S. (1989). The suicide and post-traumatic stress disorder. In D. Lester (Ed.), *Proceedings, Twenty-Second Annual Conference, American Association of Suicidology* (pp. 98–99). Denver: AAS.

Leenaars, A. A., & Wenckstern, S. (1986). Suicide postvention in a school system. In R. Cohen-Sandler (Ed.), *Proceedings, Nineteenth Annual Meeting, American Association of Suicidology* (pp. 237–239). Denver: AAS.

Lester, D., & Beck, A. T. (1976). Early loss as a possible sensitizer to later loss in attempted suicides. *Psychological Reports, 39*, 121–122.

Lindemann, E. (1944). Symptomatology and management of acute grief. *American Journal of Psychiatry, 101*, 141–148.

Mann, L. J., & Stanley, M. (Eds). (1986). Psychobiology of suicidal behavior. *Annals of the New York Academy of Sciences, 487*.

McIntosh, J. L. (1989). How many survivors of suicide are there? *Surviving Suicide, 1*(1), 1,4.

Miller, A. (1981). *The drama of the gifted child*. New York: Basic Books.

Morse, S. R. (1984). Survivors of suicide: The siblings tell their story. *Dissertation Abstracts International, 45*, 1025B. (University Microfilms No. DA8414702)

Murphy, L. B., & Moriarty, A. E. (1976). *Vulnerability, coping and growth*. New Haven: Yale.

Nagera, H. (1970). Children's reactions to the death of important objects. *Psychoanalytic Study of the Child, 25*, 360–400.

Orbach, I. (1988). *Children who don't want to live: Understanding and treating a suicidal child*. San Francisco: Jossey-Bass.

Orbach, I., & Glaubman, H. (1979). The concept of death and suicidal behavior in young children. *Journal of the American Academy of Child Psychiatry, 18*, 668–678.

Orbach, I., Gross, Y., & Glaubman, H. (1981). Some common characteristics of latency age suicidal children: A tentative model based on case study analysis. *Suicide and Life-Threatening Behavior, 4*, 180–190.

Orbach, I., Gross, Y., Glaubman, H., & Berman, D. (1985). Children's perception of death in humans and animals as a function of age, anxiety and cognitive ability. *Journal of Child Psychology and Psychiatry, 26*, 453–463.

Phillips, D. P., & Carstensen, L. L. (1986). Clustering of teenage suicide after television news stores about suicide. *New England Journal of Medicine, 315*(11), 685–689.

Pfeffer, C. R., Conte, H. R., Plutchik, R., & Jerrett, I. (1979). Suicidal behavior in latency age children: An empirical study. *Journal of the American Academy of Child Psychiatry, 18*, 679–692.

Pfeffer, C. R., Zuckerman, S., Plutchik, R., & Mizruchi, M. S. (1984). Suicidal behavior in normal school children: A comparison with child psychiatric inpatients. *Journal of the American Academy of Child Psychiatry, 23*, 416–423.

Pynoos, R. (1988, April). *The traumatized child*. Paper presented at Abbott Northwestern Hospital, Minneapolis, MN.

Pynoos, R. (1989, April). *The interplay of trauma and grief during childhood*. Paper presented at Psychiatry Grand Rounds, Albert Einstein Medical Center, Philadelphia, PA.

Richman, J. (1986). The suicidal communication system: A flight from dialogue. In J. Richman (Ed.), *Family therapy for suicidal people* (pp. 138–149). New York: Springer.

Rogan, N., & Hussey, M. (1977). *The development of a life change events scale for adolescents*. Unpublished master's thesis, University of Cincinnati School of Nursing.

Roy, A. (1983). Family history of suicide. *Archives of General Psychiatry, 40*, 971–974.

Rutter, M. (1976). *Separation, loss and family relationships*. In M. Rutter & L. Hersov (Eds.), *Child psychiatry*. Oxford: Blackwell.

Rutter, M. (1983). Stress, coping and development: Some issues and some questions. In N. Garmezy & M. Rutter (Eds.), *Stress, coping, and development in children*. New York: McGraw-Hill.

Shaffer, D. A. (October, 1986). *Preventing suicide*. Paper presented at the meeting of the American Academy of Child and Adolescent Psychiatry, Los Angeles, CA.

Shaffer, D., Garland, A., Gould, M., Fisher, P., & Trautman, P. (1988). Preventing teenage suicide: A critical review. *Journal of the American Academy of Child and Adolescent Psychiatry, 27*(6), 675–687.

Shneidman, E. S. (1971). Prevention, intervention, and postvention of suicide. *Annals of Internal Medicine, 75*, 453–458.

Shneidman, E. S. (1975). Postvention: The care of the bereaved. In R. O. Pasnau (Ed.), *Consultation-liaison psychiatry* (pp. 245–256). New York: Grune & Stratton.

Small, A. M., & Small, A. D. (1984). Children's reactions to a suicide in the family and the implications for treatment. In N. Linzer (Ed.), *Suicide: The will to live vs. the will to die* (pp. 151–169). New York: Human Sciences Press.

Smith, K., & Crawford, M. (1986). Suicide behavior among "normal" high school students. *Suicide and Life-Threatening Behavior, 16*(3), 313–325.

Stengel, E. (1969). A matter of communication. In E. S. Shneidman (Ed.), *On the nature of suicide* (pp. 74–80). San Francisco: Jossey-Bass.

Teicher, J., & Jacobs, J. (1966). Adolescents who attempt suicide: Preliminary findings. *American Journal of Psychiatry, 122*, 1248–1257.

Terr, L. (1979). Children of Chowchilla. *Psychoanalytic Study of the Child, 34*, 547–623.

Terr, L. (1983a). Chowchilla revisited: The effects of psychic trauma four years after a school-bus kidnapping. *American Journal of Psychiatry, 140*, 1543–1550.

Terr, L. (1983b). Time sense following psychic trauma. *American Journal of Orthopsychiatry, 53*, 244–261.

Terr, L. (1988, May). *A comparison of childhood and adult psychic trauma: What's alike, what's different*. Paper presented at the Annual Meeting of the American Academy of Psychoanalysis, Montreal, Canada.

Tsuang, M. T. (1977). Genetic factors in suicide. *Disorders of the Nervous System, 38*, 498–501.

van Eerdewegh, M. M., Bieri, M. D., Parilla, R. H., & Clayton, P. J. (1982). The bereaved child. *British Journal of Psychiatry, 140*, 23–29.

Victoroff, V. M. (1983). *The suicidal patient: Recognition, intervention, management*. Oradell, NJ: Medical Economics.

Walton, H. J. (1958). Suicidal behavior in depressive illness: A study of aetiological factors in suicide. *Journal of Mental Science, 104*, 884–891.

Webb, N. B. (1986). Before and after suicide: A preventive outreach program for colleges. *Suicide and Life-Threatening Behavior, 16(4)*, 469–480.

Weingarten, N., & Magran B., (1983, November). *Welcome and opening remarks*. Paper presented at the 15th Annual Conference of The Family Institute of Philadelphia, Philadelphia, PA.

Weller, E. B., & Weller, R. A. (1989, May). *Psychosocial functioning in bereaved children*. Paper presented at the annual meeting of the American Psychiatric Association, San Francisco, CA.

Werner, E., & Smith, R. (1982). *Vulnerable but invincible*. New York: McGraw-Hill.

White, R. W. (1959). Motivation reconsidered: The concept of competence. *Psychological Review, 66*, 297–333.

White, R. W. (1963). Sense of interpersonal competence. In R. W. White (Ed.), *The study of lives*. New York: Atherton.

Wolfenstein, M. (1966). How is mourning possible? *The Psychoanalytic Study of the Child, 21*, 93–123.

Wolfenstein, M. (1969). Loss, rage, and repetition. *The Psychoanalytic Study of the Child, 24*, 423–460.

Wrobleski, A. (1989). *Suicide: Why?* Minneapolis: Afterwords.

Zaw, K. M. (1981). A suicidal family. *British Journal of Psychiatry, 139*, 68–69.

Zinner, E. S. (1986). Survivor intervention strategy in the suicide of a sixth grader. In R. Cohen-Sandler (Ed.), *Proceedings, Nineteenth Annual Meeting, American Association of Suicidology* (pp. 242–243). Denver: AAS.

17

Adult Survivors after Suicide
Research Problems and Needs

Norman L. Farberow

It is primarily within the past decade that survivors after suicide have begun to receive the professional concern and research attention their difficult emotional experience has warranted. Research into the area was practically nonexistent in the 1960s, was minimal in the 1970s, and in the late 1980s has, at best, been only sparse. As a result many unanswered questions and much misinformation about the event remains. The lack of answers and information, however, has not prevented the proliferation of clinical programs both in the United States and in Canada. A survey of the literature over the past two decades revealed that of the roughly 250 publications dealing with survivorship, all but 15% describe the establishment and the functioning of group counseling programs. Most of these reports appeared in Proceedings of the American Association of Suicidology (AAS) Annual Meetings and a few appeared in the International Association of Suicide Biennial Congresses, but most often they were descriptions or summary reports containing few, if any, details. There are some indications, however, that professional awareness of the needs of survivors has begun to change. Survivors of suicide have now received official recognition from the AAS with the establishment of a permanent Committee on Survivors, the sponsoring of a National Conference of Survivors conducted for and by them, and the publication of a newsletter written for and by them.

NORMAN L. FARBEROW • The Suicide Prevention Center of the Family Services of Los Angeles, Los Angeles, California 90006.

The focus of this chapter will be on the research activities in significant areas of survivorship, especially those conducted in the 1980s with adults. A recent comprehensive overview of the field by McIntosh in 1987 outlined the need for information in such areas as epidemiological and demographic characteristics; reaction and experiences of the survivors of suicide and factors affecting them; issues in the clinical, therapeutic, and supportive efforts; education and information dissemination both to survivors and to the general public and ethical problems involved in doing such research. The last concern included such questions as when to make contact, how soon after the death is an approach for information or participation acceptable, what kind of attitudes are present in the subjects and how do they affect the data?

SIGNIFICANT RESEARCH BEFORE THE 1980s AND METHODOLOGICAL CONCERNS

Among the early research studies of survivors before 1980, a landmark report by Cain and Fast (1966) grew out of an ongoing study of 45 disturbed children who had experienced the death of a parent by suicide an average of 5 years previously. They found the remaining spouses severely negatively affected in their bereavement, especially by the "blaming" encountered and the loss of support experienced from family, friends, and community. A "conspiracy of silence" forced the survivors to deal with misconceptions and irrational guilts without adequate support. Five reaction patterns were noted in the efforts of the survivors to manage their bereavement process, several of which impeded instead of helping the course of bereavement. These included reparation by way of rescuing damaged persons; reparation by way of world-rescue plans; personal self-destructive thoughts and impulses; establishment of another marital relationship; and attraction to additional suicidal persons.

Demi's study (1978) addressed some of the major concerns about the work in this area through a carefully developed methodology. She explored the question whether there were any fundamental characteristics in the adjustment by widows after suicide (N = 20) using comparison groups of natural (N = 29) and accidental (N = 11) death survivors, controlled for age, sex, and nationality differences. She used standardized data collection instruments and a questionnaire and examined all subjects within a period of 12 to 21 months after the death of their spouse. Contrary to generally accepted beliefs, Demi's (then) startling results indicated no differences between the groups in depression, anxiety, overall symptoms of distress, and trajectory of grief over the 2-year period.

Sheskin and Wallace (1976) compared the bereavement experiences of survivors following suicide, natural, and accidental deaths by comparing the results of a study by Glick, Weiss, and Parkes (1974) of the first year of bereavement for 48 widows as a result of natural and accidental deaths of spouses with a similar year for 12 widows of a suicide death by spouses studied intensively by Wallace (1973). Although the study is flawed by different populations in terms of race, method, and frequency of data collection, the authors noted that anticipation of the death was an important factor in the adequacy of recovery of all three modes of death. Those widowed by sudden death had to make sense of a world that had lost its meaning. Those widowed by suicide were, in addition, forced to try to make sense of a self-inflicted act. There were also differences between the suicide-death survivors and the natural/accident-death survivors as a result of guilt feelings, with the former less able to use social support and having less opportunity to disclose to others. Grief, however, was a similar experience for the widows of all three modes of death.

Shepherd and Barraclough's early study (1976) of the impact of parental suicide on the children (N = 36, ages 20–17) in the family was notable for its methodology. Comparisons were made with children of nonsuicide deaths (N = 61), matched with those of suicide deaths for age, sex, marital status, and geographical area. Follow-up was by two interviews, the first 1 week after death and the second 5 to 7 years later. The researchers found that only 1 of the 36 children of suicide deaths had lived in a stable family. The age of the child was the most significant determinant of what was told to them to explain the death. For those told the truth it was 10 years mean age, for those not told it was 4 years mean age, and for those told it was something else, the mean age was 8. There were significantly more referrals for psychiatric disturbance among the suicidal death children. Among the 36 children, 16 were judged as not functioning well. The importance of marital status was indicated by the fact that these were most likely to be of parents who had been separated before the death.

The major problems in the research on survivors have been in the lack of definition of groups studied and the control of factors that may affect the results. These include factors affecting both the character and the course of bereavement, such as age; different modes of death; kinship or relationship factors between the survivor and the decedent, for example, parent, spouse, sibling, child, other family or relative, lover, friend, therapist, caregiver, fellow worker, hospital staff, and others; emotional closeness to the deceased; sex and socioeconomic status of both survivor and suicide; and time elapsed since the death. Other important research concerns include familiar methodological questions such as retrospective versus prospective data, representativeness of the sample, methods of recruitment, numbers, adequate and appropriate measuring instruments, replicability, use of control or comparison groups, clinical versus nonclinical populations, size of study populations, and whether measurements were one-time or longitudinal over time (to obtain course of bereavement) (McIntosh, 1987; Barrett & Scott, 1987).

This review focuses on the research on three major questions and the need for further study in those areas: (1) Does suicide bereavement differ from the bereavement in other modes of death? (2) Does the bereavement differ in kind and in intensity depending on the kinship of the survivors to the suicide? (3) Do the survivor programs work and if so, how?

COMPARISON OF SUICIDE VERSUS NONSUICIDE BEREAVEMENT

The first question refers to an oft-reported clinical observation about survivors of suicide that the impact of a death by suicide upon survivors has special qualities and a unique impact by its very nature, that is, a volitional termination of self that makes it different from all other types of death. The question is whether or not there are valid and unique differences from other modes of death in such aspects as kind and intensity of feelings (grief, depression, anger, anxiety, abandonment, guilt, and others); physical reactions (illness, health, stress); cognitive functioning (confusion, control, concentration, attention); behavioral actions (apathy, agitation, tension); and social reactions (isolation, withdrawal, life-style change, blame of and by others). If so, are these differences affected by developmental age as well as other demographic factors such as sex, religion, and culture?

One of the strongest convictions encountered both in the general public and among professional colleagues has been that bereavement in a suicidal death is more difficult and more emotionally disruptive than bereavement of any other kind of death. It is even more interesting that this conviction has continued despite the early study by Demi (1978) that found no differences between groups of suicide, accident, and natural death survivors in depression, anxiety, or overall symptom distress, and also none in the trajectory of grief. In more recent years, several studies have appeared that confirm Demi's early results. Williams (1985, 1986) compared 44 survivors, 6 of accidental death, 17 of sudden natural death, and 21 of suicide death by telephone interview after the deaths of their family members in an emergency hospital. Time after death was short, with three interviews, the first at 1 week and the second and third at 1 month and 2 months. No significant differences were found in any of the emotional or behavioral categories measured, such as sleeping pill use, health, medication use, daily activity levels, and others. The brief reports in the Proceedings, however, do not provide further important details, such as the relationship of the survivors to the deceased, sex, ages, and other demographic aspects.

Two well-designed studies by McIntosh and his colleagues compared survivors' reactions in suicide with other kinds of deaths. In the first, McIntosh and Milne (1986) used college students to obtain data by questionnaire and standardized scales on grief (Texas Revised Inventory of Grief), feelings (Suicide Acceptability Scale), and attitudes (Aftermath of Suicide) in the bereavement of survivors of death by suicide (N = 21), natural deaths (N = 21), and accidents (N = 12) (28 males, 51 females, mourning the deaths of 40 males and 20 females). The second study (McIntosh & Kelley, 1988) used a much larger number of college students (N = 230, of which 71 were male, 159 female) and 77 survivors of natural deaths, 92 survivors of accidental deaths, and 61 survivors of suicides. The time elapsed since death was a mean 5.39 years. The data collection instruments, in addition to those used in the 1986 study, included a suicidal behaviors questionnaire, the Impact of Event Scale, and the Revised UCLA Loneliness Scale.

In both studies, the results consistently indicated more similarities between the groups than differences. Similarities, for example, were found in such factors as perception of grief, an attitude of acceptability of suicide as a means of dealing with life's problems, and perceptions by others of families who had experienced a suicide of a member. Also, no differences were found in the early perception of guilt, shock, disbelief, embarrassment, isolation, desire to understand, the degree to which the death was put out of mind, feeling stigmatized, or the degree of upset at the anniversary of the death. All of these had been identified previously as reactions either specific to or heightened in suicide survivors. All subjects rated grief after a suicide death as most difficult, then grief after accident deaths, followed by grief from natural deaths. Both suicide and accident survivors, more often than the natural death survivors, felt less resigned, less relieved, more stigma, greater shock, and the need to understand "why." Suicide survivors did report more encounters with blaming of others, more regret for not having done more, and experiencing a greater number of stigma feelings. It was found, surprisingly, that the survivors of accidental death reported more reactions at anniversaries, more difficulties with present feelings about death, and more numbness and embarrassment after the death. In particular, the authors felt their studies refuted the declarations of Calhoun, Selby, and Abernathy (1984) that suicide survivors were characterized mainly by a need to search for explanations of the death, that suicide survivors met with less social support than survivors of other kinds of deaths, and that suicides experienced more intense feelings of guilt.

Three additional studies investigated the impact of suicide on the family survivors of the suicide deaths of spouses compared with those of other modes. In the first, McNeil, Hatcher, and Reuben (1988) compared the family functioning of 13 widows of suicide deaths with that of 13 widows of accident deaths obtained through the coroner's office several years after the deaths of their husbands. They used a lengthy structured clinical interview and standardized measures of family functioning (Family Environment Scale, Family Apgar, Life Event Questionnaire, and General Health Questionnaire). They found no differences between the groups on any of their standardized measures of family functioning. However, both groups did show a discernible level of psychiatric symptomatology. The clinical interview data suggested that the suicide survivor families experienced less intimacy, more blame by others and more feelings of guilt than the accident survivor families. The authors concluded that while there may be some increased risk of difficulty in bereavement faced by suicide survivors, there was no support for the commonly held perception of greater pathogenic impact of suicide on family functioning than from accidental deaths.

Farberow, Gallagher, Gilewski, and Thompson (1987 and ongoing) reported similar results when comparing the bereavement of spouses of elderly suicides with spouses of elderly natural deaths, and with married spouses who experienced no deaths of a spouse in the previous 5 years. Using a structured clinical interview and standardized clinical instruments (Texas Revised Inventory of Grief [TRIG], Beck Depression Inventory [BDI], Behavior Symptom Index [BSI], and 16 Personality Factors [PF]) and self-rating of mental health, spouses were interviewed four times over a period of 2 years following death, within 2 months, and at 6, 12, and 24 months. No differences between levels of grief, depression, psychiatric symptomatology, and self-rated levels of mental health appeared between the two bereaved groups at any of the time intervals. Grief, depression, and general symptomatology declined from a moderate or high level to a low level, and self-rated mental health improved over the 2 years. However, the course of decline and improvement were not the same for the suicides and the natural death bereaved subjects. Among the suicide survivors, grief and general symptomatology showed a major decline only after the 1st year, while the natural death survivors reported their grief lessened considerably in the first 6 months and then again markedly in the 2nd year. Also, among the natural death survivors, general psychological distress dropped most discernibly in the first 6 months, with relatively little decline after. Both groups showed somewhat the same course of consistent drop for depression as measured by the BDI, but not for depression as measured by the depression scale of the BSI. The latter scale indicated that depression continued high for the suicide bereaved group for the 1st year, after which the level dropped, whereas the ratings for the natural death survivors dropped mainly within the 2- to 6-month period. The BSI depression scale contains items denoting more severe aspects of depression than the Beck Scale. Self-ratings of mental health of the natural death survivors improved regularly at each period, until by the end of the 2 years there was no longer a significant difference between them and the no-death controls' ratings. Suicide survivors, however, improved in steps, with some gain in the first 6 months, then again at the end of 2 years. At that point, they still were significantly different from the normal controls, although not from the natural death survivors. The results indicated the importance of the length of time period after death when data are collected and of measures used in evaluating the results. At least for elderly survivors, whether by suicide or natural death, comparisons between the two groups will show fluctuations in the relative levels of some of the feelings and symptoms being measured that directly result from the two factors identified above.

Barrett and Scott (1987) came to a similar conclusion that the complications occurring in the bereavement course after suicide were reflections of the influence of factors other than the suicide mode itself. The researchers controlled especially for the impact of sudden death among their subjects by comparing the effects on the survivors of spouse deaths by suicide, with those by accident, anticipated natural, and unanticipated natural deaths. Data were obtained by interview from a nonclinical population. While the suicide survivors experienced more feelings of "unique" grief and rejection than all the other groups of bereaved, there were no differences in total grief, and the course of recovery was the same for all groups. Reactions to accidental deaths were most similar to suicide death reactions, while the two natural death survivor groups tended to have the more similar reactions. However, the course and quality of grief recovery was generally the same for all survivors. The authors felt that previous conclusions had been distorted by the lack of control groups; age disparities in the survivors; differences in type, quality, and duration of the lost relationships; and differences in the psychological, economic, and occupational status of the survivors.

The studies quoted above indicate the extent to which further research is needed. Comparisons of bereavement in suicide with other modes of death have shown that for the most part the widely held idea of special aspects of bereavement in suicide is not true. The qualities and characteristics of the identified similarities and differences need further intensive examination. The determination of these factors might influence considerably the response to and the treatment of survivors. There are aspects specific to suicide that remain, such as more intense feelings of rejection, and elements of stigma and shame, but there is much yet that needs to be explored in developmental age, in demographic aspects such as sex and cultural differences, and in bereavement course.

SURVIVOR REACTIONS IN KINSHIP AND CAREGIVER RELATIONSHIPS

Another widely held conviction about survivors of suicides is that there are differences in the levels of difficulties in the bereavement that are the result of the kinship of the survivors. The experience of a parent of the loss of a child by suicide has most often been considered to be the most painful, with questions of why and feelings of guilt plaguing the survivors with greater intensity than the loss of a parent, spouse, or sibling. However, several extensive researches have thrown this assumption into question and have indicated the need for continued study of this question. The following section examines the research on impact of a suicide death on different kin among the family, and looks as well at the impact of suicide on caregiver personnel and institutions.

McIntosh and Wrobleski (1988) investigated the effects of kinship in a study of 141 survivors of suicide who had attended grief counseling by subdividing them into four groups, survivors who had experienced the suicide of a child (N = 56), of a sibling (N = 37), of a spouse (N = 23), and of a parent (N = 24). In addition, the survivors of a child suicide were divided according to the age of the child, young—below 25 years of age (N = 30), and older—above 25 years of age (N = 26). Ages of the respondents ranged from 9 years to 75 years (mean = 40) and of the suicides from 16 years to 77 years (mean = 33). The time since death varied between 1 month and 500 months (mean = 40.4). With questionnaires using graded or quantified responses, the researchers found that, contrary to expectations, it was the survivors of spouse and sibling suicides who reported more problems and difficulties than the parent survivors of a child suicide. Parents reported less anger and less stigma than spouse or sibling survivors, had fewer total symptoms than all the others, worried less about their own suicide, had fewer panic attacks, experienced more forgetting that their loved one was dead, and gave fewer reports of having "seen" their deceased family member after the death. The parents did feel they encountered avoidance in talking about the death more often than the other kinds of suicide survivors. However, siblings and spouses also reported feeling people avoided talking about the death and acted as if the death had not occurred. Practically all respondents felt guilt (72% moderate to high), and nearly all felt the guilt had lessened. Anger was reported more often by the younger survivors. In general, the investigators concluded there were relatively few differences between the kinship groups in terms of the kinds and intensity of feelings reported.

When the parent-survivors were divided into those whose child died when younger than 25 versus those older than 25, the differences continued to be few. For example, no differences were found between the two groups in reports of guilt or problems with the death scene, but parents of older child suicides did indicate less anger than siblings, spouses, and child survivors. In general, the parent survivors had surprisingly fewer personal symptoms than survivors of sibling or spouse suicides, and the parents of adult suicides had significantly fewer personal symptoms than the children of parent suicides. The authors concluded that the results refuted the commonly held belief that parents of young suicides experienced the most difficult bereavement course. According to their study it was the siblings, not the parents, who reported most difficulties. The authors noted the limitations to their results in terms of subject selection (only people who had contacted a suicide survivor group), validity of instruments (questionnaires only), possible longitudinal differences (wide variation in length of time after death), and the need to compare their results with kinship factors in other modes such as accident and natural.

Solomon, Knudson, Clark, and Rubey (1987) studied 19 adolescents, aged 13 to 19, who had experienced the suicide of an older sibling to determine how the young people had reacted to the suicides and how they recovered from the loss. Of the 13 females and 6 males, 2 had lost an older sister, 17 had lost an older brother. Dividing the subjects on the basis of "making progress" (N = 10) and "unresolved" (N = 9), the researchers found no significant association between styles of communication in the families, free talking, selective talking, little or no exchange. They found a positive outcome for those who thought more about the death than for those who blocked it out. The siblings in families with little or selective communication reported they talked more to their friends. There seemed to be no significant association between anticipation and outcome, with recently bereaved adolescents reporting progress as frequently as long-term bereaved. One surprising result was the absence of any association between outcome and time after death, despite the fact that times ranged from as little as 6 months to as much as 5 years (mean = 23 months). There was no association between outcome and thinking more or less about death in general, or with more or less certainty in beliefs about afterlife. The authors felt that more longitudinal research was needed to identify the mediators and moderators of suicidal bereavement among adolescents. Also needed were comparison groups to see if the bereavement of siblings of a suicidal death was unique or different from the bereavement of sibling survivors of other forms of death. The results of this study along with the evidence from the McIntosh and Wrobleski study (1988) indicate that sibling survivors of suicide and of other deaths in general need much more attention and intensive well-designed research especially by comparison with sibling survivors of other modes of death.

The importance of the instruments used for data collection is emphasized by the differences in results reported above and those of van der Wal and Diekstra (1987) of survivors in Holland. The latter obtained a measure of the grief in bereavement (mean time after death, 3.5 months) in 91 survivors (46 male, 45 females, mean age, 44 years) of 60 suicides, divided according to their kinship relations (18 parents, 14 spouses, 35 siblings, and 24 children). The authors found that the greatest degree of grief was reported in order of difficulty by parents, then by spouses, siblings, and children. Levels of grief decreased with the age of the deceased, and females generally scored higher than males.

The differences in the levels of grief among survivors in various kinship roles between the report of this study and those reported by McIntosh and Wrobleski (1988) may lie, at least in part, in the instrument used to measure grief. The Leiden Bereavement Scale used by van der Wal and Diekstra focuses on the extent to which the bereaved has been able to separate and detach himself from the deceased, while the TRIG used by McIntosh and Kelly measures grief in terms of the kinds of behaviors engaged in and feelings experienced about the death. The parents in the Holland study were the least able of the groups studied to detach themselves from the child they had lost, especially if the loss was unanticipated. Van der Wal and Diekstra also measured the level of depression in their subjects with the BDI and found that 69% scored within the normal range, and that only 4% indicated severe depression. The researchers also noted their surprise at finding how severe the level of grief of the siblings was reported. Like McIntosh and Wrobleski (1988), van der Wal and Diekstra concluded that the general assumption of pathology and distress in survivors of suicide is not well founded, and that the level of depression in suicide did not differ much from that found in other bereavements. The study included comparison groups of natural and accident death survivors, but these data were not presented in this report.

An important finding of this review is that reactions of parents and spouses have received most attention in studies of reactions to suicide, with children following, and then siblings. Siblings have been labeled the "forgotten mourners" by Morse (1984). It is clear that this group, especially in light of reports of their prolonged and intensive grief, unresolved coping, and more problematic bereavement, needs much more research, both in quality and quantity. It is also apparent from the review that the entire area of kinship and relationship experiences needs extensive quality research. Literature review indicates only one research in the 1980s (Pfeffer, 1981) that focused on children's reactions to suicides of parents, with Pfeffer noting that the denial, distortion, and lack of open discussion that occurred on such occasions could cause psychological problems as well as hinder mourning and the child's development.

Impact on Suicide on Caregivers

Most significant survivor relationships stem from family or marital kinship. However, a special relationship arises between caregivers and their parents or clients. A mixed and often confusing state appears when a suicide of a patient occurs, arousing as it does in therapists and other caregivers both personal and professional reactions. The reactions described by Litman, 1965; Jones, 1987; Kolodny, Binder, Bronstein, and Friend, 1979; Moritz, Brouwer, van Ness, and Abraham, 1985; Bess and White, 1983; Gorkin, 1985; Goldstein and Buogiorno, 1984; and Dunne, 1987 parallel those of kinship survivors. The feelings reported are similar to those experienced by family members, such as grief, guilt, anger (at patient, families, supervisors), depression, rejection, and anxiety, in varying degrees. Mixed in with the above feelings are the professional concerns of responsibility, control, self-esteem, narcissistic injury (Gorkin, 1985), concern for colleagues' opinions, malpractice potentials, feelings of vulnerability, self-doubt, and others. Kolodney et al. (1979) emphasized the need of therapists to mourn, and not to underestimate the time required to do so.

Therapists' Reactions

Most of the studies of therapists' reactions that have appeared in the last decade have been either surveys to determine frequency or descriptions of personal experiences. That the experience is not rare is indicated by the figures quoted in some of the reports, ranging from the early prediction by Kahne (1968) that one of every four psychiatrists will experience a suicide in his practice, through estimates of as many as 16% in a residency program by Binder (1978) and 22% (of 99 psychotherapists) by Moritz et al. (1975); 38% (of 400 U.S. psychotherapists) by Lapp (1986); 43% (in a psychiatric clinic) by Holden (1978); and 51% (among 259 psychotherapists) by Chemtob, Hamada, Bauer, Kinney, and Torique (1988).

Henn (1978) interviewed 32 psychiatric residents who had been identified as having had professional contact with a patient who had committed suicide within the 12 months prior to their death. On the basis of the data, the author concluded that six such instances would occur for every 3-year residency completed. Henn decided that the suicide of a patient was a common, if not universal, part of the psychiatric residency. He urged a "morbidity and mortality" conference to be held with colleagues that would provide a productive sharing of the experience.

It is possible that the one of two estimates by Chemtob et al. (1988) is most nearly correct, based as it is on a well-done, carefully designed, extensive survey with good methodology. The study started out with a large, representative national sample of 643 names of psychiatrists and gathered information by means of a questionnaire and Impact of Event Scale, filled out twice, once for 2 weeks after the suicide and again for current feelings. Their study sample consisted of 259 respondents, 85% males, with a mean age of 51 and a mean number of years in practice of 19 years. The most notable findings were that there was no relationship between years of practice and occurrence of suicide, and that more postgraduate training was associated with fewer suicides in their practices. Age played a role in reactions, with the older therapists experiencing lower levels of guilt and social withdrawal, less loss of self-esteem, and less disruption of relationship with friends. A "striking" finding was that those therapists who experienced a suicide reported their lives felt disrupted to a considerable degree and that they experienced post-traumatic symptoms similar to those found in clinical groups seeking therapy.

Goldstein and Buongiorno (1984) surveyed 20 therapists who had experienced the loss of a patient by suicide (obtained mostly through personal knowledge and some advertising). They found the usual reactions of shock, disbelief, anger, guilt, self-blame, and loneliness. Only one therapist discontinued further work with suicidal patients and no one sought psychotherapy to help "work through" their problems. All stated they found talking to colleagues and friends most helpful. The authors felt that the therapists needed time to grieve their loss and to accept and acknowledge their feelings without a sense of additional blame. Although most of the interviewees denied the suicide had substantially affected them, the authors felt they were more distressed than they admitted.

All the researchers suggested ways in which help could be provided, such as consultation, formal reviews, support through networking, individual or group meetings, and others, but none of these has been examined systematically in terms of procedures, situations, and conditions. Differences, if any, as a result of length of time of treatment, the kind of treatment used, the closeness of the relationship between the therapist and the patient need to be evaluated. Questions about the most effective form of help need to be addressed. Should professional consultations be provided individually or in a group? What is the optimal time for a formal review, immediately after or months later? Should the therapist attend the funeral? Should the therapist meet with the family? If so, how soon? and Who should extend treatment to the family, the therapist or an uninvolved colleague?

Survivor Reactions in a Hospital

Hospitals, generally thought of as a secure, safe place for treatment of individuals who no longer can be trusted to control their self-destructive impulses, are severely affected when one of its patients or a member of its staff commits suicide. Research into such situations has been relatively infrequent and one must go back to Kayton and Freed's work in 1967 (patient suicide) and Soreff's study (staff suicide) in 1975 for studies of the impact of suicide on patients and staff. Kayton and Freed obtained the reactions of patients and staff to the suicide of a 51-year-old depressed woman who was known on a number of wards. The data came from nursing notes, charts, discussion meetings with residents and staff and from a questionnaire given to patients, nurses, and nurses aides. Soreff studied the reactions in a hospital when a staff nurse on a psychiatric ward committed suicide. Data were gathered by interviews of patients and staff 4 to 7 weeks after the death. The patients responded by mutual concern, exaggerated fears, distrust of staff, and coming together. They felt abandoned by staff, yet felt a heightened need for them. Staff had a more difficult time resolving their feelings and felt intensely longer than the patients. Staff seemed better at facilitating mourning among the patients than mourning themselves. The feelings described are similar to those named previously—initial shock, numbness, anger at the deceased, denial, guilt, despair, hopelessness, and insecurity. There were complications for the patients who may, depending on their closeness to the patient-suicide, feel either or both a marked identification with the deceased and responsibility for the death. Anger was often directed at the staff for not having prevented the death and for making them feel less secure about the protection against their own impulses. Kayton and Freed found the same reactions within each ward and different reactions between the wards. Apparently the milieu determined the reactions in part.

The same dynamics were described by Sacks and Eth (1981) in their report on the reactions of the other hospital patients to the suicide deaths of two fellow patients within a very short time of each other. For the staff there were the same feelings as those experienced by the patients, but also the "frustrations" of their personal identity as helpers and a "reactive anger toward the deceased for causing the reaction." The suggestions for addressing the feelings again called mostly for various kinds of consultations, support, and networking.

The questions raised earlier for research on suicide of patients of psychotherapists apply here, with the additional element of appraising patient-staff interaction. Should patients and staff meet together for discussion and working through of feelings or should each patient be seen separately? Measurement of the impact on the hospital will need the contributions of sociological and anthropological disciplines incorporated into the research design for comprehensive answers.

Impact on Psychiatric Residents

Much concern has been expressed about the impact of the suicide of a patient on psychiatric residents. In terms of frequency, Kahne (1968) estimated 14% of the residents, Rosen (1974) estimated 16%, while Brown, in a survey in 1987, estimated that at least 33% of psychiatrists experience a suicide during residency. Schnur and Levin (1985) describe the reactions of five psychiatric residents who had experienced the suicide of a patient, by interviewing four within 1 year and one within 2 months of the suicide. In all cases, the first reaction was of shock and disbelief, for none of the patients had been considered actively suicidal. The predominant reaction that followed was of anger, especially at staff and supervisors, but also at the patient, the patients' families, and acquaintances. Feelings also of guilt, sadness, and helplessness were reported. All the residents were uneasy about treating other suicidal patients, and consequently hospitalized their patients more readily, worried more about their own decisions, and tended more toward overcontrolling their patients. Those supervisors were considered most helpful who were most concerned about the residents' emotional turmoil.

The experience is described by Brown (1987a,b) as a very difficult one for residents because of their relative immaturity as professionals, who often had still unresolved ambivalence toward their specialty choice, who were experiencing competitive strains within the group in the fish-bowl atmosphere of a training program, and who had the desire to win approval from the faculty. In addition to the above reactions, there was often a strong need to search for the "fatal mistake," and fantasies of silent accusations from colleagues and teachers (Sacks, Kibel, Cohen, Keats, & Turnquist, 1987). Each suicide affected the entire group of residents and the institution as a whole. Brown (1987a) wondered whether residents were being asked to assume responsibilities with emotional consequences they may not have been prepared to handle. He outlined a five-step program for preparing the resident for a possible suicide of his patient. These included alertness and preparation through anticipation; response to the acute impact by involving all kinds of professional and personal support; resolution of issues of failure and blame; clarification and working through (specifically to avoid inappropriate reactions with other and future suicidal patients); and preparation for reactivation and post-training practice. Evaluation of these procedures, however, has not been systematically carried out, such as using before and after tests to evaluate changes in attitudes and skills by means of self- and other reports, comparison of various training approaches, and others.

These reports also call attention to the fact that many of the survivors group programs currently being conducted by both professional and nonprofessional volunteers (many of whom themselves are survivors of a suicide) may face a heightened risk of suicide among the participants in their groups. The reactions of the caregivers, should a suicide occur, would be expected to range through all the feelings already described, but would also be heightened by their own previous experience with a suicidal loss. Such a potential event raises concern for the provision of care and the marshalling of a supportive network unless planned for in advance. Garfield and Jenkins (1981–1982) looked at the stress and coping experience among 45 college-educated volunteers (32 females, 13 males, between the ages 24 and 34), at SHANTI, an organization providing counseling for persons dying or seriously ill. Data obtained were from a questionnaire, Moos's Social Climate Scale and Lazarus's Way of Coping Scale. Generally, the workers reported they felt most support from friends who approved of their association with SHANTI and from their contacts with other SHANTI staff. However, they more often turned to themselves or to the client when they themselves felt distressed.

Impact of Suicide of the Therapist on Patients

It is of interest to note that search of the literature for recent research (not just descriptive accounts of this event) on the impact of the suicide of a therapist on his patients yielded none. Dunne's (1987) review of relevant publications lists Chiles (1974), Ables (1974), Soreff (1975), Ballenger (1978), and Graves (1978). Of these, Chiles, Ballenger, and Soreff approached the question with somewhat of a research stance. Chiles followed five of seven patients for a year after the death of their therapists, while Ballenger interviewed five patients about 10 months after the death of their therapists. The major findings that emerged were an unrealistic assumption of responsibility for the suicide, dissatisfaction with and inability to continue with therapy, and challenges to the usefulness of therapy. Soreff interviewed inpatients in a hospital 4 to 7 weeks after the suicide death of a staff nurse and found that the patients reacted by mutual concern, reaching out, exaggerated fears, distrust of staff, and coming together. They felt abandoned and questioned the reliability of the staff, but at the same time there was a heightened need for them. The patients seemed better able to resolve the death than the staff, who still felt intensely a month or more later when interviewed. Dunne points out that for the patient survivors, already functioning at a less than optimal level, there may be severe setbacks in terms of guilt, abandonment, rejection, and grief. If there were any previous tendencies toward suicidal behavior there was a distinct increase of risk for acting out such impulses as a result of the depression, identification, and anger experienced. Dunne feels it is important to "demystify" the events and to discuss openly the anger at the therapist for having "abandoned" the patient as well as to relieve feelings of having contributed to the stress. The new therapist should prevent any efforts to "canonize" the deceased therapist, perhaps by assuring the patient that therapists have crises of their own, not necessarily related to their work and that they are not always able to meet them.

Research in this area is needed especially on procedural questions, such as how to inform the patient-survivors, who should do the informing, who should make the arrangements for transfer to the new therapist, and so on. Research is also needed on the further clinical development of those patients, short term and longitudinally, with a possible focus on how many patients were able to continue in therapy, how many were not, and how did the death affect progress in therapy?

DOES THE PROGRAM WORK?

Enthusiasm is an inadequate criterion for the determination of the efficacy of survivors groups. As Schuyler (1975) pointed out in an early article, there are a number of psychotherapeutic issues that arise in dealing with suicide survivors. The survivor is searching for an understanding of the act that preserves his own self-worth and provides some answer to the search for meaning; the survivor needs to be able to express his feelings in a nonrejecting atmosphere; the survivor needs to complete the mourning process, which involves life without the deceased, and coming to terms with the suicidal nature of the death; the survivor needs to be monitored for possible suicidal feelings; and the survivor needs to overcome any feelings of shame or stigma that may be attached.

Both professional and public interest and involvement in bereavement groups is evident in the number of programs reported in the past 8 years. However, the number objectively evaluated for efficacy is distressingly small, and many questions continue to press for an answer. Heilig's survey of survivor groups reported in the 1985 annual AAS meeting in Toronto (41 questionnaires returned from 70 programs contacted) indicated a wide variety of formats used in terms of leadership, 65% with some professional training, 25% with none; community affiliation, 80%; co-leaders, 76%; variable frequencies for time-limited versus unlimited number of meetings (only 7 had a set number), and open-ended versus closed membership. Discussion was mostly around the pros and cons of mental health professional participation, a question still raised. The major problems identified were lack of community support and leader burnout.

Two comprehensive reports of program evaluation have appeared, the first by Rogers, Sheldon, Barwick, Letofsky, and Lancee (1982), and the second by Battle (1984). Rogers et al. described their Toronto program, which met with survivors within 2 years of the suicide, used trained volunteers to lead groups, some of them survivors, some not, and used a time-limited format of 8 weekly meetings, 2 hours in length, with a specific focus for discussion in each. Four additional subsequent biweekly meetings were available. All volunteers were given eight training sessions focusing on understanding participant needs, communications, sharing bereavement experiences, resources, and supervision. Pre- and post-course data were gathered with a questionnaire and a standardized symptom scale (SCL-90). Follow-up was 4 to 6 weeks after the termination of the last meeting. Responses from 33 survivors indicated they felt they got perspective on suicide (97%); found a safe place to express their feelings (71%); and could talk about the suicide (70%). The program was generally perceived as helpful and the symptom scale was much lower at follow-up. Important points made were that the use of volunteers was actually expensive in terms of cost of supervision and training, the mix of survivors with nonsurvivors in the volunteers worked well, and the participants preferred the structured sessions.

The group format described by Battle (1984) was different from the Rogers et al. (1982) procedure in that the clients entered the group an average of 2 months after the suicide and the group was open-ended. Among the 36 survivors who were subjects in the study (78% female), most left after 12 sessions. Most survivors, 61%, felt they were helped, 27% did not feel the group could help them further, and 12% reported no help. Before and after questionnaires compared the group with 13 survivors who did not attend a group and with 31 nonbereaved who were in psychotherapy. The usual differences between bereaved and nonbereaved were found in terms of significantly more feelings of guilt, self-blame, and intensity of feelings reported by the survivors. Significantly, 50% of the survivors reported having felt so miserable that they had suicidal feelings themselves while none were reported by the nonsurvivor group.

Farberow (in press) evaluated the Survivors after Suicide program conducted at the Los Angeles Suicide Prevention Center by comparing 60 clients, 70% female, who completed the 8-week closed-end, once-a-week sessions and who completed pre- and post-course questionnaires, with 22 controls, of which 17 were females. The latter had applied for admission to a group but did attend. They also completed pre- and post-questionnaires within the same 2- and 3-month interval as the participants. All groups were led by the professional and a survivor-facilitator who had completed the 8-week sessions and had undergone a period of training and supervision. Sessions were semi-structured with reading material and suggested discussion topics distributed at each meeting. Age and sex differences were not significant, with most, approximately 77%, of both groups in the young adult and mid years. Kinship of losses were 35% siblings, 23% children, and 20% parents for the participants; and 27% parents, 27% spouse, and 18% for both children and siblings for the controls. Time lapse between the death and the application for admission was within the first 6 to 8 months for 77% of both participants and controls. For both groups, change of residence was indicated as the most common major change in their lives since the death, about 18% for the participants and 32% for the controls.

Comparisons of self-ratings of specific feelings were obtained from both groups at 3 points in time, Time 1 (retrospectively) just after death; Time 2 at point of application for the group, and Time 3 at 2 to 3 months later, that is, when the participants had completed the sessions and when a similar amount of time had passed for the controls. Feelings rated were depression, grief, anxiety, shame or stigma, guilt, anger at self or others, anger at the decedent, puzzlement, and suicidal feelings. No significant differences among any of the feelings appeared between the participants and the controls in the self-rated level of feelings at Time 1, just after the death. At Time 2, just before the groups started, the participants rated themselves significantly higher in grief, shame and guilt than did the controls. At Time 3, after the sessions were completed, each of these feelings had diminished for the participants to the degree that there were no longer any significant differences between them and the controls. However, at Time 3, significant differences appeared in the ratings of two other feelings, depression and puzzlement, with the high ratings among the participants dropping to a moderate level, and the moderate ratings among the controls dropping to the low level.

To note the impact of the group experience itself on the feelings, the changes in the ratings of the feelings for each group between Time 2 and Time 3 were determined. For the participants significant changes occurred for all the feelings except one (suicidal feelings), with the changes indicating a significant diminution of the intensity of each of the feelings. Apparently the level of suicidal feelings among both groups had diminished to such a degree between Time 1 and Time 2 that the little further decrease that occurred between Time 2 and Time 3 did not reach a significance level. Among the controls, however, no significant differences appeared between the ratings at Time 2 and Time 3 for any of the feelings except for anxiety, which saw a decrease of some of the high ratings to moderate and low. The participants indicated that what they had most often gained from the group was the opportunity to share in an atmosphere of acceptance and understanding.

One of the most important needs supplied by participation in survivors groups is that of support. Most people usually have a variety of sources of support available to them in times of great stress but many of these supports seem to be lost when a suicide occurs. An elaborate schema conceptualizing the elements in the social support was constructed by Mitchell (1969) and seems to offer many opportunities for research into the role of this factor in bereavement. Walker, MacBride, and Vachon (1977), for example, found Mitchell's characterization highly relevant for identifying an individual's support structure in bereavement. The basic elements in social support were identified as size, or the number of people with whom there is contact; strength of ties, including emotional intensity and intimacy; density, or the extent to which the individual's network knows and has contact with each other independently; homogeneity of membership, the degree to which members share social attributes and attitudes, such as demographics aspects, social class, and life-styles; and dispersion of membership, or the ease with which network members can make face to face contact. These characteristics interact and affect each other, resulting in varied networks that are differentially supportive for different types of crises and at different times within a crisis. In the course of their bereavement, survivors need to maintain a social identity, emotional support, and to obtain material aid, services, information, and new social contacts. Social identities are more easily maintained when the network is small in size, but correspondingly strong in ties, with a high density, cultural homogeneity, and low dispersion. Density and homogeneity increase the likelihood of material aid and services. The need for information, on the other hand, may be most readily met by a network with somewhat weak ties so that new social contacts can occur and can provide new information to meet the requirement of new activities and changed roles.

In the bereavement process the needs change as the phases of bereavement change. First, there is the strong need for empathy and emotional support that gives permission to expression of deep feelings. When the role of widow is clear, a dense, homogeneous network is most useful. Later, the survivor needs assistance in returning to a normal social life, sometimes involving a radical reorganization of social roles. At this point, new social contacts and more information is needed. A close-knit network can actually, in theory, become a disadvantage in limiting access to new information and new contacts.

The characteristics outlined above may provide a theoretical basis for many of the questions raised for research and evaluation of survivor groups. The question whether groups should be homogeneous in terms of age, type of kinship loss, sex, and socioeconomic status may be examined with new insights when these variables are arranged or modified to emphasize the most desirable network factor. The interaction of these factors with optimal time after death for entry into the group, the most effective leadership, time-limited versus unlimited, open-ended versus closed, and so on might be more profitably explored. The possibility of different types of groups being formed for different information needs at different phases of bereavement holds intriguing possibilities.

Much research in evaluating the usefulness of the bereavement group programs needs to be done; questions remain. Who profits from the group? who does not? Do the young? Do the elderly? Does the developmental age of both survivor and suicide make a difference? Does the type of loss make a difference? Are homogeneous groups more effective than heterogeneous in terms of age, kinship loss, sex, and socioeconomic status? What is the optimal time to enter group? What is the most effective leadership arrangement? How do results using time-limited groups compare with no time-limit? Open-ended compared with closed groups? Structured versus nonstructured in content? What are the most valid criteria for evaluation of recovery? Are we on the right track?

REFERENCES

Ables, B. S. (1974). The loss of a therapist through suicide. *Journal of the American Academy of Child Psychiatry, 13*, 143–152.

Ballenger, J. C. (1978). Patients' reactions to the suicide of their psychiatrist. *Journal of Nervous and Mental Disease, 166*, 859–867.

Battle, A. O. (1984). Group therapy for survivors of suicide. *Crisis, 5*(1), 48–58.

Barrett, T. W., & Scott, T. B. (1987). Suicide versus other bereavement recovery patterns. In R. Yufit (Ed.), *Proceedings of the 20th Annual Meeting of the American Association of Suicidology*, San Francisco, CA.

Bess, D., & White, S. B. (1983). Care for the caregivers. In C. F. Vorkoper & K. Smith (Eds.), *Proceedings of the 16th Annual Meeting of the American Association of Suicidology*, Dallas, TX.

Binder, R. (1978). Dealing with patients (Letter). *American Journal of Psychiatry, 135*, 1113.

Brown, H. N. (1987a). Patient suicide during residency training (1): Incidence, implications and program response. *Journal of Psychiatric Education, 11*(4), 201–216.

Brown, H. N. (1987b). The impact of suicide on therapists in training. *Comprehensive Psychiatry, 28*(2), 101–112.

Cain, A., & Fast, I. (1966). Legacy of suicide. *Psychiatry, 29*, 406–411.

Calhoun, L. G., Selby, G. W., & Abernathy, C. B. (1984). Suicide death: Social reactions to bereaved survivors. *Journal of Psychology, 16*, 255–261.

Chemtob, C. M., Hamada, R. S., Bauer, G., Kinney, B., & Torigue, R. Y. (1988). Patients' suicides: Frequency and impact on psychiatrists. *American Journal of Psychiatry, 145*(2), 224–228.

Chiles, J. A. (1974). Patient reactions to the suicide of a therapist. *American Journal of Psychotherapy, 28*, 115–121.

Demi, A. S. (1978). Adjustment of widows after a sudden death: Suicide and non-suicide survivors compared. University of California Library, San Francisco Medical Center, San Francisco, CA.

Doyle, P. (1978). Grief counseling for the survivors of suicide. In H. Z. Winnick & L. Miller (Eds.), *Proceedings of the 8th International Congress on Suicide Prevention* (pp. 155–164). Jerusalem: Jerusalem Academic Press.

Dunne, E. J. (1987). Surviving the suicide of a therapist. In E. J. Dunne, J. McIntosh, & K. Dunne-Maxim (Eds.), *Suicide and its aftermath: Understanding and counseling the survivors*. New York: W. W. Norton.

Farberow, N. L., Gallagher, D. D., Gilewski, M. J., & Thompson, L. W. (1987). An examination of the early impact of bereavement on psychological distress in survivors of suicide. *Gerontologist, 27*, 592–598.

Farberow, N. L., Gallagher, D. D., Gilewski, M. J., & Thompson, L. W. (in press). Course of psychological factors in bereavement of elderly suicide survivors. *Psychiatrica Fennic*.

Farberow, N. L. (in press). Survivors after suicide: A group bereavement program. *Crisis*.

Garfield, C. A., & Jenkins, G. J. (1981–1982). Stress and coping of volunteers counseling the dying and bereaved. *Omega, 12*(1), 1–13.

Glick, I. O., Weiss, R. S., & Parkes, C. M. (1974). *The first years of bereavement*. New York: Wiley.

Goldstein, L., & Buongiorno, P. (1984). Psychotherapists as suicide survivors. *American Journal of Psychotherapy, 33*(3), 392–398.

Gorkin, M. (1985). On the suicide of one's patient. *Bulletin of the Menninger Clinic, 49*(1), 1–9.

Graves, J. S. (1978). Adolescents and their psychiatrist's suicide. *Journal of the American Academy of Child Psychiatry, 17*, 521–532.

Heilig, S. M. (1985). Survey of 41 suicide groups. In R. Cohen-Sandler (Ed.), *Eighteenth Annual Meeting of the American Association of Suicidology* (pp. 110–113). Toronto, Canada.

Henn, R. F. (1978). Patient suicide as part of psychiatric residency. *American Journal of Psychiatry, 135*(6), 745.

Holden, L. D. (1978). Therapist response to patient suicide: Professional and personal. *Journal of Continuing Education In Psychiatry*, *39*, 23–32.

Jones, F. A. (1987). Therapists as survivors of client suicide. In E. J. Dunne, J. McIntosh, & K. Dunne-Maxim (Eds.), *Suicide and its aftermath: Understanding and counseling the survivors*. New York: W. W. Norton.

Kahne, M. J. (1968). Suicide among patients in mental hospitals: A study of psychiatrists who conducted their psychotherapy. *Psychiatry*, *31*: 32–43.

Kayton, L., & Freed, H. (1967). Effects of a suicide in a psychiatric hospital. *Archives of General Psychiatry*, *17*, 187–194.

Kolodny, S., Binder, R. L., Bronstein, A. A., & Friend, R. L. (1979). The working through of patients' suicides by four therapists. *Suicide and Life-Threatening Behavior*, *9*(1), 33–46.

Lapp, G. E. (1986). Therapists' response to client suicide (Doctoral dissertation, California School of Professional Psychology, Berkeley). *Dissertation Abstracts International*, *47*, 2622B.

Litman, R. E. (1965). When patients commit suicide. *American Journal of Psychiatry*, *19*, 570–576.

McIntosh, J. L. (1987). Research therapy and educational needs. In E. J. Dunne, J. McIntosh, & K. Dunne-Maxim (Eds.), *Suicide and its aftermath: Understanding and counseling the survivors*. New York: W. W. Norton.

McIntosh, J. L., & Kelley, L. D. (1988). Survivors reactions: Suicide versus other causes. In D. Lester (Ed.), *Proceedings of the 21st Annual Meeting of the American Association of Suicidology* (pp. 89–90). Washington, DC.

McIntosh, J. L., & Milne, K. L. (1986). Survivors reactions: Suicide versus other causes. In R. Cohen-Sandler (Ed.), *Proceedings of the 19th Annual Meeting of the American Association of Suicidology* (pp. 136–138). Atlanta, GA.

McIntosh, J. L., & Wrobleski, A. (1988). Grief reactions among suicide survivors: An exploratory comparison of relationships. *Death Studies*, *12*, 21–39.

McNeil, D. E., Hatcher, C., & Reuben, R. (1988). Family survivors of suicide and accidental death: Consequences for widows. *Suicide and Life-Threatening Behavior*, *18*(2), 137–148.

Mitchell, J. C. (1969). The concept and use of social networks. In J. C. Mitchell (Ed.), *Social networks in urban situations*. Manchester, England: Manchester University Press.

Moritz, B. J. M., Brouwer, W. A., van Ness, J. O., & Abraham, R. E. (1985). Psychotherapists as survivors of suicide. *Thirteenth Annual Congress of the International Association for Suicide Prevention* (pp. 515–518). Vienna, Austria.

Morse, S. R. (1984). Survivors of suicide: The siblings tell their story. *Dissertation Abstracts International*, *45*, 1025B.

Pfeffer, C. R. (1981). Parental suicide: An organizing event in the development of latency age children. *Suicide and Life-Threatening Behavior*, *11*, 43–50.

Rogers, J., Sheldon, A., Barwick, C., Letofsky, K., & Lancee, W. (1982). Help for families of suicide: Survivors support program. *Canadian Journal of Psychiatry*, *27*, 444–449.

Rosen, D. H. (1974). *Mental stresses in residency training and opportunities for prevention*. Paper presented at 12th Annual Meeting of the American Psychiatric Association, Detroit, MI.

Sacks, M., & Eth, S. (1981). Pathological identification as a cause of suicide on an inpatient unit. *Hospital and Community Psychiatry*, *32*(1), 36–40.

Sacks, M. H., Kibel, H. D., Cohen, A. M., Keats, M., & Turnquist, N. (1987). Resident response to patient suicide. *Journal of Psychiatric Education*, *11*(4), 217–226.

Schnur, D. B., and Levin, E. H. (1985). The impact of successfully completed suicides on psychiatric residents. *Journal of Psychiatric Education*, *9*, 127–136.

Schuyler, D. (1975). Counseling suicide survivors: Issues and answers. *Omega*, *4*(4), 313–321.

Shepherd, D. M., & Barraclough, B. M. (1976). The aftermath of parental suicide for children. *British Journal of Psychiatry*, *129*, 267–276.

Sheskin, A., & Wallace, S. E. (1976). Differing bereavements: Suicide, natural and accidental death. *Omega*, *7*(3), 229–242.

Solomon, M. L., Knudson, G., Clark, D. C., & Rubey, C. (1987). A study of sibling survivors of suicide. In R. Yufit (Ed.), *Twentieth Annual Meeting of the American Association of Suicidology* (pp. 209– 211). San Francisco, California.

Soreff, S. M. (1975). The impact of staff suicide on a psychiatric inpatient unit. *Journal of Nervous and Mental Disease*, *161*(2), 130–133.

Van der Wal, J., & Diekstra, R. F. W. (1987). Grief reactions of survivors of suicide: Results of a sample survey. In R. Yufit (Ed.), *Twentieth Annual Conference of the American Association of Suicidology*, San Francisco, CA.

Walker, K. N., MacBride, A., & Vachon, M. L. S. (1977). Social support networks and the crisis of bereavement. *Social Sciences and Medicine*, *11*, 35–41.

Wallace, S. (1973). *After suicide*. New York: Wiley.

Williams, M. (1985). Use of a concluding process for suicide survivors. In R. Cohen-Sandler (Ed.), *Proceedings of the 18th Annual Meeting of the American Association of Suicidology*, Toronto, Canada.

Williams, M. (1986). Comparing responses of sudden death survivors. In R. Cohen-Sandler (Ed.), *Proceedings of the 19th Annual Meeting of the American Association of Suicidology* (pp. 139–141). Atlanta, GA.

VI

Preventing Suicide

As shown in this volume, it is an unarguable advantage to come to the topic of suicide informed by a developmental perspective. This understanding has direct implications and applications for prevention. Part VI consists of two parts: a discussion of prevention in the young and a similar presentation on prevention in adults.

18

Developmental Perspective on Prevention and Treatment of Suicidal Youth

Pamela Cantor

Each year 5,200 adolescents commit suicide in the United States and 500,000 attempt suicide. This is a national health problem that is selectively affecting our youth.

Over the past 20 years, the mortality rate of every age group in the United States has improved, except for the group aged 15 to 24 (see Chapters 5 and 6, this volume).

The two types of death that are largely responsible for this increase are suicide and homicide. Both of these have doubled in the past 20 years and both reflect social factors more than any other cause of death.

What can be done to reduce these alarming statistics? How do we *treat* the problem of suicide?

SOCIETY'S RESPONSIBILITY: THE BROAD VIEW

The issue of treatment can be viewed on two different levels. There is the broad social view and more narrow, traditional individual perspective. In the larger

PAMELA CANTOR • Department of Psychiatry, The Cambridge Hospital, Harvard Medical School, Cambridge, Massachusetts 02138.

social view, treatment might be interpreted as an epidemiological approach. This approach would encompass two major aspects: education and environmental risk reduction.

Education means programs in positive mental health, for students, teachers, and parents. Children as young as kindergarten age could be taught to identify emotions such as sadness, joy, and rage, and learn how to enjoy or modulate these feelings. Youngsters in junior high might talk about self-confidence and how to be a friend. High school students could learn how to reduce stress and deal with peer pressure.

To make the point that education is a form of prevention and treatment—a treatment that can save lives—here is an example.

Bruce was a high school student in Massachusetts. He came into school one morning and went to the nurse's office to call a crisis intervention center. He called because he was feeling suicidal. He spoke for a half an hour and then hung up because school was starting. He walked to his classroom, gathering students along the way saying "Follow me, you don't want to miss the most sensational act of the century. You don't want to miss this!" He walked into his classroom, opened his desk, took out a gun, and shot himself. Half the kids stayed to watch, half ran. After a few agonizing days in the intensive care unit, Bruce died. You can imagine the repercussions.

If anyone had known that missing school a lot and missing work, or coming into school with bruises on his neck from previous attempts at hanging himself, or that not handing in homework and telling his teacher not to worry about it because he wouldn't be around anymore, or giving away his favorite records and tapes, or writing about suicide, or calling a hot line, were clues to suicide, his death might have been avoided. If anyone, the nurse, the students, the teacher, had been aware of the warning signs and knew how to intervene, Bruce would be alive today (see Chapter 8, this volume).

Educational intervention is difficult to evaluate because of the absence of data. However, over a period of years, education would appear to have a great potential for decreasing self-inflicted mortality. I will use the analogy of sanitation and its effects of infectious diseases to make the point. More lives have been saved by preventive sanitation than by antibiotics. Based on studies of the effects of public education in the areas of child abuse, discrimination, and drunk driving, self-inflicted mortality for children and adolescents could be reduced by about 20% through public education.

A second aspect of the epidemiological approach to prevention is the limitation of the availability of lethal agents. The increase in suicide among young people can be accounted for almost entirely by firearms. Guns account for more suicides than all other methods combined: 65% of all teenager suicides are committed with firearms. An environmental risk-reduction strategy would call for the decreased availability of handguns. Some 25 million households have handguns and one-half of these keep their handguns loaded. Adolescents are impulsive and having a loaded gun in the house is an invitation to disaster.

I recognize that mandatory safety training on the dangers of guns, or eliminating guns entirely, would not resolve the underlying problem that drives our young people to suicide, yet it could result in fewer deaths. Here, I use the analogy of mandatory seatbelts: Seatbelts do not make people better drivers, but they do improve the chances of surviving a collision.

Studies estimate that 70% of gun victims could not have obtained them if there had been handgun regulations. Fifty percent of these individuals might have used another method. Thus, a reduction in firearm accessibility could save the lives of approximately 20% of our youngsters. Prevention, in this case, means education and the cooperation of police and parents to reduce firearm accessibility.

When highly lethal methods of suicide are less available, there is evidence to show that individuals do not necessarily switch to other means. When the English converted their home heating gas from deadly coke gas to low-lethality natural gas, their suicide rate dropped 33%. This low rate has remained constant despite the bleak economic picture in England, which would ordinarily be expected to lead to an increase in the suicide rate.

Poisoning, usually with prescription medicine, is the second most common method of suicide, and accounts for 11.3% of all suicides. The availability of lethal drugs could be limited by restricting the number of tablets permitted with each prescription. This kind of legislative restriction on sedative and hypnotic drugs is thought to be largely responsible for the decline in the suicide rates in Australia in the 1960s and 1970s. In addition, the tricyclic antidepressants could be sold with an emetic or antidote. If a teenager overdosed and changed his mind, or was found, an antidote could be given and a life could be saved. The projection is that this could save approximately 3% of all teenage suicides per year.

Thus, the prevention strategies that would appear to have the greatest impact on youth suicide are the limitation of the availability of firearms and medications together with education programs in positive mental health.

THE CLINICIAN'S RESPONSIBILITY: THE NARROWER VIEW

In the more traditional view, the treatment of the suicidal young person requires making an appropriate diagnosis and planning beneficial treatment.

In making a diagnosis the clinician might first divide mental illness into two admittedly limited and crude groups: organic brain syndromes and nonorganic syndromes. Unfortunately, many of the problems a clinician treats do not clearly fall into one category or another. Encephalitis is certainly an organic problem. Schizophrenia and manic-depressive illness were long thought to be of nonorganic origins and have only recently been clearly attributed to biochemical dysfunctions.

Depressive personality, obsessive compulsive disorders, or phobias have been—perhaps wrongly—considered nonorganic whereas character disorders, such as borderline or narcissistic disorders or problems in self-esteem, are considered nonorganic. Diagnosis is in a state of flux.

The important point to remember among all this controversy is that suicidal behavior is a *symptom* and not a disease entity; thus, it can appear in any of these diagnostic categories.

THE CHOICE OF TREATMENT

Treatment—the final step in helping a young person cope with the conflicts that generate a suicidal crisis—might take any one of the following forms: supportive psychotherapy, insight-oriented therapy, psychoanalytic psychotherapy, psychoanalysis, brief time-limited psychotherapy, family therapy, or group therapy.

In my opinion, the most appropriate choice for treatment of suicidal adolescents is supportive psychotherapy, followed by insight-oriented psychotherapy or family therapy.

Let's discuss the three forms of therapy. Supportive psychotherapy reinforces the patient's defenses and helps control disturbing thoughts and feelings by such measures as reassurance, suggestion, inspiration, and persuasion. Unlike psychoanalytic therapy, it focuses on present difficulties and avoids probing into the past or the unconscious. It is limited in therapeutic objectives rather than in duration.

It is most effectively used when a youngster is experiencing extreme stress or turmoil (as in most suicidal situations) or when a person with psychotic potential becomes overtly psychotic or goes into acute decomposition with psychotic overtones. Thus, the therapist uses supportive psychotherapy in response to a patient's dealing with a life crisis or regressive episodes.

In diagnostic terms, the therapist can use supportive psychotherapy most effectively with psychotic and borderline adolescents. The therapist can also use this as the initial approach with patients who have neurotic difficulties or character disorders. With fragile youngsters a supportive approach may be all that can be accomplished. Also, it may be the best initial treatment for those with less fragile organization, but who are experiencing extreme stress, which reduces their capacity to cope.

Thus, while a therapist using an insight-oriented approach fosters regression by undermining the patient's resistances and probing the unconscious, the therapist using supportive psychotherapy moves in the opposite direction.

In supportive psychotherapy, the therapist assumes an active role to promote an alliance and minimize regression. He is a constant source of support. He, however, avoids premature reassurance, which the teenager might see as a lack of understanding of the intensity of pain.

The therapist might use medication to relieve anxiety or to decrease depression. He might use hospitalization to control the patient's behavior and ease the strain. Medication and hospitalization can act as a protection between the patient and overwhelming anxiety and allow the family a chance to regroup their emotional resources.

In supportive treatment the therapist is friendly, actively involved, protective, and constant. The therapist tolerates the youngster's needs for dependency and attachment. The quality of the alliance differs, therefore, from psychoanalytic psychotherapy.

Once the goals of supportive psychotherapy are achieved—those of stabilization—the therapist can move to insight-oriented psychotherapy. This is done gradually, all the while testing the patient's capacity to sustain the more insight-oriented approach with techniques closer to those of psychotherapy.

While supportive psychotherapy focuses on the patient's defenses, and psychoanalysis focuses on the relationship between analyst and patient, insight-oriented psychotherapy focuses primarily on the patient's life situation and secondarily on the therapeutic relationship. Psychoanalytic or insight-oriented psychotherapy focuses on the resolution of symptoms and the functioning of the patient. This form of therapy is best suited to those patients with neurotic conflicts and reactive depressions. It is also suitable for some patients with borderline personality disorders, although the management of regressive periods will require some supportive therapy as well.

Family therapy is used when an adolescent's difficulties reflect ongoing difficulties with the family. It is also useful when there is identifiable pathology in other members. Traditionally, clinicians have been taught that the initial diagnostic session with parents should occur *before* seeing the adolescent. Contrary to this teaching, I think that it is advantageous to see the adolescent *first*, perhaps for two or three sessions, before seeing the parents. This increases the chances that the adolescent will see the therapist as his ally and not as an emissary of his parents. I also always invite the adolescent to be present at the initial session with the parents so that there is not a question of a breach of confidentiality.

Generally, the initial diagnostic session with parents should include *both* parents. Too often therapists underestimate the importance of fathers to the psychological disturbances of their adolescents and are dissuaded from requiring their participation. The mother reports over the phone that the father really is not very involved with the children, the father protests about the inconvenience of coming to an appointment, and they both agree that the mother can give all the necessary information about the child. In fact, however, the mother cannot provide all the information, let alone give us a feeling for the father's personality or attitude. By excusing the father from treatment, the therapist may be giving tacit permission for the father's exclusion from family affairs and may be helping to excluding him from the life of the child.

The difficulties encountered are those of keeping both parents, the patient, and the patient's siblings in therapy. Frequently, one parent will pressure all into treatment, intensifying resistance in other family members. Typically, the father won't come at all, or the father and other family members will attend a few sessions and then drop out, leaving the therapist with the patient and his or her mother.

In theory, I was taught that if any family member could not come, the session must be canceled. While it is ideal for all family members to be involved, this can be a problem in families with more than one child. In practice, I continue even if only a fragment of the family is present because as all parents know, there is rarely 1 week in 1 year when one child is not sick!

In family treatment the focus is on the family *process* and not on the individual. The goal is to help the family become aware of the underlying emotional configurations and to open up the potential for change.

HOW TREATMENT IS CONDUCTED WITH SUICIDAL ADOLESCENTS

Having discussed by bias regarding the three treatment modalities I would use to work with suicidal adolescents, I will now state another bias. It is that *how* treatment is conducted is much more important than the specific choice of treatment.

In discussing the "how's" of treatment I will take a psychodynamic orientation because it reflects my background, because it is what is taught at most training centers and because it is the major perspective outlined elsewhere in this book. The discussion of the how's of therapy will, I hope, illuminate a few of the differences between therapeutic work with nonsuicidal and with suicidal adolescent patients.

The first difference I call "aloof versus warmth." The attitude of the therapist toward all patients, suicidal or not, is usually one of respect. It is one of recognition that the patient is under stress, confused, embarrassed, or humiliated. In other words, we know he deserves more consideration than under normal social interactions. The patient deserves some physical contact, such as a handshake to set him at ease, and convey warmth and respect. This, I believe is one time not to follow the analytic model where the physician never touches his patient.

To the adolescent, the physician may appear to be an awesome stranger who will probe the most intimate aspects of a teenager's life, who is seen as an authority over life and death and, often more importantly, of declaring sanity versus insanity. When working with suicidal adolescents I go beyond this gesture of physical contact and I work at making my patients feel "at home." My office is attached to my house, although in separate quarters, and I have made it look like a home rather than an office. Frequently, my patient and I will eat or drink something together. I sit across from my patient and we share a foot ottoman. There is an attitude of our being in this together, which removes some of the aura of omnipotence.

The key in working with suicidal adolescents is to be warm and responsive without being familiar or effusive. And this is a most difficult line to walk. This is the second problem for the therapist of an adolescent patient—the risk of blurring the boundaries between a professional and a social relationship. In therapy it is a *must* for the patient to remain a patient and not become a social friend. Therapy is *not* social. It is to evaluate and treat the conflicts that brought the patient to seek help. But with suicidal adolescents I *do* blur the lines. I *believe* that this leads to my success with adolescents who are suicidal. I *know*, however, it also leads to most of the problems I have in maintaining any degree of order or sanity in my personal life.

The focus of the professional relationship with the suicidal adolescent is on evaluation and treatment of the patient—just as it is in a regular treatment relationship. But, I believe, it should go further and involve the therapist in the patient's life and the patient in the therapist's life, but *not* in the therapist's needs. A regular professional relationship is a somewhat constrained relationship, focused on evaluation and treatment, focused on the needs of the patient, *never* on the needs of the therapist. A social relationship is focused on the needs of *both* parties, and the therapeutic relationship is not social. The patient should see the therapist as a friend, someone strongly for him, an ally in a common struggle, For example, I frequently attend weddings, graduations, rites of passage, concerts, and school plays.

Another question that a therapist must confront is when to intensify emotion. In therapy with nonsuicidal adolescents, the therapist might purposely choose to increase anxiety and see how the patient reacts under stress. With a suicidal adolescent, I never try to increase anger or anxiety.

Some therapists are aloof and unresponsive in order to assure distance. This, I believe, is *never* beneficial to a suicidal adolescent. Analytic anonymity *does* have a purpose. The purpose is to allow the patient to project, onto the therapist, feelings he has about significant people in his life. In therapy with a nonsuicidal adolescent, if he asks me where I am going this weekend, I might turn the question around and ask "Why do you ask?" I would not do this with a suicidal adolescent. This technique certainly has its place, but a suicidal adolescent who *is* sensitive to adult rejection to begin with can interpret analytic anonymity as rejection and alienation from the therapist. When working with a suicidal adolescent, if I want to know how he feels about his mother or his father, I will ask him. Usually, he will have no difficulty in telling me *just* how he feels. What I may sacrifice in my understanding of the patient's dynamics, I gain twofold in developing a closer relationship.

In most therapeutic situations, the therapist will wait for the patient to open conversation. With suicidal adolescents, often I do not wait. I might ask a question such as, "Did you have any difficulty getting here?" I use words to fill space and allay anxiety, but not to focus the session. I just break the silence. I will not meet silence with silence, nor will I try to provide answers for the patient. I will just try to open conversation and allow the patient to explore his own feelings with free association. This is a nonjudgmental way to open feelings.

Many patients see their therapists as a powerful source of wisdom. Otherwise why would they come to us? But many suicidal adolescents want to see their therapists as more than powerful. They want to see them as omnipotent. I very quickly tell my patients that I am not omnipotent. I tell them that as much as I want to help them, and as much as I will try to be there when they need me, I cannot be with them 24 hours a days, and it may be that I cannot be there at precisely the moment that they may be counting on me to intervene. I care, but I have human limitations.

One young woman was contemplating suicide. On the night of her attempt she called everyone she knew, even long distance. She cried "Why weren't they there? Why weren't they home? If they were I would not have done it." This is a narcissistic response of someone who expects someone else to be there and to save her. This is typical. Many patients call on Saturday night at 8 o'clock and expect me to be there and get angry if I am not. The example of this young woman also shows the fragile balance between the decision for life or for death, a balance that you may not be able to tip to the side of life at that precise moment you are wanted.

In treatment with a nonsuicidal patient one must keep quiet, keep the spotlight focused on the patient, be responsive and insightful, avoid judgments, and wait patiently through silence and tears. With suicidal adolescents, one must do all of that, and more. The therapist must do active listening as well as passive listening. For example, it is hard enough to wait through tears with a nonsuicidal adult patient, but with a suicidal adolescent it is excruciating to wait through pain before offering some solace. So I don't. I think of some way to actively show that I hear the suffering without saying anything that could interrupt the flow of thoughts or emotions. For instance, I may get up, hand tissues to the patient, and sit down.

Fatigue is a problem for all therapists. Sitting physically inactive while mentally active, listening to emotional material, hour after hour, is exhausting. Freud said that a physician who sees 10 patients a day is exposing a concealed attempt at suicide. I don't do it. I see a few suicidal patients a day. That is all I can handle. I may see 2 in the morning and 2 in the later afternoon and do something else in between (in my case, it is often car pools, or jogging around the supermarket).

Another obstacle to listening to any patient is impatience. All therapists are eager to make a diagnosis and find a solution. If we are active we feel that we are doing something. Our impatience may cause us to ask too many questions. We may bombard a suicidal youngster with "When did you attempt suicide? How did you do it? And are you going to do it again? With a nonsuicidal patient this is not too damaging, but with a patient who is suicidal this kind of impatience really defeats our purpose of exploring his actions and it blocks any catharsis.

What about the issue of countertransference? Some therapists feel it is unfair to begin therapy with a patient they do not like. Most people have some quality that others do not like such as aspects of immaturity or defects of character. The careful clinician makes distinctions between symptoms of the patient he does not like, and the person himself, and will try to understand and help the patient. If, however, negative feelings of the therapist are strong—even if they stem from the therapist's unconscious rather than reality—I would recommend that the therapist *not* work with the patient. Adolescents, and particularly suicidal adolescents, are especially sensitive to hypocrisy. Working with them with underlying negative feelings will do more harm than good.

Regardless of the treatment choice, or even the "how's of treatment," the optimal sequence of treatment should be the following:

First, establish a warm and caring relationship, which the adolescent and his family can accept. Second, allow dependency through support. In essence, you are encouraging regression and family support. Third, foster emotional growth and self-sufficiency. And last, help the adolescents detach from the therapist and establish better parent and peer relationships.

In sum, first you are establishing a dependency-gratifying relationship with the youngster. Then you are stimulating emotional growth, including the task of helping the adolescent to become more self-sufficient without stirring fears of abandonment. Then you are lessening the dependent aspects of the relationship at a pace consistent with the adolescent's maturation, accepting that some patients will need some degree of support indefinitely. Thus, the patient is actually repeating the developmental tasks of infancy, childhood, adolescence, and early adulthood with the guidance of a supportive parent-therapist.

The first goal of therapy is to establish enough of a relationship to allow the adolescent to communicate with the therapist and to want to come again. Each therapist develops his or her own techniques to accomplish this elusive task, but the principles remain the same for all. More than anything, adolescents are looking for someone they can trust and who will be consistent. They mistrust authority and bureaucracy, and tend to be intimidated by clinics, physicians, psychiatrists, psychologists, and rituals of appointment-making and form-filling. Those in helping roles are often seen by young people as too old, too formal, too inflexible, too powerful, and too unavailable.

In fact, the theorist has cautioned, "If you insist on adopting the unsuccessful methodology of traditional psychotherapeutic intervention, you will exclude yourself from having much relevance for the young." This may be a bit of an overstatement, but a point made so strongly is difficult to ignore. The most important clinical guideline in working with young people is how well one learns to listen to them and to what is going on around them.

In the initial meeting it is usually unproductive to ask an adolescent to explain *why*, he thought about or attempted suicide. Such a question will often be heard as an accusing one. It is better to ask about the circumstances of his life, school, work, family, dates, friends. This will convey interest in the whole person and not just in the suicidal event. What we want to do is to help the adolescent to be comfortable, to talk with him about more than the superficial and the obvious, and to get him to acknowledge his own role in the treatment process. What we don't want to do is to embarrass him at having been brought for help to a "shrink," or to give him any excuse for deciding that therapy is irrelevant to his needs, or that we are insensitive to his problems.

In the treatment process we are building a dependent relationship and then trying to decrease the dependent relationship we tried so hard to build. This will involve very stormy periods. The adolescent's intense dependent-independent conflicts, as well as negative feelings about parents can be turned on the therapist with such strength that the therapist is sure that the adolescent is more intent on making the therapist miserable than on using his help. Fears of dependency may make it difficult for the adolescent to express gratitude or affection and may lead instead to criticism and demanding behavior and broken appointments. All of these behaviors leave the therapist feeling incompetent and ready to turn his efforts to some other profession. Or what may be worse, the therapist may become hostile or defense toward the adolescent. This is generally an invitation to further disruptive or suicidal behavior. The course the therapist has to steer between giving in to excessive demands for affection, attention, and flexibility—and empathetic responses to the young person's despair, require all the combined magical skills of King Arthur's Merlin and Cinderella's fairy godmother. The therapist's ability to walk this tightrope is probably the most important and difficult aspect of the treatment process.

There are other special problems for the therapist in working with suicidal adolescents. I wish to mention a few.

In therapy with nonsuicidal patients there are infrequent phone calls. With suicidal adolescents there are incessant phone calls from the adolescent and from his family, with little regard to the time of day or night or the dinner hour.

In therapy with nonsuicidal patients you are needed to a degree. With suicidal adolescents you are purposely fostering dependency. Thus, when adolescents do try to become independent, they often attack. It is easier to separate when angry. That is how they separate. One clinician says that he often feels that the goal of the suicidal adolescent, in therapy, is to make the therapist miserable.

In therapy with any adolescent, the adolescent is usually brought to treatment by the parent, and the parent is in the position to disrupt therapy. Often an adolescent's parents will disrupt treatment precisely when the adolescent is *most* involved because parents see this relationship as threatening to them. The parents become jealous and sabotage therapy when the adolescent most desperately needs the alliance. This break or threatened loss can precipitate a suicide threat or attempt.

In therapy with nonsuicidal patients the therapist generally has an understanding regarding appointments. With suicidal adolescents the therapist needs to be flexible and allow for manipulation. This makes the therapist's life totally unmanageable.

In therapy with nonsuicidal patients, the therapist can take vacations. With suicidal adolescents, it is difficult to go further than a phone call or a car ride away because, while there may be coverage, in a crisis, a different therapist is not an adequate substitute.

When a nonsuicidal patient experiences anxiety, the response of the therapist, while important, is not crucial. When extreme anxiety is present, as in the case of the suicidal adolescent, the therapist's response *is* crucial. Unfortunately, the therapist's response to the patient's anxiety, is usually anxiety. If the therapist handles anxiety with talk, he will block the patients. If he handles it with silence, he may appear rejecting. If he offers premature reassurance, he may give the impression that he doesn't really understand the seriousness of the symptoms. For example, if the therapist is made anxious by the thought a youngster has of killing himself he may respond, "Don't worry, thoughts are not the same as actions" and quickly change the subject. Thus, he blocks the expression of underlying conflicts.

In general, in therapy, the age of the therapist does not matter. With suicidal adolescents, I think, age may matter. If it is true that it is the "how's of therapy" that matter as much, if not more than experience, then young therapists may be more effective. The younger therapist usually has fewer constraints, fewer time conflicts, can be seen more as an ally and peer, less a feared authority figure, and may have more strength and exuberance. He may be less skilled but more giving. For example, years ago I took calls, even encouraged them, from patients at all times of the day or night, as *they* needed me. Now *I* need my rest.

In therapy with nonsuicidal patients, giving medications is relatively safe. With suicidal adolescents there is always the fear of overdose. Medications can be lethal if kids are stockpiling them without the therapist's knowledge. Medications have been found to be of special use in suicidal states only insofar as they are indicated for an underlying disorder, such as manic-depressive psychosis, or decreased serotonin levels. In situations of depression, the benefits must be weighed against the risks of stockpiling a lethal dose and the potential for exacerbating problems of self-image and drug dependency. If the parents are depressed, giving them the antidepressants may help the youngster more.

With nonsuicidal patients the question of hospitalization is based on the patient's needs. With suicidal adolescents it is, as often, based on the families' needs. Hospitalization should be considered if a suicide attempt or gesture has been made and if the family atmosphere is not supportive. A period of hospitalization affords the therapist the time to evaluate the adolescent and the family situation before making treatment plans. It also allows the parents a safety net and a respite in their constant vigilance of a suicidal youngster. Brief use of a hospital can serve to assure the young person that his cries for help have been taken seriously and not dismissed as an attention-getting maneuver. On the other hand, hospitalization can be depersonalizing and punitive experience. This depends on the unit available and the staff. If the situation seems too equivocal, a consultation can help resolve the dilemma. One difficult problem is when a suicidal adolescent says, "I'll commit suicide if you put me in a hospital" and you are fearful that he will commit suicide if you don't. The hospital can be a frightening proposition. If a hospital is not used, an extensive support system must be made available. This includes frequent therapy appointments, the support of family and friends, and the removal of all lethal weapons from the house, including kitchen knives, sleeping pills, and cars.

Motto (1985) said, in a paper he wrote 5 years ago, that treating suicidal adolescents is a most difficult task, and that no therapist should handle more than three or four suicidal patients at any one time. As I wrote this chapter and reflect on what I actually do each day, I am convincing myself that this job *is* almost impossible. If I did not love what I do so much, I would certainly choose another less demanding profession. Treating suicidal adolescents is not the earliest way to earn a living. In my next life I am going to manufacture underwear. It is something that people always need; the factory will keep producing, even while I am on vacation in the Caribbean. And there are no emergency calls on Saturday nights.

BIBLIOGRAPHY

Cantor, P. (1975). The effects of youthful suicide on the family. *Psychiatric Opinion, 12*, 6–11.

Cantor. P. (1977). Suicide and attempted suicide among students: Problem, prediction and prevention. In P. Cantor (Ed.), *Understanding a child's world: Readings in infancy through adolescence*. New York: McGraw-Hill, 433–443.

Cantor, P. (1982). Suicide and depression: A case study, "too sad to live." In M. Schwarz (Ed.), *TV and teens: Experts look at the issues* (pp. 175–186). Reading, MA: Addison-Wesley.

Cantor. P. (1983). Depression and suicide in children. In C. E. Walker & M. C. Roberts (Eds.), *Handbook of clinical and child psychology* (pp. 741–759). New York: Wiley.

Hendin, H. (1982). *Suicide in America*. New York: W. W. Norton.

Husain, S. A., & Vandiver, T. (1984). *Suicide in children and adolescents*. New York: Spectrum Publications.

Motto, J. (1985). Treatment concerns in preventing youth suicide. In M. L. Peck, N. L. Farberow, & R. E. Litman (Eds.), *Youth suicide* (pp. 91–111). New York: Springer.

Nicholi, A. M., Jr. (1978). The adolescent. In A. M. Nicholi, Jr. (Ed.), *Harvard guide to modern psychiatry* (pp. 519–541). Cambridge, MA: Harvard University Press.

Weeks, E., & Mack, J. (1978). The child. In A. M. Nicholi, Jr. (Ed.), *Harvard guide to modern psychiatry* (pp. 519–541). Cambridge, MA: Harvard University Press.

Weiner, I. (1970). *Psychological disturbance in adolescence* (pp. 157–197). New York: Wiley-Interscience.

19

The Prevention of Suicide in Adults

John T. Maltsberger

Were it not for the fact that the great majority of those who set out to commit suicide are ambivalent about it, writing (or reading) a chapter about suicide prevention would be a waste of time. The subject invites attention, however, because most would-be suicides are not at all sure they wish to go all the way over the edge. For every person who successfully commits suicide, a hundred will attempt it. Most patients who become seriously suicidal do not remain so for very long periods—self-destructive fever ameliorates. Only a small fraction remain continuously and seriously suicidal over many months or years. Because most patients are not at all sure they wish to do away with themselves, they are likely to involve others in their self-destructive enterprises, and to make us a part of their struggle in the choice between living and dying. The majority of would-be suicides are prepared to accept our preventative interventions, with whatever mixture of feelings. A discussion of suicide-prevention makes sense because for the very great majority of patients suicide is a permanent solution to a temporary problem (as Ed Shneidman is fond of reminding us); these patients commonly thank us for interfering with their lethal designs and activities once their psychological distress has been ameliorated. For a small and resolute minority, therapeutic efforts at suicide prevention will fail; some of these will have been more or less intent on dying from the beginning. Some others incline more and more toward death with the passing of time despite all outside efforts to reverse the lethal trend.

JOHN T. MALTSBERGER • **Boston Psychoanalytic Society and Institute, Boston, Massachusetts 02108.**

Community psychiatrists have borrowed the terms primary, secondary, and tertiary prevention from colleagues in public health. For the purposes of this chapter, it will be convenient to discuss suicide prevention under these rubrics. Primary suicide prevention refers to measures to prevent the development of significant suicide intent. Secondary suicide prevention addresses those measures undertaken to stop the suicidal process once it has begun from moving forward to a lethal culmination, and to reverse it so that the patient will be relieved of the pressure to commit suicide. Tertiary suicide prevention refers to measures to reduce impairment and suicide probability in the minority of individuals who tend to remain suicidal over many months and years, that is, those who have become chronic suicide cases.

PRIMARY SUICIDE PREVENTION

Broad social measures that would diminish child abuse, minimize the breakdown of families, reduce the rates of alcoholism and drug addiction, lower the poverty level, and decrease the isolation of elderly individuals would expectably lower the prevalence of many disorders, including suicide. The contribution of alcohol abuse to suicide and to suicide attempts is enormous; drug abuse is increasingly abetting suicidal behavior, among older patients as well as among adolescents and younger adults. The correction of these broader social ills, however desirable, cannot be extensively discussed here. Some public health concerns bearing on primary suicide prevention can be outlined, nevertheless, if we limit ourselves to goals more practically attainable and bearing specifically on the suicide problem.

Education of Physicians, Nurses, Clergy, and Teachers in Recognizing Depression

We know that about 60% of patients who commit suicide make a medical contact shortly before their deaths (Inwood & Anderson, 1964; Yessler, Gibbs, & Becker, 1961). And we know, too, the commonplace fact that the majority of those about to commit suicide make an unequivocal threat of suicide in the month before their death (Barraclough, Bunch, Nelson, & Sainsbury, 1974); even more make veiled threats and references. It is plain, therefore, that primary care physicians are particularly well situated to recognize and to treat (or to refer for treatment) depressed patients and depressed patients who are moving in a suicidal direction. Yet physicians frequently fail to diagnose and treat depression in general, and the danger of suicide in particular. There are a number of reasons why this is so.

The psychiatric education of the ordinary physician in the United States is sadly deficient in this sector. Although medical students are still carefully taught in early diagnosis courses to ask about everything from double vision to joint swelling, systematic inquiry as to a history of depression is not ordinarily routine. At a major Eastern medical school, not one lecture on suicide is included in the curriculum, and such education as the students may obtain on this subject is left to chance in the various clerkships to which they may be assigned. This regrettable state of affairs is quite common, although suicide is the leading cause of death after accidents in young people.

The bias of most physicians is in the direction of diagnosing and treating physical ailments. The patient who complains of difficulty sleeping is likely to receive a prescription for a benzodiazepene; another, complaining of weight loss, will be subjected to a barium enema or an upper gastrointestinal investigation. Patients, especially older patients, are not likely to complain of depression as such, although they may present with vague complaints involving a variety of different organ systems, and mention fatigue and loss of energy as such. Any mention of one of the common depressive symptoms should prompt physicians to ask about the others—difficulty sleeping or sleeping too much, loss of interest, guilty preoccupations, diminished energy, difficulty in concentrating (or remembering), loss of appetite, weight loss, overeating, psychomotor agitation or retardation, and suicidal ideas. But all too often they do not.

Failure to ask about suicidal thoughts is particularly frequent. In two separate studies of suicide carried out 14 years apart, it has been shown that only one of six physicians had known of the suicidal preoccupations of their patients who took their lives, even though information about self-destructive ideas was readily obtainable from others (Murphy, 1975; Robins, Gassner, Kayes, Wilkinson, & Murphy, 1959).

Some physicians may be reluctant to ask about suicidal ideas because they are embarrassed, even though they have been carefully schooled when they were students about the importance of asking about any history of sexually transmitted diseases. I suspect that many others do not ask because they do not wish to hear about depressive symptoms, preconsciously fearing that a depression will be uncovered. Older patients with multiple vague complaints may be perceived as wasting the physician's time. The discovery of suicidal preoccupations may be even more unwelcome. Such patients are likely to evoke a sense of helplessness or fear in medical personnel, and trigger aversive responses (Maltsberger & Buie, 1974).

Physicians and surgeons need to keep on the alert for signs of dementia in elderly patients. Not only are some forms of dementia treatable in themselves, depression may sometimes masquerade as a dementing illness. Rigorous clinical investigation of these cases is always indicated, often with psychiatric and neurologic consultation. In doubtful cases, sophisticated neuropsychological testing will often help in the identification of depressive pseudodementia (McCallister, 1983; Wells, 1982) (see Chapter 12, this volume).

That delirious patients have a high suicide risk often goes unappreciated on general medical and surgical wards. Elderly patients in particular may become confused and excited in unfamiliar surroundings, occasionally throwing themselves out of high hospital windows when panicked and disoriented.

The increasingly litigious climate in the United States makes it important for all physicians to be aware of the malpractice implications of failure to diagnose and treat depressive illness. A suicide arising from an undiagnosed depression is an ever-present likelihood, and makes it all the more important to include routine questions about depression and suicide in ordinary medical and surgical visits.

Heath care in the United States is changing rapidly with the increase of health maintenance organizations (HMOs), and it is likely to become even more impersonal in the future because of the heavy demands on physicians' time. Frequently, the first person the patient encounters in the HMO setting will be the triage nurse whose responsibility it commonly is to make suggestions for symptomatic treatment or to refer to the appropriate specialist. Nurses in these organizations are taking on many of the responsibilities once assumed by general practitioners. Their training in the recognition of depression is increasingly essential. School nurses also need this training.

Many depressed and potentially suicidal patients will take their difficulties to the clergy. Good seminary education in the recognition and treatability of depression is an important primary preventative of suicide.

Training of physicians, their assistants, nurses, and clergy in the use of depression rating scales and in suicide rating scales would be easy. A strong case can be made for the wide administration of these tests outside the consulting rooms of psychologists and psychiatrists. The encouragement of their general use would in itself serve to alert caregivers to the ubiquity and hazards of depression, and very likely lead to the treatment of many depressed patients who otherwise might go unnoticed. Physicians in particular could be encouraged to make use of Beck's "hopelessness" scale, a measure of a patient's despair. By now it has been well established that the depth of hopelessness is much more highly correlated with suicide danger than depression as such (Beck, Weissman, Lester, & Trexler, 1974; Beck, Kovacs, & Weissman, 1975).

Gun Control

Whether gun control legislation can be effective in lowering the suicide rate is unclear. There is some support for the idea that strict gun control laws may reduce the incidence of suicide by firearms, but those states where firearms are strictly controlled are likely to have a higher rate of suicide by other means.

Nevertheless, the overall suicide rate is likely to be lower in states with strong gun-control legislation (Lester & Murrell, 1980). Hitherto most of what has been published about this subject has been unsupported opinion. Different jurisdictions and countries are difficult to compare because their gun-control laws differ, as do their cultures. Furthermore, there are differences in how rigorously gun-control statutes are enforced. Future studies will perhaps shed light on the utility of gun-control legislation as a primary suicide preventative (Lester, 1989).

Suicide Prevention Centers

Lester (1989) has reviewed the literature reporting on comparative suicide rates in cities of the United States with and without suicide prevention centers and has found much of it scientifically flawed. He therefore undertook a study of the suicide rates in 24 American cities for the year 1969, studying three samples: those with suicide prevention centers established by 1967, those with centers established by 1969, and those without centers. Shifts in suicide rates from 1960 to 1969 were determined for each of the samples, and the cities were matched according to populations. He concluded that when population size in cities is controlled for, the suicide prevention centers do not appear to have a statistically significant effect on suicide rates.

He is careful to point out that studies such as his need to be repeated in future years, because the suicide prevention centers were comparatively new, and may not have had an opportunity as yet to exert an ameliorative effect.

Lester's findings are congruent with those of others who studied cities in England, matching them for ecological similarity (Barraclough, Jennings, & Moss, 1977; Jennings, Barraclough, & Moss, 1978)—suicide prevention centers were not found to alter the suicide rate.

At variance with these studies is the recent report by Miller, Coombs, Leeper, and Barton (1984) who compared counties in the United States with and without suicide prevention centers. They found that the centers appear to have a beneficial impact on the suicide rates of young white females, but no other group.

SECONDARY SUICIDE PREVENTION

When we deal with patients who are not only depressed but presuicidal, our concerns are those of secondary prevention. Patients who have entered the suicide zone require specialized treatment, all the details of which cannot be addressed here. But certain difficulties and problems that suicidal cases present do merit special mention, inasmuch as patients are lost from time to time because these points are overlooked.

Inadequate Treatment of Depression

A recent review of 30 follow-up studies with patients with depressive illnesses has emphasized what has long been the consensus in the psychiatric literature—that 15% of depressives, whether classified as endogenous, neurotic, psychotic, or otherwise, will ultimately die by suicide (Miles, 1977). Furthermore, we know that between 40% and 60% of patients who complete suicide suffer from a depressive illness (Sainsbury, 1986). Despite these facts, the depression that is the primary destructive force in many suicidal patients is sometimes inadequately treated. Furthermore, the suicide rate among English and Dutch psychiatric inpatients has increased with the introduction of more liberal regimens in hospitals (Sainsbury, Baert, & Jenkins, 1978; de Graaf, 1976).

At least in the United States the tendency is to treat all depressions with antidepressant drugs, even though the illness may be profound, and the patient quite suicidal. There are three difficulties with this approach, especially in suicidal cases. First, many days and weeks may pass before a therapeutic effect is obtained. Commonly, several different compounds must be tried because the first one or two are found to be ineffective, or because the patients cannot tolerate side effects the drugs occasion. Much time is lost during which the more dangerous patients may destroy themselves. Second, although some amelioration of the depression may be obtained in time because of drug action, the depression may remain only partially relieved and inadequately treated. Some patients improve only enough to regain enough psychic energy to mobilize themselves into suicidal action. Third, we overlook what it costs our patients in terms of depressive suffering as they drag themselves through a succession of hideous days, waiting for the drugs to take effect.

If antidepressant drugs are the primary method employed to treat a suicidal patient, the psychiatrist should not rest until he is sure the depression relief he seeks is full and adequate. This may require the administration of drug combinations and expert psychopharmacological advice. However common such a treatment plan may be, I do not support it. For suicidal patients it is likely to offer too little too late.

By far the best course for treating suicidal patients with major depressive illnesses is to admit the patient to a closed psychiatric unit and to administer a course of electroconvulsive treatment forthwith, reserving the antidepressant drugs until after the treatments have been finished. Then it is important to prescribe the drugs prophylactically against the reoccurrence of the illness. In this way, quick recovery from the dangerous suicidal phase is almost always assured, with good depression relief and quick relief of suffering.

Many psychiatrists fail to appreciate that the more severe suicidal depressions may require more electroconvulsive treatments than is the case with simpler depressions. Lesse (1988) argues that 5 or 6 treatments may be necessary just to blunt the suicidal drive, and that 10 or 15 treatments are usually necessary to complete the series. "I do not subscribe to statements purporting that suicidal patients may require only five or six treatments," he writes. "This concept is fallacious and dangerous and too often results in avoidable exacerbations." After all symptoms of depression have cleared Lesse begins to taper the treatments to 2 per week for another week or more, and then gives 1 each week for 1 or 2 more weeks. Other psychiatrists experienced in the treatment of suicidal cases will agree with these recommendations, and so do I.

Management in the Recovery Phase

The postdepressive recovery phase is well understood to be a high-risk time for suicide. Fawcett et al. (1987) showed that of nearly a thousand patients with major affective disorder, a third of those who would go on to commit suicide did so within 6 months of admission to their study, and half did within the year following their admission. (The average time of follow-up was 4 years.) Roy (1982) found that among a diagnostically mixed group of 94 patients, 65% of the suicides took place within 6 months of hospital discharge. No patient who has been suicidal receives adequate treatment unless prolonged outpatient follow-up is provided after the acute episode has passed.

The recurrence of depression can be watched for during weekly follow-up visits so that it can be treated early and vigorously. Patients should be maintained on appropriate antidepressant drugs for a year at least after recovering from a suicidal crisis. Coppen, Noguera, and Bailey (1971) have reported a prospective clinical trial of lithium carbonate prophylaxis in patients with manic-depressive illness and demonstrated its usefulness in preventing the recurrence of depressive episodes. Barraclough (1972) believes that were lithium prophylaxis used widely enough, a reduction of the suicide rate should result.

It is a clinical commonplace that severely ill patients, especially those who have been psychotic, are particularly prone to rely heavily on denial as a defense. In the process of recovering from a serious depression, these individuals are likely to make up their minds that all is well, that their dark days are forever past, and that continuing outpatient visits are not necessary. No small number will even refuse to take important prophylactic antidepressant medicines.

It is at this point that the quality of rapport between the patient and his psychiatrist will be most severely put to the test. If a good therapeutic relationship is to be formed (a good relationship may spell the difference between life and death for the patient), the clinician must set about building it from the very beginning. If he and his patient have been engaged in a struggle for control from the beginning of hospitalization, he can hardly expect to reshape the relationship into one of collaboration and trust at the moment of hospital discharge. Countertransference acting-out on the part of psychiatrists and nursing staff have been shown to contribute to patient suicide, especially when depressed patients also bear the diagnosis of borderline personality disorder (Kullgren, 1988; Kullgren, Renberg, & Jacobsson, 1986; Maltsberger & Buie, 1974).

When a suicidal patient resists treatment recommendations, refuses to cooperate with his caretakers, or, as so commonly is the case, will not consent to voluntary hospitalization and must be committed, those responsible for his care should consider establishing a therapeutic-administrative split. The clinician responsible for continuing monitoring, including post-discharge contacts, and for psychotherapy, is then relieved and making decisions that affect the patient's freedom to come and to go, and in this way may avoid becoming the target of anger and devaluation to a considerable extent.

There is a general tendency to make decisions concerning hospital discharge primarily on the basis of improvement in a patient's mental status. The depressed patient, commonly having received a course of antidepressant medication, will be seen to be substantially if not completely improved, and at this stage may deny that his suicidal ideation continues. A decision may at that time be made to allow the patient to go home. Suicide then follows in a few days.

Close review of a number of such cases over the past several years has shown that the patient's increase hopefulness has depended on the support and care provided by the ward staff and the hospital environment, as well as removal from stressful circumstances that contributed to the development of the suicidal crisis in the first place. It is essential that decisions about hospital discharge (and admission, for that matter) not be made on the basis of mental status examination alone. Such decisions need to be based on a careful assessment of the patient's inner life, what reasons he has for hope, what life may offer to help him want to go on living, and what forces may be at work in his social environment that are suicide promoting. That is to say, clinical decisions should be made on the basis of the case formulation (Maltsberger, 1986).

> Mrs. R., a 30-year-old mother of two small children, one aged 6 months, the other, 2 years, was admitted to the psychiatric department of her local hospital when she developed a psychotic depression characterized by persecutory delusions and powerful suicidal impulses.
>
> She had recently moved to New England from a distant state, leaving behind her extended family and her mother, on whom she had been particularly dependent. The care of her children was overwhelming to her, and she had grown increasingly convinced that she was an inadequate mother without whom they would be better off. Her husband, though he loved his wife, was struggling to keep abreast of the demands of his new job, and was not able to lend much support. He appeared to resent his wife's tears and her wish to visit her mother so often—Mrs. R. was incurring expensive telephone bills that the couple could ill afford by calling across the country several times a day.
>
> The patient was assigned to an unlocked unit (the hospital had no other) and given a course of imipramine and haloperidol, all the while being carefully watched by the staff. She improved somewhat in her mood; her delusions abated, and she no longer reported feeling suicidal. She felt very distressed by the fact that her children were being cared for temporarily in a foster home, and pleaded to be discharged so she could go home and take care of them. Because she seemed so much better, the staff agreed and she was allowed to go home, with a good plan worked out for post-hospital aftercare.
>
> Two days later she was found dead, having hanged herself in the basement.

This case illustrates the importance of case formulation in making discharge decisions. Here we find a failure to appreciate that the patient could not sustain herself without significant support, support that her mother and other family members had offered her at home before she moved away and was overwhelmed by the demands of family life. Her husband could not provide all the support she needed, and resented her tears and complaints. With the support of the hospital staff and the antidepressant medicines, she felt somewhat better, but was still somewhat depressed and guilty, if not completely despairing and obviously psychotic. The loss of support that discharge cost her, plus the reimposition of the stresses of mothering two children in diapers, was more than she could bear.

It illustrates other points as well. There is a general tendency at present to underestimate the danger of major depressive syndromes when complicated by psychosis. It has nevertheless been shown that deluded depressed patients are five times more likely to commit suicide than those without delusions (Roose, Glassman, Walsh, Woodring, & Vital-Herne, 1983). The use of antidepressant drugs, or combinations of antidepressant and antipsychotic agents, as the primary mode of treatment in such cases cannot be defended clinically, inasmuch as response may be delayed for many days or weeks, and the response may not be complete. Should suicide occur, as it did here, legal defense against a malpractice action would be very difficult indeed. Electroconvulsive treatment was what Mrs. R. needed, and it was dangerous to treat her in an unlocked unit. In the event that patients or families refuse electroconvulsive treatment, as they may do from time to time, especially if the psychiatric staff is ambivalent about its use, it is essential that the refusal be fully documented in the hospital record. From time to time, it may be necessary to have a guardian appointed for a patient in order to obtain permission to give life-saving treatment.

TERTIARY SUICIDE PREVENTION

The tertiary prevention of suicide concerns those patients who remain, as it were, on the suicidal brink more or less continuously, or intermittently, over months and years.

The schizoaffective and the depressed schizophrenic patient population is a particularly troublesome one that may require complex interventions. This population has, furthermore, a highly uncertain prognosis. Electroconvulsive treatment may be necessary from time to time. Such patients are also likely to do better when treated prophylactically with drug combinations.

Drug Combinations and Electroconvulsive Therapy

A recent review of retrospective studies of more than 800 patients has demonstrated that delusional depressed individuals do not respond well to tricyclic antidepressants alone, and that they respond better to combinations of tricyclic and antipsychotic agents (Roose & Glassman, 1988).

Schizoaffective patients have been shown to fare far better when treated with electroconvulsive treatment (ECT). Tsuang, Dempsey, and Fleming (1979) followed up 74 schizoaffective patients admitted to the hospital between 1934 and 1944 and found that 55 of these were still alive in 1975. Comparisons between the 24 who had received electroconvulsive treatment and the 50 who had not showed a significant difference in mortality between the two groups—only 8% of the ECT patients were deceased at follow-up, but 34% of those who had not been treated with ECT had died.

"Modified Narcosis"

Although modified narcosis combined with ECT and antidepressant drugs is unknown in the United States, it is sometimes used in Europe as a treatment for intractable depression. Modified narcosis is obtained by giving combinations of chlorpromazine or other sedative compounds with the goal of keeping the patient asleep for 16 of 24 hours. The sleep treatment is continued for 4 to 6 weeks, and ECT is given twice a week during this period (Walter, Mitchell-Heggs, & Sargant, 1972).

Neurosurgical Treatment of Suicidal Patients

The neurosurgical treatment of intractable depression is also largely unknown in North America. So-called psychosurgery has been abandoned in all but a few centers, although it offers hope for some of the sickest patients.

The original Freeman and Watts leukotomies were, of course, unsatisfactory. About 4% of the patients subjected to that procedure died, a comparable fraction developed severe personality problems having to do with social disinhibition, and some became epileptic. The procedure furthermore was found to be ineffective as a treatment of schizophrenia. The increasing public distrust of all institutionalized authority that emerged during the 1960s became concentrated on neurosurgical treatments for mental illness, and those who carried them out were widely perceived to be sadistic and Nazi-like. This prejudice has infected many psychiatrists as well who remain unaware of the more recent and effective surgical interventions that can help correctly chosen patients whose depression does not yield to other treatments (Sweet, 1982).

Ballantine, Levy, Dagi, and Guirinas (1977) have reported a series of chronically disabled mental patients whose illnesses had crippled them for many years, 10 on average. Of 204 patients who received anterior stereotactic procedures, 84 were followed-up carefully for 7 years after the series concluded. Of these patients 80% had significantly improved, none had died, and none had developed serious complications (including personality alterations).

More recently, Ballantine, Bouckoms, Thomas, and Guirinas (1987) reported a prospective study of almost 200 psychiatric patients who received stereotactic cingulotomies, all of whom had previously failed to respond to other treatments. Of these patients 61% had affective disorders, and 72% had attempted suicide. The patients were followed up for almost 9 years on average. Although there were 18 suicides in this group, 62% had substantially or very substantially improved, none had died of surgical complications, none had developed lasting neurologic or behavioral problems, and some had improved on intelligence testing.

While neurosurgical treatment may not offer hope to all patients who are chronically suicidal, there is good reason to believe that it can help many, and that it is, furthermore, recommended too infrequently.

The Calculated Risk

Despite every therapeutic effort a small minority of patients will remain suicidal, even though they have received psychotherapy, psychoactive drugs, electroconvulsive treatment, and possibly even neurosurgery. After extensive consultation and many trials of treatments, singly and in combination, the psychiatrist may have to face the fact that the only way to preserve the patient's life is to enforce lifelong custodial care.

There may be no other choice in those rare cases when the patient remains floridly psychotic. But in most others, there is another choice. The patient may be given back some of the responsibility of the choice about living or dying, responsibility that may long ago have been taken away from the patient by involuntary hospitalization. A strong argument can be made to the effect that we are not justified in abridging a patient's freedom unless there is good reason to believe that his suicidal pressure can be relieved by the treatment he may not welcome, and that in the future he will thank us for it.

The threat of malpractice or other legal action makes many psychiatrists reluctant to allow known suicidal patients outside an institution, but, morally speaking, there comes a point in time when enforced hospitalization becomes meddlesome.

Outright discharge when all treatment has failed would seem to invite suicide, because patients may perceive such dismissal from the hospital as a rejection—it conveys a message of hopelessness from the psychiatrist who could be seen as abandoning the patient.

The preferable alternative is to allow chronically suicidal patients who have not been relieved of their suicidal pressure by all available treatments to leave the hospital from time to time, for increasingly long intervals, up to and through the point of discharge, but all the while offering continuing supportive help and occasional rehospitalization should the patient wish it. Under these circumstances some patients may hang on to life for many years, while others, electing to endure their painful and incurable illnesses no more, may choose to take their own lives.

REFERENCES

Ballantine, H. T., Jr., Levy, B. S., Dagi, T. F., & Guirinas, I. E. (1977). Cingulotomy for psychiatric illness: Report of 13 years' experience. In W. H. Sweet (Ed.), *Neurosurgical treatment in psychiatry, pain and epilepsy* (pp. 333–353). Baltimore: University Park Press.

Ballantine, H. T., Jr., Bouckoms, A. J., Thomas, E. K., & Guirinas, I. E. (1987). Treatment of psychiatric illness by stereotactic cingulotomy. *Biological Psychiatry, 22*, 807–819.

Barraclough, B. M. (1972). Suicide prevention, recurrent affective disorder and lithium. *British Journal of Psychiatry, 121*, 391–392.

Barraclough, B., Bunch, J., Nelson, B., & Sainsbury, P. (1974). A hundred cases of suicide—clinical aspects. *British Journal of Psychiatry, 125*, 355–373.

Barraclough, B. M., Jennings, C., & Moss, J. R. (1977). Suicide prevention by the Samaritans. *Lancet, 1*, 237–239.

Beck, A. T., Weissman, A., Lester, A., & Trexler, L. (1974). The measurement of pessimism: The hopelessness scale. *Journal of Consulting and Clinical Psychology, 4*, 861–865.

Beck, A. T., Kovacs, M., & Weissman, A. (1975). Hopelessness and suicidal behavior: An overview. *Journal of the American Medical Association, 234*, 1146–1149.

Coppen, A., Noguera, R., & Bailey, J. (1971). Prophylactic lithium in affective disorders. *The Lancet, 2*, 275–279.

De Graaf, A. C. (1976). Zelfmoord in Psychiatrische Zeikenhuizen, *Tijdschrift Psychiatrie, 18*, 11–12.

Fawcett, J., Scheftner, W., Clark, D., Hedeker, D., Gibbons, R., & Coryell, W. (1987). Clinical predictors of suicide in patients with major affective disorders: A controlled prospective study. *American Journal of Psychiatry, 144*, 35–40.

Inwood, E. R., & Anderson, M. (1964). Suicide and the family physician. *GP, 30*, 130–133.

Jennings, C., Barraclough, B., & Moss, J. (1978). Have the Samaritans lowered the suicide rate? *Psychological Medicine, 8*, 413–422.

Kullgren, G. (1985). Borderline personality disorder and psychiatric suicides, *Nordisk Psychiatrisk Tiddskrift, 39*, 479–484.

Kullgren, G. (1988). Factors associated with completed suicide in borderline personality disorder. *Journal of Nervous and Mental Disease, 176*, 40–44.

Kullgren, G., Renberg, E., & Jacobsson, L. (1986). An empirical study of borderline personality disorder and psychiatric suicides. *Journal of Nervous and Mental Disease, 174*, 328–231.

Lesse, S. (1988). *What we know about suicidal behavior and how to treat it* (p. 202). Northvale, NJ: Jason Aronson.

Lester, D. (1989). *Can we prevent suicide?* New York: AMS Press.

Lester, D., & Murrell, M. (1980). The influence of gun control laws on suicidal behavior, *American Journal of Psychiatry, 137*, 121–122.

Maltsberger, J. T. (1986). *Suicide risk: The formulation of clinical judgement*, New York: New York University Press.

Maltsberger, J. T., & Buie, D. H. (1974). Countertransference hate in the treatment of suicidal patients, *Archives of General Psychiatry, 30*, 625–633.

McCallister, T. W. (1983). Overview: Pseudodementia. *American Journal of Psychiatry, 140*, 528–533.

Miles, C. P. (1977). Conditions predisposing to suicide: A review. *Journal of Nervous and Mental Disease, 16*, 231–246.

Miller, H., Coombs, D., Leeper, J., & Barton, S. (1984). An analysis of the effects of suicide prevention facilities on suicide rate in the U.S. *American Journal of Public Health*, *74*, 340–343.

Murphy, G. E. (1975). The physician's responsibility for suicide: II. Errors of omission. *Annals of Internal Medicine*, *82*, 305–309.

Robins, E., Gassner, S., Kayes, J., Wilkinson, R. H., Murphy, G. E. (1959). The communication of suicidal intent: A study of 134 consecutive cases of successful (completed) suicide. *American Journal of Psychiatry*, *115*, 723–733.

Roose, S. P., & Glassman, A. H. (1988). Delusional depression. In A. Georgotas & R. Cancro (Eds.), *Depression and mania* (pp. 75–85). New York: Elsevier.

Roose, S. P., Glassman, A. H., Walsh, B. T., Woodring, S., & Vital-Herne, J. (1983). Depressions, delusions and suicide. *American Journal of Psychiatry*, *140*, 1159–1162.

Roy, A. (1982). Risk factors for suicide in psychiatric patients. *Archives of General Psychiatry*, *39*, 1089–1095.

Sainsbury, P. (1982). Depression and suicide prevention. *Biblothetica Psychiatrica*, *162*, 17–32.

Sainsbury, P. (1986). Depression, suicide and suicide prevention. In A. Roy (Ed.), *Suicide* (pp. 73–88). Baltimore: Williams & Wilkins.

Sainsbury, P., Baert, A., & Jenkins, J. (1978). Suicide trends in Europe: A study of the decline in suicide in England and Wales and of the increase elsewhere. A report to the World Health Organization Regional Office for Europe, Copenhagen.

Sweet, W. H. (1982). Neurosurgical aspects of primary affective disorders. In J. R. Youmans (Ed.), *Neurological surgery* (pp. 3927–3946). Philadelphia: W. B. Saunders.

Tsuang, M. T., Dempsey, G. M., & Fleming, J. A. (1979). Can ECT prevent premature death and suicide in schizoaffective patients? *Journal of Affective Disorders*, *1*, 167–171.

Walter, C. J. S., Mitchell-Heggs, N., & Sargant, W. (1972). Modified narcosis, ECT and antidepressant drugs: A review of technique & immediate outcome. *British Journal of Psychiatry*, *120*, 651–662.

Wells, C. E. (1982). Refinements in the diagnosis of dementia. *American Journal of Psychiatry*, *139*, 621–622.

Yessler, P., Gibbs, J., & Becker, H. (1961). On the communication of suicidal ideas. *Archives of General Psychiatry*, *5*, 12–29.

VII
Concluding Remarks

Our attempt has been to introduce the reader to a developmental view of suicide. We now see that the suicidal process—despite its commonalities across the life span—can be conceptualized from time-lines. Part VII presents a few brief final comments derived from the volume itself.

20

A Life Span Perspective of Suicide

Antoon A. Leenaars

Suicide is probably best understood as a multidimensional malaise. It would seem most accurate to define suicide as an event with biological (including biochemical), sociocultural, interpersonal, psychological, and personal philosophical/existential aspects. It is also possible, as we believe this volume has shown, to attempt to structure suicidal phenomena from a developmental point of view.

INTRODUCTION

There are various ways in which life's—including the suicidal person's—time-lines can be conceptualized. Though suicide is in many ways the same across the entire life span, understanding suicide from a developmental perspective is productive. These final comments are a brief summary of the findings that arose from this volume, though there is no intent to be exhaustive.

Part I consisted of four chapters. The first, by John Benjafield, presented a meta-outline of the developmental process as open-ended. The concept of development, as Benjafield notes, "is ambiguous, and that ambiguity allows for both positive and negative outcomes as people struggle to define the meaning of devel-

ANTOON A. LEENAARS • Private Practice, 880 Ouelette Avenue, Suite 702, Windsor, Ontario, Canada N9A 1C7.

opment in their own lives. The only thing we can be reasonably sure of is that the end of development will be a central issue in people's lives." Suicide is—all too often—one such end.

The second chapter, by David Lester, presented a brief review of the time-lines (or stages) of development. A division of the time-lines is presented, mainly through Erik Erikson's model: Infancy (age:0–2); Preschool Years (age:2–6); Middle Childhood (age:6–12); Adolescence (age:13–18); Young Adulthood (age:18–25/30); Middle Adulthood (age:25–55/60); and Late Adulthood (age: 55/60 and older). Lester, however, shows us that defining such stages is difficult. There are fine distinctions. This, of course, is an inherent problem in developmental psychology itself since no developmental period can be rigidly defined.

In Chapter 3, Ronald W. Maris provided a developmental perspective of suicide. He states that "The suicidal act is a process, a convergence of many factors over time. . . . suicide is not one thing and is not the simple product of an acute crisis." He argues that the person's history (or "career" as he terms it) is always relevant to that person's self-destruction.

In Chapter 4, Edwin S. Shneidman outlined the commonalities of suicide across the life span. He argues that although it may be useful to group suicides under "adolescent or adult, or middle age or old," there is only suicide: "There is only human suicide and all of it is to be understood in terms of the same principles."

EPIDEMIOLOGY

An American dies by his or her own hand on the average of every 17 minutes. However, this differs depending on the time-line/age (as well as other major demographic factors, sex, gender, race/ethnicity, and so on).

Part II presented three chapters on the epidemiology of suicide across the life span. The first, by John L. McIntosh, presented the epidemiology of suicide in the United States. There are approximately 30,000 annual suicide deaths; yet, McIntosh shows us that the rate of suicide varies depending on developmental age. The second chapter by David Lester looked at international trends and illustrates that there are different rates of suicide for different ages in different countries. In the third chapter, David P. Phillips and Daniel G. Smith provided a study of suicide at symbolic ages. They show us, for example, that—in a California sample—peaks occur at age 40 and 65 and conclude that the data are consistent with the hypothesis that symbolic birthdays are stocktaking occasions that can prompt suicidal behavior.

Part II, we believe, raises a number of questions including: "Why should the rate of suicide be higher at one developmental age (or symbolic age) than at other ages?"

SUICIDE BY TIME-LINES

Developmental ages (or time-lines) have their unique—despite commonalities—psychological issues. In line with the epidemiological findings that there are different rates of completed suicide across the life-span—and such rates differ from country to country—research and clinical findings, indeed, show that there may well be unique psychological issues at different ages for the suicidal person.

Part III consisted of five chapters. The first two chapters addressed suicide in children and adolescents. The first of these chapters by Antoon A. Leenaars and Susanne Wenckstern presented both some important observations about suicide in youth—such as definition, concept of death, depression, learning disabilities, physical disabilities, precipitating events, and the role of the family—and some common clues to suicide, that is, overt behaviors that the child or adolescent may exhibit. Alan L. Berman wrote the second chapter on children and adolescents. Berman, noting the value of both the nomothetic and the idiographic in understanding suicide, writes that "Ultimately, the true understanding of suicidal behavior must rest on more idiographic methods, through intensive study of unique and individual suicidal cases." Both of the above chapters allow us to understand the enormous complexity of suicide in youth and how important it is to structure developmentally the end of their short time-line.

The third chapter, by Leenaars, provided a discussion of suicide in the young adult, utilizing suicide notes. Noting that research regarding suicide in the young adult is scarce, Leenaars demonstrates that young adults' suicide notes and, by implication, their suicides are psychologically different from other adults. Despite similarities with older adults, differences can be noted in such areas as intimacy, identification-egression, identity, indirect expressions, inability to adjust, long-term instability, and ego. He concludes "There appear to be differences in such psychological issues as 'I love you'; 'This is me'; 'I am caving-in'; 'I want to be gone'; 'I am weakened'; and 'This is the only thing I can do.' "

The next chapter in Part III, by W. D. G. Balance and Leenaars, presented a discussion of suicide in middle adulthood. Utilizing Sigmund Freud's model of suicide, Balance and Leenaars show that the suicide of middle adults is quite different from those who have been only drawn to simulate it. Loss/rejection is shown to be important in suicide. Demonstrating that suicide—in the United States—is moderately higher after midlife, they show that superego processes in the suicidal individual appear to be more important before midlife than after midlife.

The final chapter, by Joseph Richman, offered a discussion of suicide in the elderly. Richman shows us that suicide in the elderly is not to be understood primarily or even solely to being old. As in other age groups, suicide in the elderly is viewed as a multi-factored event. Since elsewhere, suicide notes are provided for different ages except the elderly, a sample of such notes is presented here in Figure 1.

1. *Sue*

Im heartsick. First granma the Bill—then my home—my car—my eyesight—now my apartment. The last few days my sight is getting worse. I can only write by (one word)

Love

Mary

Thanks for everything to everyone
Alice & George: so long to two good friends.

Mary

2. *I'm tired of the pressure for so long*
I'm too old to fight any longer
I'm sick

3. *If you don't make sure I succeed this time—you can't say I haven't* tried

If you are honest within yourselves—you know you are anxious to get-on with your lives

I know you all have loved me—but this has nothing to do with that—keep on loving me.

With all the brains between you surely you can help me if my efforts fail. I've been sharp enough to help you all (cash) through some tough spots—now it's your turn

Ask yourself—just "what does she have to live for in this world?"

If you will put your "seal-of-approval" on what I have tried to do with my life—I'm ready for the next step with joy + anticipation. One step at a time.

Do help me get my act together if need be!

Mother

There is a little money which will repay you for the bother.

4. *Dear Bill, Mary + Family—*

Since the doctors diagnosed my illness, I have been contemplating this act. Life is absolutely miserable for me and I do not want to live. My only bright spots have been when you are around to cheer me a little and help me with the things I needed done. I know that I no longer want to be a burden on you and I'm sure I will be better off. I want to thank you for all the kind help you have been to me. All my love to the whole family and I hope no one grieves for me—we are all better off this way

All my love and Gods blessing to
you all.

Dad

Figure 1. A sample of suicide notes of the elderly.

The fourth note was written by an elderly person with terminal cancer. All of the notes allow us to understand what it was like for these individuals (in late adulthood) in the last minutes of their lives.

CORRELATES OF SUICIDE

As we have seen, suicide is, indeed, probably best understood as a complex event. Suicide is a dynamic phenomenon. There is not just one cause for suicide. The behavior is not just psychological. There are multiple (conscious and unconscious) pushes and strains, both inner and outer, on an individual who defines an issue for which suicide is perceived as the best solution. Not only can one structure suicide from a psychological perspective, but it would seem most accurate to define suicide as an event with biological aspects, sociological aspects, anthropological aspects, and so on.

Part IV consisted of three chapters: one on biological correlates, one on sociological correlates, and the other on anthropological correlates.

In the first chapter by Jerome A. Motto and Victor I. Reus, the biological correlates of suicide across the life span were outlined. The possible markers include urinary 17-hydroxycorticosteroids (17-OHCS), cortisol in plasma and cerebrospinal fluid, cerebrospinal fluid 5-hydroxyindoleacetic acid, tritiated imipramine binding, 3-methoxy-4-hydroxyphenylglycol and homovanillic acid, urinary norepinephrine:epinephrine ratio, and thyroid-stimulating hormone response to thyrotropin-releasing hormone. However, although there has been a recent flood of information regarding such biological observations related to suicide, Motto and Reus conclude that "It seems clear that the concept of biological correlates across the life span is premature." This conclusion is, in fact, embedded in the larger state of this science "that relatively little knowledge regarding the neurobiology of aging in humans is presently available."

The next chapter, by Steven Stack, presented the social correlates of suicide by age. Stack states that "correlates of suicidal behavior that vary by age include the position of the age group in society's institutional structure: the economy, religion, and family." He shows us that there are different correlates depending on age such as the high divorce rates for young adults, the disproportional investment in motherhood by middle-aged females, and physical illness in the elderly. Stack goes on to show the impact of the media on the rate of suicide at different ages.

The final chapter, by Dorothy Counts, illustrated the importance of the cultural context in understanding the meaning of suicide for different ages in a particular society. She elucidates, utilizing field data, that "people invest their actions with meaning that is based on stereotyped cultural models that are communicated to members of the society in ways that range from child's play to mythic tradition, models that are widely known and clearly understood." Like the psychological, biological, and sociological correlates, the anthropological correlates of suicide must be understood as we define or conceptualize suicide across the life span.

SURVIVOR ISSUES

Loss of a loved one due to suicide is a traumatic event. Reactions vary depending on one's age. Indeed, it is a myth that children and adolescents do not truly experience the pain associated with such a loss. A developmental perspective is essential in understanding these young people and any survivor.

Part V consisted of two chapters. The first, by Bonnie Frank Carter and Allan Brooks, discussed survivorship in children and adolescents. They address directly the myth that children cannot truly experience mourning because of their developmental age or more specifically their incomplete understanding of death. Carter and Brooks, in fact, note that a suicide death poses for children and adolescents one of the highest possible stresses, often resulting in post-traumatic stress disorder. Acknowledging the developmental age of the individual allows us to see how the distress is expressed. Utilizing research and case illustrations, Carter and Brooks allow us to know what it is like for these young survivors, including that they themselves now become at greater risk for suicide.

The next chapter, by Norman L. Farberow, presented survivorship in adults. Farberow begins his chapter noting that professional concern and research attention into adult (and child) survivorship after suicide began primarily within the last decade. He exposes—although further research is needed—a number of myths; for example, "Comparisons of bereavement in suicide and other modes of death have shown that for the most part the widely held ideas of special aspects of bereavement in suicide is not true." As another example, he throws into question the widely held conviction that there are differences in levels of difficulties in the bereavement that are the result of the kinship of the survivor.

In line with the current text, Carter, Brooks, and Farberow raise many questions. Is survivorship the same or different in the child from that of the elderly? Young adult? Is the bereavement of suicide versus nonsuicide affected by developmental age? And so on. In addition, regarding prevention, they raise even more questions: Do support groups help? The young? The late adult? Both chapters on survivorship in this book suggest that much greater attention is needed on survivorship across the life span.

PREVENTING SUICIDE

As shown in this volume, it is an unarguable advantage to come to the topic of suicide informed by a developmental perspective. This understanding has direct implications and applications for prevention.

Part VI consisted of two chapters addressing suicide prevention. The first, by Pamela Cantor, presented a discussion of prevention in the young. Cantor suggests at least two avenues of prevention: the social view and the traditional individualistic view. The social approach would encompass education and environmental risk reduction (such as the limitation of the availability of firearms). The individual approach is psychotherapy. Cantor makes note that the understanding of the developmental age is important in diagnostics and treating the young, especially the suicidal young: "The course the therapist has to steer between giving in to excessive demands for affection, attention, and flexibility . . . and emphatic responses to the young person's despair, require all the combined magical skills of King Arthur's Merlin and Cinderella's fairy godmother."

The next chapter—and final chapter in the volume—offered by John T. Maltsberger, provided a similar presentation on prevention in adults. Maltsberger writes "Because most patients are not at all sure they wish to do away with themselves, they are likely to involve others in their self-destructive enterprises, and to make us a part of their struggle in the choice between living and dying." We can involve ourselves in primary prevention (or prevention), secondary prevention (or intervention), and tertiary prevention (or postvention), all having a place in assisting in the struggle. Psychotherapy is seen as a key for many adults, including those in late adulthood. Maltsberger goes on to illustrate the use of medication, hospitalization, and other modes of preventing the event in the adult.

We see the insights by Cantor and Maltsberger as a fruitful beginning to addressing suicide prevention across the life span. Much greater clinical and research endeavors are needed. We, following the findings that are presented in this volume, need to know how can we best assist the suicidal young? Young adult? Middle adult? And late adult?

CONCLUDING REMARKS

As we have seen, understanding the time-lines in the suicidal process has a pivotal place in the study of the suicidal person. Much greater attention by the clinician and researcher alike is needed. This book, we hope, may assist in understanding—and hopefully preventing—suicide across the life span.

Index